Community Recreation and Persons with Disabilities
Strategies for Integration

Stuart J. Schleien, Ph.D.
and
M. Tipton Ray, M.Ed.
Division of Recreation, Park, and Leisure Studies
School of Physical Education and Recreation
University of Minnesota
Minneapolis

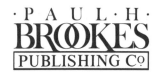

·P·A·U·L·H·
BROOKES
PUBLISHING CO.

Baltimore • London • Toronto • Sydney

Paul H. Brookes Publishing Co.
Post Office Box 10624
Baltimore, Maryland 21285-0624

Typeset by Brushwood Graphics Inc., Baltimore, Maryland.
Manufactured in the United States of America by
The Maple Press Company, York, Pennsylvania.

Cover illustration drawn by William Olfson.

Library of Congress Cataloging-in-Publication Data
Schleien, Stuart J.
    Community recreation and persons with disabilities: strategies for integration
Stuart J. Schleien and M. Tipton Ray.
        p. cm.
        Bibliography: p.
        Includes index.
        ISBN 0-933716-95-8
        1. Handicapped—United States—Recreation.   2. Handicapped—Services for—
United States.   3. Recreation centers—United States.   I. Ray, M. Tipton.
II. Title.
GV183.5.S35   1988   87-21300
790.1′96′0973—dc19   CIP

Contents

Foreword

*C*ommunity Recreation and Persons with Disabilities: Strategies for Integration *is the first text that provides both the conceptual framework and the specifics of application relative to integrated leisure life-styles for persons with disabilities. As such, it responds to an issue that will become an increasingly important social priority as the 21st century approaches.*

The conceptual foundation for this text rests on the interrelated aspects of the least restrictive environment and environmental or ecological models for active participation in recreation. Given this foundation, concepts discussed in the text may be readily applied to the challenge of developing programs that are meaningful and accessible for *all* people—not just individuals with disabilities.

The least restrictive environmental approach to program development requires an identification of the functional strengths of the potential participant and the provision of an environment, modified only to the minimal degree necessary, that corresponds to the abilities of the participant. Nondisabled persons, for example, utilize least restrictive environments by skiing on beginner ski slopes, or by scoring handicaps at the golf course or at the bowling alley. Integration of the person with a disability into the life-style of the community involves a process that differs only minimally from the generic social integration process utilized by society as a whole.

The environmental or ecological model for program development addresses the milieu of activity involvement instead of the prevailing pattern of myopic attention to the activity. Again, the issues are common to society as a whole, and are not unique to individuals with disabilities. Transportation, fees and charges, the skill demands of an activity (as determined by activity analyses), dress codes, levels of competition, and so on, are as exclusionary to activity participation for the "normal" population as for persons with disabilities.

Based upon this conceptual foundation, authors Stuart J. Schleien and M. Tipton Ray have provided a clear and valid application of the process approach to the integration of persons with disabilities within the spectrum of community leisure services. Following a thorough presentation of the planning process, the authors address the innovative issues of environmental assessment and modification, behavioral analysis and functional growth, and the evaluation process, with specific attention to the cognitive, affective, and psychomotor domains. A key strength of the text is the closing chapter, which provides a series of case studies that clearly illustrate the application of concepts and approaches in a community setting.

The excellent balance achieved by the authors between conceptual issues and the application process is a testament to the expertise of Schleien and Ray in the development of integrated community-based programs. Dr. Schleien's professional career has been heavily focused, both as a practitioner and as an educator, in the area of community integration of persons with disabilities. The texts and journal articles authored by Dr. Schleien have made significant contributions to the fields of therapeutic recreation and special education. Similarly, Mr. M. Tipton Ray, who is in the final stages of his doctoral program at the University of Minnesota, has a sound, unique, and varied background of practitioner experiences that contributes substantially to the conceptual-application balance in the text.

Human services face a multitude of challenges as the 21st century approaches. In this excellent textbook, Schleien and Ray have provided a framework for service delivery that has not only generic application to all populations but also has basic relevance to all human services providers—whether they are social workers, special educators, doctors, nurses, or therapeutic recreators.

Fred Humphrey, Ph.D.
University of Maryland

Preface

L ife, Liberty, and the Pursuit of Happiness. These are the inalienable rights of citizens of the United States. This does not imply that only those citizens "of sound mind and body" are protected by our country's constitution. *All* American citizens have these rights, and therefore, every citizen should have access to all of the programs and services available in the community—medical, religious, educational, and recreational. The purpose of this book is to provide a practical and philosophical basis for including children and adults with disabilities in community leisure services.

The following circumstances support the existence of integrated leisure services in the community. First, current legislation mandates the provision of special education and related services, including recreation, for all individuals with disabilities in the *least restrictive environment* (LRE). Second, there are large numbers of persons with disabilities living and working within community environments who wish to make use of community services. Third, barriers or obstacles to participation by persons with disabilities in community leisure environments are no longer insurmountable.

This book represents the culmination of almost 10 years of work involving the integration of persons with disabilities into community environments. Its major focus is on integrating existing services versus merely developing or providing additional segregated programs. The authors understand and accept the place for separate, "handicapped-only" recreation programs within the continuum of leisure service delivery. However, for persons wtih disabilities, these segregated programs must be considered only as second priority alternatives.

The following eight chapters in this book grew out of the relative dearth of specific information on the development, implementation, and evaluation of integrated community leisure services. Efforts have been made to provide information and guidelines on issues and topics most commonly sought by community recreation professionals, careproviders, and teachers. These topics and issues include:

Why should community leisure services be accessible to everyone?
What are the roles and responsibilities of educators, recreation professionals, and families in the recreation integration process?
How does one implement recreation programs that meet the needs of participants both with and without disabilities?
How are these programs evaluated?
Do model programs exist that could be replicated in leisure settings?

The subsequent chapters in this book address these concerns directly in a succinct and informative manner.

Chapter 1 establishes the rationale and philosophical basis for the provision of community leisure services and for the inclusion, or integration, of persons with disabilities into these programs. This chapter includes a definition and brief historical overview of community leisure services and special populations. Much of the discussion focuses on segregated versus integrated services, and on the impact of mandatory legislation on the educational and leisure services provided to persons with disabilities. The advantages of integrated leisure services to all citizens are examined.

In Chapter 2, a program planning process is presented that systematically produces guidelines for planning integrated community leisure services. A *diamond analogy* depicting the nature of community leisure services is provided. The planning of the ideal program, the truly accessible recreation program, is delineated as the final component of the continuum of service model. A process of accessible leisure services designating the tasks to be accomplished by community recreation professionals is discussed in detail.

In Chapter 3, an integrated community leisure services planning and implementation model is presented that defines the roles and responsibilities of professionals, careproviders, and other "key players." In order to conduct a "shared responsibility delivery system" of leisure services, a networking matrix displaying these players' collaboration in the system is examined. Also, general strategies that could be employed by a municipality to promote integrated leisure services are outlined. These strategies include the conducting of architectural accessibility surveys of community-based facilities, the establishment of Community Advisory Boards, and the provision of inservice training to existing staff at these sites.

An *Environmental Analysis Inventory* is presented in Chapter 4; this provides a systematic approach for studying environments and for overcoming obstacles to participation in community recreation programs. This inventory is used as an initial screening device for future participation and as a means of identifying necessary skills for participation in the environment or activity. This fundamental tool assists the program planner in the identification of modifications to enhance participation by persons with disabilities.

Programmatically, the common philosophical thread in the design of the most innovative community leisure services encompasses emphases on ecological and behavioral perspectives. Teaching procedures, instructional arrangements, and special considerations proven effective in the provision of integrated community leisure services are addressed by Dr. Richard Amado, Psychologist, in Chapter 5. In the authors' opinion, the principles of applied behavior analysis are not yet fully understood by professionals and paraprofessionals currently working in community leisure settings. Therefore, Dr. Amado has enumerated a variety of behavioral strategies and solutions to problems typically faced by the recreation professional.

Chapter 6 contains vital information on participant and program evaluation. This chapter presents instrumentation and easily followed, step-by-step, procedures on conducting evaluations in the agency. An added feature of this section is the inclusion of all forms necessary for the evaluation process.

To determine the quantity and quality of community leisure services for special populations and to identify major obstacles to physically and socially integrated programs, the outcomes of two surveys are reported in Chapter 7. These surveys help clarify the perceived and real barriers to integrated community leisure services. Specific solutions to common barriers are suggested.

The final chapter of the manual, Chapter 8, provides the reader with a wealth of information regarding six exemplary programs. These successful programs illustrate the types of viable procedures that may be implemented in a variety of recreation/leisure environments. The reader may discover a situation in one of these programs that closely parallels his or her own situation and may perhaps glean some specific suggestions from the information contained in this chapter. We believe that these exemplary programs are potentially replicable by other agencies. One might argue that successful major systems changes are unique to the municipality, and that any attempt to disseminate strategies for change (e.g., segregated to integrated programs) are difficult and useless. We believe that by disseminating these model programs, other agencies could make any necessary modifications to their services, and could anticipate similar obstacles in future program endeavors.

An appendix of references and resources, including blank forms for use by the reader, are provided. This detailed appendix should prove to be a valuable resource for community recreation professionals, careproviders, and teachers who are attempting to integrate recreation programs. Also, an annotated bibliography of the most current and relevant literature concerning integrated community leisure services is provided.

This book represents the efforts of a group of professionals in community recreation, therapeutic recreation, special education, and psychology. Also represented are the efforts of careproviders and students who are promoting integrated community leisure services. These individuals have taken a proactive approach to ensuring that existing leisure services become accessible to children and adults with and without disabilities. No longer can society afford to exclude people from programs based on their special needs. Professionals and families must continue to work toward total accessibility and consequent full participation through the structuring and restructuring of recreational environments and activities. It is the authors' intent to share what we have learned about integrated community recreation and persons with disabilities in order to reach these goals. We wish you much success in your endeavors!

Acknowledgments

We would like to express our appreciation to a number of individuals who participated in the research and development of this book. We are grateful for their creative efforts and generous cooperation. We wish to give special thanks to members of the Special Interest Committee on the Handicapped and to all the center directors and administrators of the Minneapolis Park and Recreation Board for their daily involvement, commitment, and leadership in the integration of persons with disabilities in community leisure services.

In appreciation for their professional knowledge, expertise, and moral support, we thank Dale Johnson of the Minneapolis Park and Recreation Board, Dr. John Rynders, Dr. John Schultz, and Dr. Michael Wade, of the University of Minnesota. A word of gratitude is due Dr. Gene Hayes, University of Tennessee, for assisting in the initial conceptualization of this text. We are extremely grateful to Dr. Fred Humphrey, University of Maryland, for his contribution of the Foreword. We trust this text is an adequate reflection of the efforts he pioneered in the area of community recreation and persons with disabilities.

The work of Angela Larson, Tina Rutten Moenkedick, Carla Slick, and Diane Bjorkman, Graduate Research Assistants of PIRC: Project for Integrated Recreation in the Community, in the planning and development of this manuscript, was an essential component to the successful completion of this book. We express our appreciation for their contributions and effort.

We especially wish to thank Theresa Mustonen, Graduate Research Assistant of the Minnesota Consortium Institute for the Education of Severely Handicapped Learners for her significant contribution to Chapter 1, and Jennifer Cameron, Graduate Research Assistant of Therapeutic Recreation, University of Minnesota, for her assistance in the development of this book.

Special thanks are also extended to Donna Shear, Production Editor for Paul H. Brookes Publishing Co., for her editing of the manuscript.

We would also like to thank Kay Lowinske for her diligent efforts and outstanding work in typing and preparing the manuscript. The graphics and artwork, which added clarity and interest to the text, were created by Dana Kuller and Ann Ray, and we are grateful for their assistance.

Most importantly, we wish to express our appreciation to all the key players who had the courage and foresight to move beyond the traditional approaches to community leisure service delivery. The creativity of consumers, careproviders, professionals, volunteers, advocacy agencies, and students of the University of Minnesota has enabled persons with and without disabilities to benefit from each other's presence in the community.

We wish to dedicate this book
to our lovely and supportive partners,
Dana and Ann.

Chapter 1

Community Recreation
and Persons with Disabilities

Participation in leisure and recreation activities is an important aspect of life in our society. When such activities meet the needs of individuals, they promote physical health and conditioning, provide opportunities to develop social relations, and lead to the development of new skills. Unfortunately, leisure services have had relatively low priority in programs for persons with disabilities; only recently have specific recreation and leisure skill educational techniques (Schleien, Kiernan, & Wehman, 1981; Voeltz, Wuerch, & Wilcox, 1982) and leisure curricula (Bender & Valletutti, 1976; Wehman & Schleien, 1981; Wessel, 1976; Wuerch & Voeltz, 1982) been developed. The neglect of relevant programming and services for persons with disabilities is particularly unfortunate because appropriate participation in leisure activities is an important factor in successful community adjustment (Bell, Schoenrock, & Slade, 1975; Cheseldine & Jeffree, 1981; Eyman & Call, 1977; Gollay, 1981; Hill & Bruininks, 1981). Furthermore, participation in leisure activities is associated with the development of collateral skills (Newcomer & Morrison, 1974; Schleien, Kiernan, & Wehman, 1981; Strain, Cook, & Apolloni, 1976) and the reduction of maladaptive behaviors (Adkins & Matson, 1980; Flavell, 1973; Schleien, Kiernan, & Wehman, 1981; Voeltz & Wuerch, 1981).

Even though the short- and long-term benefits of participation by disabled persons in recreation activities have been established, there is room for improvement in the quality of services to persons with disabilities. For persons with disabilities to maximally participate in community recreation activities, specific recreation and leisure skill training in home and school environments must be available, and specific efforts by communities to incorporate these persons into recreational activities should be made.

The rationale for the development of recreation opportunities for persons with disabilities in community settings has been well established from both a theoretical (i.e., normalization) and a practical (i.e., deinstitutionalization) standpoint. Recreation participation in community settings offers the disabled individual the opportunity to develop a positive self-concept through successful experiences and satisfying relationships with peers. Channels for self-expression, opportunities to interact with the environment, and the establishment of a more personally fulfilling way of life are other positive results of integrated, community leisure participation by individuals with disabilities.

Federal legislation, including Public Law 94-142, the Education for All Handicapped Children Act, and its amendments (PL 98-199; PL 99-457), Section 504 of the Rehabilitation Act of 1973, and other recent mandates, prohibit discrimination against individuals with disabilities. These initiatives have facilitated the movement of large numbers of persons with disabilities into community living situations, consequently placing the responsibility of recreation programming upon community agencies. This legislation has paved the way for persons with disabilities to live, learn, and engage in recreation activities in settings with their nondisabled peers.

However, providing services in least restrictive environments, such as community leisure settings, for persons with and without disabilities, requires a great deal of preparation by recreation professionals, careproviders, and the participants themselves. Many fundamental skills must be acquired by the professionals and the concerns of community recreation personnel must be anticipated if these programs will indeed meet the leisure and recreation needs of all citizens of a given locale. Thus, the service delivery system in recreation programming that includes individuals with disabilities must be comprehensive and community-based.

HISTORICAL OVERVIEW

> But what then am I? A thing which thinks. What is a thing which thinks? It is a thing which doubts, understands, conceives, affirms, denies, wills, refuses, which also imagines and feels (Descartes, 1955).

What then is an individual with a disability? Too often such a person is considered to be one who does not think, feel, or imagine, but rather one who exists at the will of society. He or she is thought of as one who exists in a condition of dependency totally determined by other members of society, a condition generally regarded as disgraceful and often despicable. Individuals with disabilities have generally been ignored by society; until recently, society has not considered individuals with disabilities worthy of membership (Repp, 1983).

Historically, persons with disabilities were not provided with opportunities to participate in recreation programs and activities. Prior to 1800, for example, people were apparently aware of the existence of individuals with disabilities but did little in the way of systematic study, treatment, or care of them. Between 1800 and 1950, an interest in the problem of educating persons with disabilities began. Systematic programs of sensorimotor training were developed, institutional care for disabled persons was initiated in the United States, and the first compulsory school laws were passed. Also, laboratories were developed for training teachers to work with disabled people. The late nineteenth century saw the rise of professional organizations for those who worked with disabled individuals. More recently, however, individuals with disabilities have been given these opportunities because of various legislative acts at the local, state, and federal levels. Since 1950, there has been more interest in, and activity on behalf of, individuals with disabilities than during any other period of time. In order to provide the reader with a better understanding of the role of recreation in the lives of individuals with disabilities, a brief historical overview of the treatment of disabled persons follows. A summary of community leisure services is also provided.

Evidence of cruelty toward individuals with disabilities may be found as far back as the Spartans of ancient Greece, who eliminated anyone who was disabled. In Rome, persons with disabilities were used as fools or court jesters, and later, in France and Germany, deformed and retarded persons were used as buffoons. As centuries passed, disabled individuals were occasionally provided with food, clothing, and shelter, but they did not receive treatment, and did not enjoy the rights of other, nondisabled citizens. During the first part of the medieval era, individuals with disabilities were looked upon with superstitious reverence. Evidence shows that crude surgery on the skull, purgation, and rituals of exorcism were practiced during this period as attempts to "drive out the devil." In the middle of the seventeenth century, homeless, outcast, and bodily and mentally infirm persons were placed in asylums. Once institutionalized, these individuals received no treatment, rehabilitation, or education, and they were provided with only custodial care.

However, there were isolated events in the treatment of individuals with disabilities that showed that better things were to come. In 1794, Philipe Pinel went into an asylum and abolished treatment utilizing whips, chains, and stocks, and replaced it with kind, gentle, and effective methods of treatment. In 1785, Valentine Haüy founded a school in Paris for the education of blind persons. Also at this time, in Germany and in France, work was being done to educate persons with hearing impairments.

The real beginnings of therapeutic treatment took place in the early 1800s when education and political reform became widespread. The first successful public residential institutions for disabled persons were established. Schools throughout Germany, France, and the United States were begun; by 1898, a total of 24 state schools were being operated in 19 states.

Role of Recreation

Recreation did not play a large role in the lives of individuals with disabilities until the 1900s. In 1906, the Playground Association of America, later to be known as the Playground and Recreation Association and known still later as the National Recreation Association, was formed. As a service organization, it promoted the cause of community recreation for more than half a century. The recreation and park organizations declared from the beginning that their services were for all people, including those persons who had been discriminated against because they possessed physical disabilities.

During the 1920s and 1930s, public schools began offering after-school recreation programs for persons with disabilities. This practice still exists today; the Emerson After-School Program sponsored by the Minneapolis Park and Recreation Board is one example of such a program. (See Chapter 7 for a description of this and five other programs.)

During World War II, the National American Red Cross was active in providing recreation opportunities for military personnel. It was not until the late 1940s that recreation programs began to appear in public hospitals. The Veteran's Administration, which provided therapeutic recreation services to emotionally disturbed populations in hospitals and state institutions, was a pioneer in this effort.

In the 1940s, the idea of using outdoor or wilderness areas as therapeutic environments became popular. Therapeutic wilderness programs can be defined as any variety of outdoor activities that take place in wilderness environments and that are designed to improve the emotional and behavioral skills of the participants engaging in that activity (Gibson, 1979). Such therapeutic programs may range from half-day outings to year-round operations, and can include such activities as: backpacking, mountaineering, rock climbing, canoeing, camping, and cross-country skiing.

The origin of therapeutic wilderness programs in the early 1900s in the United States was chronicled the *American Journal of Insanity* during the early 1900s. Caplan (1967) stated that "tent treatment" for hospitalized psychiatric patients began in 1901 when the hospital administrator at Manhattan State Hospital East in New York City placed patients in tents on the hospital grounds to relieve overcrowding and to avoid the spread of tuberculosis. When the hospital staff noted improvements in both the physical and mental health of these patients, the tent treatment became a regular practice. By 1910, an additional therapeutic wilderness/outdoor education program was established when another state hospital in New York began a summer camp program for adult psychiatric patients.

Summer camps for children and adolescents first appeared in the United States in 1861, but it was not until the 1940s that camping became popular as a service delivered to meet the needs of persons with disabilities. In the camping programs of the 1940s, efforts were made to meet the needs of individual campers, and new ways of meeting those needs were explored. Today, several national organizations exist that provide camp and recreation experiences to individuals with disabilities. These organizations include: the National Easter Seal Society for Crippled Children and Adults (residential camping), Lighthouse (New York Association for the Blind recreation and camping programs), the New York Service for Orthopedically Handicapped Persons (integrated program of recreation activities), the United Cerebral Palsy Associations, Inc., the Muscular Dystrophy Association, the National Multiple Sclerosis Society, the Goodwill Industries, The Joseph P. Kennedy, Jr. Foundation, the American Foundation for the Blind, Inc., and the Association for Retarded Citizens of the United States (ARC-US).

Early Legislation

Since 1920, many of the problems confronting citizens with disabilities have been addressed in legislation and in programs initiated at the federal level. During the 1930s, for example, federal legislation to expand the rights of persons with disabilities was implemented. The Social Security Act of 1935 provided federal grants-in-aid to states for maternal and child health and welfare, and for services to crippled children.

In the late 1950s, congressional action provided increased funding for various research, educational, and vocational training projects addressing the needs of individuals with disabilities. In the Cooperative Research Act of 1957 (PL 83-531), for instance, Congress provided $675,000 to support research concerning the education of children with disabilities. During the next year, PL 85-926 was enacted to provide aid to universities and colleges to prepare teachers and professionals to work in the field of mental retardation. PL 88-164, passed in 1963, extended PL 85-926 to include training of professionals to work with children with all types of disabling conditions. PL 89-313 amended PL 89-10, the Elementary and Secondary Education Act, and expanded the definition of "disadvantaged" to include school-age persons living in state residential institutions or state-supported private schools (Repp, 1983).

Recent Legislation

Group segregation is not necessarily a deliberate maneuver; to the contrary, it usually occurs through thoughtlessness or inaction. Inaccessible buildings and lack of communication segregate the walking, hearing, and seeing population from persons who have disabilities. Today, state and federal legislation have made discrimination against individuals with disabilities illegal. The Architectural Barriers Act of 1968 (PL 90-480) requires that buildings and facilities designed, constructed, altered, or leased with federal funds must be accessible and useable by individuals with physical disabilities. This legislation excludes buildings built by private capital, without government contributions. The Architectural and Transportation Barriers Compliance Board (ATBCB) under Section 502 of the Rehabilitation Act of 1973 (PL 93-112), was created by Congress to enforce the Architectural Barriers Act. This act enables individuals with disabilities to participate in programs that are available to the general public. (Written complaints about inaccessible facilities or architectural barriers in buildings constructed or altered since passage of the Architectural Barriers Act should be sent to the ATBCB).

The 1970s may be remembered as the "Decade of the Disabled," for during this decade, monumental civil and human rights advances by disabled people were achieved. These historic gains produced a firm foundation for new achievements in the marketplace. The 1973 Rehabilitation Act (PL 93-112), as amended in 1974 (PL 93-516), is one of the most significant landmarks in the struggle for equality for individuals with disabilities. Section 504 of the Rehabilitation Act, entitled "Nondiscrimination Under Federal Grants," or the "Civil Rights Act for the Handicapped," stated that:

> No otherwise qualified handicapped individual in the United States, as defined in section 7(6), shall, solely on the basis of his handicap, be excluded from the participation in, be denied the benefits of, or be subjected to discrimination under any program or activity receiving Federal financial assistance. (p. 794)

In effect, the Rehabilitation Act makes it illegal for any agency or organization that receives federal funds to discriminate against a disabled person solely on the basis of his or her disability.

All public and private organizations receiving federal monies must take special steps (including making programs and facilities accessible) to make it possible for persons with disabilities "to learn, work, and compete on a fair and equal basis (PL 93-112)." Noncompliance with the provisions of this act by an agency or organization can result in the cutoff of all federal support to the agency or organization. The Rehabilitation Act also requires that all programs receiving federal funds must be accessible to persons with disabilities. Existing programs and new facilities constructed after June, 1977 must be designed to meet the standards of the American National Standards Institute. It is important to note that every building need not be remodeled, since emphasis is placed on *program* accessibility. For example, an existing program may be considered accessible *if the portion of the facility used by persons with disabilities meets the standards of ANSI,* or if other steps are taken to make the program accessible, such as assigning students to alternative accessible facilities or using aides to assist the students. The regulations stipulate that such modifications cannot result in the segregation of disabled persons from nondisabled persons who are also involved in the program.

PL 94-142, the Education for All Handicapped Children Act, was signed into law in 1975 by President Gerald R. Ford. The Act provided equal educational opportunity to all children who have disabilities.

> It is the purpose of this Act to assure that all handicapped children have available to them a free and appropriate public education and related services designed to meet their unique needs, to assure that the rights of handicapped children and their parents or guardians are protected, to assist States and localities to provide for the education of all children, and to assess and assure the effectiveness of efforts to educate handicapped children. (Sec. 601 [3] [c])

Any handicapped child living in Minnesota, for example, age 4–21, is entitled to a free and appropriate educational program. The service is progressive and is available at the discretion of the local school district for children from birth through 3 years of age. Many districts currently provide programs for preschool-level children with disabilities such as vision and hearing impairments. All districts must identify, assess, plan for, and monitor all preschoolers who have potentially handicapping conditions.

PL 94-142 also addresses the use of related services in least restrictive environments. Related services are those additional services, such as transportation, that are necessary for the child to benefit from special education instruction. Related services might also include developmental, corrective, and other support services such as: speech pathology and audiology, psychological services, physical and occupational therapy, medical and counseling services, and recreation.

In October, 1986, President Ronald Reagan signed PL 99-457 into law, thus amending the Education for All Handicapped Children Act. The major feature of PL 99-457 is that it specifically addresses the needs of disabled infants and toddlers (from birth through age 2) and preschoolers (ages 3 through 5). Under Part H of the act, a new program was established to provide early intervention services to meet the special needs of young children with disabilities and their families in least restrictive environments.

The least restrictive environment (LRE) concept suggests that children with disabilities are to be educated, to the maximum extent possible, alongside their nonhandicapped peers. In the past, many children with disabilities were separated from their nondisabled peers and were educated in special classrooms throughout their school years. These children were segregated solely on the basis of their disability. They missed opportunities for learning and development because they were categorized by what they were unable to do, rather than by their abilities and strengths. The principle of LRE seeks to correct this by enabling individuals with disabilities to participate in community leisure services alongside their nondisabled peers.

These laws have advanced the movement for deinstitutionalization of persons with disabilities and have championed the principle of normalization. Deinstitutionalization is a procedure that involves removing as many people as possible from institutions and subsequently integrating them into community settings. The philosophical position informing this process is the normalization principle. This principle advocates that persons with disabilities should be placed into communities where the residents are nondisabled persons. Such placement results in a normal routine of life whereby schooling occurs in one place, residency in another, and recreation in several others, rather than all activities taking place in one location. The normalization principle will continue to play a major role in the lives of individuals with disabilities in such areas as employment, living alternatives, and recreation and leisure pursuits.

NEEDS ASSESSMENT OF COMMUNITY LEISURE SERVICES

Schleien, Porter, and Wehman (1979) addressed the topic of community-based leisure services in their survey of community agencies and programs in the state of Virginia. The purpose of the investigation was to assess the roles of various agencies in providing for the leisure needs of developmentally disabled persons. The sample included county and regional parks and recreation departments, special education coordinators of public school systems, community mental health and mental retardation service boards, state hospitals serving mentally ill and mentally retarded persons, and other programs funded by the Virginia Developmental Disabilities Unit. The investigators found that 69% of the agencies offered some form of recreation service to their developmentally disabled clients, but 31% of the agencies did not, indicating a need for more ongoing (rather than sporadic) recreation services. Among the respondents providing inadequate recreation programs, 66% reported that improvements could be generated if professional expertise and appropriate instructional materials were made available. Fifty-eight percent of the agencies expressed the need for a relevant leisure skills curriculum on which to base programs.

Austin, Peterson, Peccarelli, Binkley, and Laker (1977) distributed questionnaires to municipal park and recreation departments and health care and correctional facilities in the state of Indiana to determine the current status of therapeutic recreation services in that state. Of the 50 responding parks and recreation departments, 80% believed that their agencies should be providing recreation services to special populations. Although 76% of the departments offered some form of therapeutic recreation service, in only two cases (5%) was the individual in charge of the program a therapeutic recreation specialist. The type of assistance cited as necessary by 92% of the departments for establishing a program for special populations was the presence of a specially trained staff member. The data revealed that existing programs were not extensively developed and that a majority of municipal park and recreation departments were not serving special populations adequately.

To determine the quantity and quality of recreation programs and services throughout the state of Minnesota, Schleien and Werder (1985) conducted a needs assessment inventory to survey park and recreation departments, community education agencies, and schools. Data from the inventory, at a 73% return rate, enabled the authors to identify perceived responsibilities and the degree of coordination among agencies. The authors were also able to determine the scope and nature of special recreation services currently offered, and the extent of integration of disabled and nondisabled participants. This study revealed not only several weaknesses and needs in recreation services throughout the state, but also ideal opportunities for future growth in service provision. Based on Schleien and Werder's results, five recommendations for future special recreation programming were developed:

1) A clear network of communication across agencies must be delineated to reduce duplication and complement resources.
2) Activity offerings must be expanded.
3) Integration of disabled individuals into recreation programs with nondisabled participants should be encouraged.
4) Support should be generated for increasing the number of specially trained personnel across agencies.
5) Accessibility and availability of special recreation programs should be improved.

Several other studies have been conducted throughout the country to evaluate the status of recreation services available to individuals with disabilities. Edginton, Compton, Ritchie, and Vederman (1975) and Lancaster (1976) identified lack of funding, poorly trained professional personnel, and lack of awareness of the need for community and municipal recreation services for special populations as the major factors inhibiting widespread provision of these services.

In addition to inadequately trained recreation professionals, lack of training program materials and funds, and lack of awareness of the need for services, studies reveal the additional problem that no appropriate recreation service delivery model has been developed at the community level. That is, there is no community-based leisure service delivery system addressing the total life and leisure needs of disabled persons living in communities (Compton & Goldstein, 1976). Thus, although the delivery of therapeutic recreation services is legally mandated, and although many communities have accepted the responsibility for providing those services, the necessary personnel, methods, and procedures to implement the mandate have not been adequately developed.

NORMALIZATION AND INTEGRATED COMMUNITY LEISURE SERVICES

The integration of children and adults with disabilities into community leisure services and facilities may be viewed as an outgrowth of the normalization principle and the resulting movement toward community placement. Normalization, a concept defined by Nirje (1969), involves making the same societal patterns and conditions of everyday life that are enjoyed by nondisabled persons available to persons with disabilities. Wolfensberger (1972) expanded upon his definition to include the "use of means which are as culturally normative as possible, in order to establish and/or maintain personal behaviors and characteristics which are as culturally normative as possible." According to Lakin and Bruininks (1985) normalization involves placing a high value on the life, rights, and dignity of citizens with disabilities. Normalization is maintained by the belief that disabled people should be accepted as members of the community and should be permitted to participate in the activities enjoyed by other members of society.

Although the normalization principle has been a guiding force behind efforts to integrate persons with disabilities, adherence to this philosophy by human services professionals does not guarantee that disabled persons will be less socially isolated than they would have been had they been living in institutions. Providing opportunities for people with disabilities to live in neighborhoods occupied by nondisabled residents, to work, or to go to neighborhood schools is consistent with normalization, but opportunities alone do not ensure that social integration into a community will take place. All too often, disabled persons living in a community facility have minimal contact with nondisabled people in their neighborhoods (Salzberg & Langford, 1981). Additionally, persons with disabilities generally spend little time working or residing in community environments (Crapps, Langone, & Swaim, 1985), and may actually decrease their involvement in community activities over time (Birenbaum & Re, 1979). The extent of social integration into a community may be measured by the way people with disabilities are viewed by nondisabled people, by the social environments they share with nondisabled people, and by the participation of disabled persons in social interactions that parallel those of nondisabled persons (Meyer & Kishi, 1985). Salzberg and Langford (1981) suggested that true social integration has been achieved when regular and friendly contacts take place between nondisabled citizens and citizens with disabilities.

Normalization and the social integration that accompanies it provide support for the inclusion of individuals with disabilities in community recreation programs. Although the scarcity of segregated programs would appear to suggest that normalization efforts have thus far been successful, the fact that segregated programs still exist at all leads the authors to question the success of their efforts. Reasons for the continued existence of segregated programs, despite the growing belief that such programs are not consistent with normalization, must be examined.

Evolution of Segregated Programs

In years past, segregated services were often initiated by parents of disabled children. Ross (1983) stated that voluntary parent associations are established to meet the need for support services for disabled children. Faced with a lack of programs for disabled persons or with the reluctance of regular program providers to accept their children, parent associations (e.g., the Association for Retarded Citizens) began providing segregated services. Meyer and Kishi (1985) studied the concerns expressed by parents regarding the quality, benefits, and safety of integrated services and found that these concerns were best understood in the context of the parents' previous experiences with agencies. For example, parents who invested great amounts of time and financial support to provide needed services for their children were understandably hesitant to turn their children over to the very agencies that were once unwilling to provide for them.

Social attitudes have also been mentioned as a reason for the existence of segregated programs. Wilkenson (1984) cited comments of personnel from a variety of agencies serving people with disabilities. Respondents reported that parents of disabled children were concerned that if their children were integrated into regular programs, the children would suffer physical harm and isolation. The attitudes and misconceptions of those parents were also cited as a barrier to integration (Wilkenson, 1984). For example, several respondents mentioned that parents, concerned that their child would "catch" a disability or have a less valuable experience, had withdrawn their nondisabled children from integrated programs.

Perceived Responsibilities

Municipal park and recreation departments are also responsible for the continued existence of segregated programs. It is possible these departments continue to offer segregated programs because, as Richler (1983) pointed out, segregated services have become the models for serving people with disabilities, and have thus come to be viewed as the norm. According to Wilkenson (1984), some municipal agencies believe that special associations have the responsibility for dealing with disabled people. Other respondents to Wilkenson's survey attributed their own failure to offer integrated activities to a scarcity of requests for such programs from disabled citizens. The inefficiency of agency staff with little experience in serving people with disabilities was also cited by Wilkenson as a barrier to the implementation of integrated programs. McGill (1984) and Schleien and Werder (1985) suggested that the reluctance of recreation program staff to share responsibility for the integration of regular programming is understandable when one remembers that programs serving persons with disabilities tend to rely upon trained specialists to staff their programs. Voeltz et al. (1982) recommended that special educators seek to remove the mystique surrounding people with disabilities by de-emphasizing their need for special programs and facilities by encouraging their use of generic services.

The responsibility for failing to fully integrate community leisure services and facilities must be shared by disabled citizens and their families or careproviders as well. Several studies have shown, for example, that people with disabilities do not utilize community programs. Visually impaired adult respondents to a survey by Sherrill, Rainbolt, and Ervin (1984) reported that they desired acceptance into community recreation and neighborhood athletic programs. However, only 10% of the subjects participated in community recreation programs, and 47% did not even know what programs their communities offered. Despite this desire to become involved in existing integrated community activities, several of the subjects were instrumental in originating segregated activities such as beep baseball or blind bowling leagues for visually impaired people.

Residents of a large community facility for mentally retarded adults who had previously resided in state institutions also reported a desire for more independence and community involvement (Birenbaum & Re, 1979). However, 83% of these adults were found to spend much of their leisure time in passive residential activities. Community activities led by staff members declined over the 4–year longitudinal study and were not replaced by ventures into the community alone, with friends, or with family members. In another study, mentally retarded residents of group homes and intermediate group residences were found to spend the majority of their leisure time in their homes, relying almost completely on their supervisors for trips into the community (Crapps et al., 1985). Birenbaum and Re (1979) speculated that this decline in community involvement may have been due to the fact that residents lacked the skills necessary for engaging in community activities, or possibly to their reluctance to travel in what they considered to be a "dangerous community."

Crapps et al. (1985) differentiated between passive integration (e.g., a situation wherein a disabled person participates in a community activity planned and implemented by a supervising adult) and active integration (e.g., a situation wherein an environment and/or activity is selected by a disabled person). Lack of skills may limit a disabled individual's involvement in the community to passive integration experiences unless that individual receives training in specific skills related to the use of community recreation environments. Voeltz et al. (1982) noted that when an individual lacks the skills to participate in leisure options, the range of those options become meaningless in light of his or her skill deficits.

INHIBITORS AND FACILITATORS OF LEISURE PARTICIPATION

Environmental barriers, long a concern to people working with individuals with disabilities, have been brought to the attention of the general public by legislation and consumer advocates. Successful functioning within our society requires the ability to understand, to interpret, and to act appropriately upon signs, symbols, and communications in the environment. Functioning successfully also requires the ability to influence external forces, to have access to resources, to move about with minimal difficulty, and to assimilate and learn from experiences.

Children and adults with disabilities are greatly hampered in their daily activities by subtle emotional obstacles as well as obvious, physical barriers. Often, persons with disabilities do not recognize the causes of their frustration or the reasons for their limited participation in normal human activities; it may take a degree of awareness and exposure for them to realize that they are missing experiences that others have. Availability of transportation, access into, and mobility within recreation areas and facilities are features that must be present in a program in order to promote recreation participation by persons with disabilities. Additionally, lack of knowledge and education in the use of recreational services, inaccessibility of services due to physical or geographic impediments, and the presence of architectural barriers will inhibit travelers who have disabilities (Laus, 1977). When these individuals are prevented from traveling about the community independently, they may suffer from boredom and, subsequently, may turn to an inappropriate use of free time that results in minimal community participation.

Children and adults with disabilities often are excluded from many recreation options due to the limitations imposed on them by their physical impairments. In general, community recreation programs do not provide the types of modifications necessary to accommodate such individuals. For example, special equipment and materials, activity space and facilities, the scheduling of activities, suitable rules and regulations, and the employment of special instructors are all required for programs seeking to overcome the many existing barriers to participation. Thus, it is important to ascertain what disabled individuals perceive as obstacles to participation in regular recreation programs and to determine how these obstacles can be removed or overcome.

Federal legislation has played an important step in the removal of environmental barriers. The 1968 Architectural Barriers Act, for example, requires that any structure built or renovated with public funds must be physically accessible to individuals with disabilities. For the law to be effective, however, strict enforcement of the act is essential. In addition, architects, urban planners, and transportation engineers should be made aware of the needs of persons with disabilities. Medical technology and engineering can also contribute to increasing the participation of disabled persons in activities by designing safe and effective appliances that facilitate mobility and correct physical impairments.

MacNeil (1977) identified three major obstacles to the delivery of cultural arts opportunities for persons with disabilities: the lack of trained personnel, architectural barriers, and attitudinal barriers. These obstacles prevent access to various public and private recreation services in the community as well. Yet, consumers of goods and services in the community who have disabilities have the right to expect certain levels of service from providers of recreational opportunities. Austin and Powell (1981), for instance, identified consumer representation to the service provider, economic feasibility, clearly stated user fees and charges, and an accessible environment as levels of service expected by all consumers. Furthermore, Wolfensberger (1972) recommended that at least one-half of any governing or advisory board should consist of consumers representing the special group to be served.

The professional literature cites a variety of issues that hinder professionals seeking to integrate persons with disabilities into community leisure services. Concerned with inadequate or inferior programs, voluntary service organizations providing segregated programs may be hesitant to relinquish their participants to agencies that had previously rejected them. Similarly, parents of nondisabled children may express opposition to integrated programs. Persons with disabilities and parents and careproviders of disabled individuals often express the desire to be integrated into generic programs, yet they fail to make their desires known to the right people, or may fail to participate in the integrated programs available to them for any of a variety of reasons. One reason for this may be that skill deficits can limit the involvement of persons with disabilities in community recreation programs. Also, general recreation program staff who were previously led to believe that they did not possess the expertise to work effectively with disabled people may question their own abilities to conduct integrated programs.

Katz and Yekutiel (1974) reported that parents discouraged their mentally retarded children from participating in segregated activities. Disabled adults and parents of disabled children who were interviewed in regard to mainstreaming recreation and leisure services identified a preference for integrated recreation programs (Howe-Murphy, 1980). Sherrill, Rainbolt, and Ervin (1984), for example, reported the results of interviews with a sample of 30 adults with visual impairments. While 72% of the subjects reported negative experiences pertaining to acceptance and integration in their communities during adolescence, as adults, the subjects still desired acceptance into activities in their neighborhoods and communities.

The Leisure Information Studies (1976) suggested that the provision of recreation services for disabled individuals should be provided at the community level in anticipation that the majority of institutionalized persons will eventually return to the community. The reason for this proposal is that discharged patients are frequently left stranded between institutionalized recreation programs and community agencies without proper preparation and education to make the necessary adjustment.

GUIDELINES FOR COMMUNITY
LEISURE SERVICES AND SPECIAL POPULATIONS

The principle of normalization demands the phasing out of segregated programs in favor of integrated programs. According to Richler (1983), the salient issue for people who are disabled is not simply gaining full access to community resources; the issue is the ability to become a full participant in community life. An individual with a disability can take advantage of community resources through a segregated program without ever experiencing the benefits of social integration, an essential component of normalization. Segregated programs have been defended as a way to prepare individuals with disabilities to engage in community programs. However, Salzberg and Langford (1981) note that while segregated programs for disabled individuals are preferable to isolation, the practice of segregation is inconsistent with the principle of normalization. Such special programs usually favor the lowest skill common to the group rather than maximizing each individual's skills. Segregated program activities also tend to be characterized by large numbers of participants, a situation not typical of the more solitary adult leisure pursuits of nondisabled individuals. Such groupings also tend to discourage interactions with nondisabled persons who are also using the community facility (Certo & Schleien, 1982; Certo, Schleien, & Hunter, 1983).

All too often, persons with disabilities remain in segregated programs because they are not judged to be ready for participation in regular activities. The segregated program was intended to be a "stepping stone" to participation in integrated activities; instead, it has become the only type of program many disabled persons ever experience. An acceptable alternative to special and segregated programs is to provide individual skill instruction to a participant with a disability. Instruction may be provided at a separate time apart from the activity, or during the time the activity is occurring. Separate, individualized skill instruction, rather than group instruction in a special, segregated program, is the preferred way of promoting social integration.

In 1981, Reynolds summarized the major premise and corollaries of the normalization principle. He also listed the common misconceptions that hinder its implementation, and discussed normalization as it relates to recreation programming. He identified a substantial shift in the roles and orientations of therapeutic recreation specialists and educators and discussed trends that illustrate several new service functions and challenges. The following five trends were described:

1. Large group diversional activities and coordinated special events will be decreased in favor of individualized leisure and educational programming.
2. The medical model will be replaced by programming oriented toward leisure services.
3. Behavior techniques can and will be reconciled with the principle of normalization.
4. Recreation and special education personnel will adopt rules as advocates and as community liaisons to ensure that the rights of disabled persons to participate in community leisure opportunities are respected.
5. The problem of transfer of training and generalization will be addressed by teachers of leisure skills.

Bates and Renzaglia (1979) discussed a number of areas pertinent to developing and successfully conducting community recreation programs. They were searching for a systematic approach to providing community leisure services for special populations. The areas they examined included program planning, assessment, training and skill development, maintenance and generalization of recreational skills, and future research needs.

The National Therapeutic Recreation Society (NTRS), a branch of the National Recreation and Park Association, approved guidelines and suggested solutions to alleviate the problems encountered by persons with disabilities. These guidelines were recommended for use by public park and recreation agencies in developing community-based recreation programs serving members of special populations (Vaughan & Winslow, 1979). Transportation was identified as the major problem hindering the establishment of a special recreation program in the community. Possible solutions to this problem included car pools, use of federal grant monies (e.g., Federal Aid Highway Act of 1973, PL 93-87) available to community recreation and park agencies for the purchase of transportation vehicles, involvement of service clubs and social service agencies (e.g., American Red Cross, Kiwanis Clubs), and contractual agreements with schools, health agencies, and private organizations.

A project was funded by the U.S. Department of Education, Office of Special Education, to devise a comprehensive inservice education system to promote the development, delivery, and advocacy of leisure services for persons with disabilities in New Jersey communities (New Jersey Office on Community Recreation for Handicapped Persons, 1980). As a result of the project, a handbook was prepared for the administrator of the public recreation agency outlining objectives to guide public agencies wishing to initiate or expand community recreation services for disabled persons.

Certo et al. (1983) developed an inventory to enable therapeutic recreation specialists and other educators to develop functional, age-appropriate instructional leisure skills. The authors believed that this approach, coupled with longitudinal planning, would increase opportunities for individuals with severe disabilities to actively participate in normalized recreation activities in integrated community settings. The inventory was divided into three interrelated areas: skill selection and skill/facility description, component skills and adaptations for full or partial participation, and supportive skills.

BENEFITS OF INTEGRATION

Integrating persons with disabilities into community recreation environments can be beneficial to all participants. The opportunity to learn from and to socialize with nondisabled peers has been cited as one benefit for individuals with disabilities participating in integrated programs. For example, moderately retarded teenagers increased their frequencies of appropriate social interactions with nondisabled teenagers who volunteered to teach them playground skills; the retarded teenagers also showed an increase in appropriate playground behavior (Donder & Nietupski, 1981). A second benefit was observed by McGill (1984), who noted that integrated play opportunities are stimulating and highly motivating experiences for disabled children, offering them opportunities to imitate and model the play behavior of nondisabled peers. Stainback and Stainback (1985) supported the notion that nondisabled students provide disabled students with models of age-appropriate dress, language, gestures, and leisure behavior. The presence of nondisabled peers may also provide more opportunities for social interaction.

In a study by Brinker (1985), the social interactions of severely retarded students in segregated and integrated settings were compared. Brinker concluded that integrated groupings promoted more social behavior than did the segregated groupings. Severely retarded subjects interacted more often with nonretarded peers in integrated settings than they did with their severely retarded peers in either the integrated or segregated settings. Brinker's findings support the observation of Katz and Yekutiel (1974) that people who are mentally retarded tend to shy away from the company of others who are also mentally retarded. While these findings should not be extended to account for the behavior of all people with disabilities, they do provide support for the belief that integrated activities prove more beneficial than segregated activities. The findings also suggest that many individuals with disabilities prefer integrated activities.

Benefits to Persons without Disabilities

Participation in integrated environments is also believed to be beneficial for the nondisabled participants. Attitudes of nondisabled children toward their disabled peers have been extensively studied in recent years. McHale and Simeonsson (1980) found that the nondisabled children in their study expressed overwhelmingly positive attitudes both before and after play sessions with playmates who were autistic. The nondisabled children also displayed a more accurate conception of autism after contact. Voeltz (1982) administered a survey to elementary school students to measure their attitudes toward peers with severe disabilities. More positive attitudes were expressed by students in schools that included severely disabled students than by students who attended schools without the presence of severely disabled students. Students in a school that sponsored a peer interaction program for severely disabled and nondisabled children expressed the most positive attitudes of all groups studied. Sixth graders involved in a peer tutoring program with moderately and severely retarded peers showed an increase in positive attitudes toward their disabled peers (Fenrick & Petersen, 1984). In a study by Donder and Nietupski (1981), integrated activities were found to be very enjoyable by the participants without disabilities. The authors reported anecdotal data from a study in which nondisabled teenagers volunteered to teach playground skills to moderately retarded peers. The nondisabled teens commented that they enjoyed their recess period and playground activities more when they were acting as peer tutors than they had prior to becoming tutors. The results of these studies help dispel the notion that nondisabled participants "lose out" when programs are integrated. The evidence that activities could be just as enjoyable for nondisabled persons when people with disabilities are included provides additional support for integration.

The integration of persons with disabilities into community recreation programs is essential if the process of normalization is to be completed. Successful integration requires that the key players involved in service delivery adopt a philosophy and value system consistent with the principle of normalization. Of central importance in this philosophy is the recognition that people with disabilities are valuable as individuals and that they thus possess the right to participate in the same programs in which nondisabled citizens participate. Agencies committed to normalization must articulate and practice a policy of inclusion into existing programs rather than providing only special segregated programs. A belief that the creation and provision of segregated programs is exclusionary and results in the removal of a person with a disability from the rest of society is a vital component of this philosophy. Commitment to the integration of programs also requires that agencies actively recruit participants with disabilities to their facilities.

Personnel Preparation

Community recreation agencies also have a responsibility to ensure that personnel in their agencies are prepared to share the responsibility for integrating participants with disabilities. Effective integration requires that general program staff and therapeutic recreation specialists begin working collaboratively. An emphasis must be placed on the utilization of generalists, rather than specialists, to facilitate and implement integrated programs. The use of specialists as support personnel will assist integration efforts by de-emphasizing a disabled person's need for specially trained staff and special programs. Lord (1983) offered important advice that is useful for personnel involved in recreation integration efforts. Lord stated that instead of asking the question "Is this person ready for integration?", it makes more sense to ask, "What support does this person need to be involved and to participate?"

SUMMARY

Lord's advice should be a guiding principle in all efforts to integrate people with disabilities into community recreation programs. Acceptance of the normalization principle means endeavoring to include individuals with disabilities into all aspects of society. It is not enough to merely accept these individuals into integrated programs. Recreation and human services professionals must go further to recruit and encourage the participation of persons with disabilities by providing them with successful mechanisms of support.

Integration is not something that can be avoided by the rationalization that segregated programs are for preparation of future integration. Integration is characterized by the dichotomy "all or nothing." Unless the philosophy of normalization is embraced, and the physical and social integration of individuals with disabilities is effected, the right and privilege of disabled persons to lead truly normal lives will continue to be denied.

Not all leisure experiences in least restrictive environments need to be successful, but the privilege to achieve or fail is part of a learning process that for too long has been denied individuals with disabilities. In the final analysis, it is up to disabled consumers, parents, and community recreation professionals to ensure the continued availability of community recreation programs to members of special populations and the continual experimentation of participation in least restrictive environments. Making additional opportunities available for participation in integrated programs by disabled persons will increase the probability that individuals with disabilities will live their lives as normally and as meaningfully as possible. The purpose of this book is to examine the planning and development, the implementation, and the evaluation of integrated community recreation programs for individuals without and with disabilities.

Chapter 2

A Plan for Creating Opportunities in Community Recreation

The organized movement for municipal park and recreation services has a distinctive and widely documented history (Chubb & Chubb, 1981; Meyer & Brightbill, 1964). Much of the organization of public recreation services centers today, as it did during its formative years, on the provision of leisure services that reflect broad neighborhood or community interests. Developing organized and publicly funded recreational services was a way for local governments to address the health and well-being of its constituency in a manner that was consistent with the prevailing belief that recreation participation contributed to the quality of one's life (Sessoms, 1984). As one of the larger components of the community's leisure service delivery system, municipal park and recreation agencies have, as a general mission, the public interest in mind.

It is typically the policy of municipal park and recreation agencies to establish, to expand, and to improve leisure opportunities and facilities that citizens cannot supply themselves. To this end, the agency may adopt objectives similar to the following:

1. It shall be the agency's policy to establish and multiply those leisure opportunities which will be personally satisfying, consistent with the varied interests, needs and competencies of the changing population regardless of age, sex, race, creed, social or economic status. Insofar as it is able, leisure opportunities will be directed toward developing the physical, social, educational, and cultural self-potential and expression of the individual; and respect for the dignity, autonomy, and self-determination of each person will be paramount.

2. Recognizing that the harmonious relationship of man to nature is critical to human life, an equally important objective is to conserve nature and make natural beauty paramount. Thus, the agency will do everything within its power to encourage and provide opportunity for people to enjoy, appreciate, protect, and strengthen their ties with the natural

and aesthetic values of the neighborhood, community, and urban environment in which they live.

3. The agency's services and resources will be evaluated primarily in terms of their worth to humans.
4. Social, physical, educational, and cultural development, including sports, outdoor living, the performing, graphic and plastic arts, and all of the major leisure interests of people will be encouraged and multiplied.
5. Proper attention will be given to individual need for privacy and solitude.
6. Primary focus will be upon opportunities in leisure for the full personality development of all citizens particularly special populations (i.e., persons with disabilities, minority groups).
7. The agency recognizes that its services do not stand alone, that they are closely related to urban and regional planning, to housing, to health and welfare, to the business, political, cultural and spiritual community, to education in all of its settings, and to all of the functions of government; and, therefore, it shall be the continuing policy of the agency to seek the cooperation and assistance of all such interests, and to make the public a continuing partner in its work. (Minneapolis Park and Recreation Board, 1984)

The goals relating to the above objectives and applying specifically to the municipal park and recreation agency's recreation division may include the following:

1. To provide positive recreational experiences which contribute to the growth and development of every individual.
2. To provide a comprehensive, year-round recreational program for all city residents.
3. To strengthen cooperative efforts with other agencies in order to maximize capital, human, and financial resources.
4. To develop a qualified staff which will promote and expand interest in leisure activities. (Minneapolis Park and Recreation Board, 1984)

Municipal leisure services have become, in essence, a mandate of the community. These services are expected to mirror the leisure and recreational needs, desires, and expectations of a constituency whose tax dollars they require. And, with increased pressure from private or commercial recreation concerns with whom they compete, municipal park and recreation agencies must make an objective and comprehensive appraisal of their niche in the community leisure service delivery system, along with the management and planning systems they employ (Edgington, Compton, & Hanson, 1980; Russell, 1982; Sessoms, 1984). An appropriate place to begin this appraisal is by identifying a process model that provides the recreation professional with a systematic approach toward delivery of community leisure services.

IDENTIFYING A PROCESS FOR ACCESSIBLE LEISURE SERVICES

In order to identify and address the needs of its community, a municipal park and recreation organization often develops a model of service delivery based upon a general social planning process (Edginton, Compton, & Hanson, 1980; Russell, 1982) such as the model depicted in Figure 2.1. Models of this type help municipal park and recreation personnel to organize services around a central, philosophical mission. A simply expressed mission reflecting the objectives noted above might read: "To provide leisure opportunities that contribute to the social, physical, educational, cultural, and general well-being of the community and its people" (Sessoms, 1984, p. 19). The program plan, its implementation, and subsequent evaluation are considered within the overall mission of the agency. This model assumes interaction between all components (i.e., tasks I–VI), representing a process that is both active and open to constructive change.

However, this model, while useful for a general analysis of social systems, may appear to be too vague to the community recreation professional. This individual might

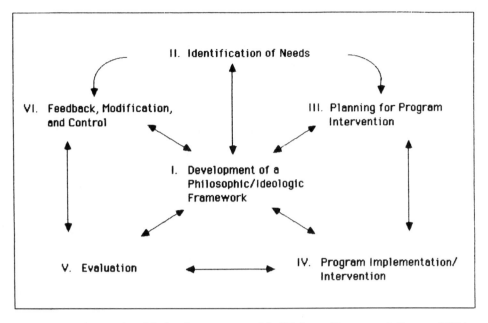

FIGURE 2.1.   A general social planning process model. (Edginton, Comptom, & Hanson, 1980.)

need a more specific picture of the leisure service delivery system in which she or he is expected to operate, not some idealized flow model. It is likely that many municipal park and recreation departments already have adapted various model processes and strategies for meeting the leisure needs of their constituents, including persons with disabilities. However, some of these models may not provide the recreation professional with a reliable, comprehensive, or logical approach to total community leisure service delivery. The following continuum models and "diamond" analogy are introduced to illustrate planning processes currently in use. Included among these models is a process that is practical and functional, and that provides reasonable assurance that community leisure services will be accessible to everyone, including persons with disabilities.

When persons with disabilities enter into programs offered at community recreation settings, they do so with varying levels of ability, knowledge, skills, and interests. It is quite probable that the nature of their disabilities will limit successful participation in recreation activities with nondisabled peers. For example, a young person whose mobility is impaired and who uses crutches will be unable to keep pace with other participants actively playing kickball. Another example would be the dependency of persons with cognitive impairments (e.g., persons with mental retardation) upon group home staff to locate, plan, and lead outings into the community because they are unaware of other, more independent options. This may be due to insufficient leisure education or to the lack of opportunities to make independent choices about preferred leisure activities. Other persons may find themselves left out of recreational activities and programs, thus inhibiting their ability to practice or to improve the skills they do have. An example would be the visually impaired cross-country skier who learns to ski at an out-of-town event only to find, upon arriving home, that there is no one qualified to guide him or her on local ski trails. Also, all persons, regardless of ability, vary in their degree of interest and motivation prior to and during participation in a recreational activity. The person with a hearing impairment may find increased strength, fitness, and self-worth while participating in a volleyball league. However, his or her teammates may be more interested in the socialization that occurs, the competition among teams, the escape from life's pressures, or in simply appreciating the elements of the game. However, these examples are not necessarily "handicap-specific:" many nondisabled participants of recreation programs enter into programs with varying levels of skills or experience. It is important, therefore, that the community recreation professional be aware that there exist individual differences in skills, abilities, knowledge, and interests of persons both with and without disabilities.

A major responsibility of the community recreation professional is to adequately assess the needs, interests, and preferences of potential recreation participants from the community prior to selection and implementation of specific programs and services. Failure to do so may hinder the ability of disabled persons living in the community to have satisfying leisure experiences within community recreation environments. When a society fails to provide for the needs of individuals with disabilities, "barriers of omission" result (Kennedy, Austin, & Smith, 1987). Barriers of omission occur when a leisure service agency fails to provide opportunities for persons with disabilities to express their needs and to assist in program selection and development. An example of this type of barrier occurs when a municipal park and recreation agency fails to involve representatives of a large group residence serving youths who are mentally retarded in the planning of a new neighborhood playground. Other barriers of omission result when recreation professionals fail to acquire the necessary skills to make recreation programs accessible. The following chapters in this text, in particular, the staff training and development section in Chapter 3, identify the most pertinent and relevant skills and knowledge needed by the recreation professional. Without these skills, recreation professionals must depend on others (e.g., advocacy groups, care providers) to provide meaningful leisure experiences for persons with disabilities. This "barrier of omission" prevents persons with disabilities from participating in mainstream, integrated recreation programs. It has been demonstrated that persons with disabilities can be successfully integrated into community recreation programs and settings where they can actively participate alongside their nondisabled peers (Schleien, Olson, Rogers, & Mclafferty, 1985; Schleien & Ray, 1986). Failure to provide individualized adaptation to enhance the participation and the enjoyment of these individuals keeps them from receiving equal opportunities to utilize community leisure services.

Hutchison and Lord (1979) have noted that leisure service agencies may not consider it their responsibility to respond to the needs of all members of the community. This idea seems contrary to the stated mission and goals of such agencies. This apparent dichotomy of mission is not without foundation, however. In his introductory text for students entering the leisure service profession, Sessoms (1984) suggested that consideration of priorities is a primary issue in programming services. Sessoms stated that the assumption that public recreation programs should be open to all individuals is now being challenged due to limited fiscal resources of human services agencies. Discrimination against various special population groups that results from limiting services is apparently not the concern. Agencies must necessarily be concerned with efficiency and management of scarce resources but they must endeavor to continue providing accessible leisure services as much as possible. Unfortunately, Sessoms offered few specific guidelines to assist the professional in establishing priorities, particularly those pertaining to fiscal resource management and service provision for persons with disabilities.

In all fairness to park and recreation agencies and the professionals they employ to provide services, it is quite doubtful that barriers of omission are a result of deliberate discriminatory practices. In fact, the obstacles that prevent or inhibit persons with disabilities from receiving community leisure services are more often due to administrative oversight or poor program planning rather than to discrimination. These obstacles, and specific suggestions on how to overcome them, are comprehensively addressed in Chapter 7. Whatever the cause, persons with disabilities have not, as a whole, been receiving adequate leisure services. Perhaps the reason is that community leisure professionals have gotten into the practice of assigning blame somewhere other than on themselves and their agencies (Hutchison & Lord, 1979). This and a variety of other familiar excuses assail the ears of those advocates wishing to open and to integrate generic recreation programs to include persons with disabilities. Common excuses that have been encountered by human services professionals include:

"Our doors are always open, but . . ."
"That's not really our responsibility."
"It will hold back other people."
"We are committed but we don't have the finances right now."
"Our mandate is only to provide programs."
"We can't make exceptions for two or three people."
"You must demonstrate that it works before we can commit any funds or resources."
    (Hutchison & Lord, 1979, p. 17)

A CONTINUUM OF LEISURE SERVICES FOR PERSONS WITH DISABILITIES

Two concerns become immediately apparent when one considers the necessity for developing accessible community leisure services. First, leisure service providers must eliminate barriers of omission if they are to effect the movement of persons with disabilities out of the "basement of noninvolvement." Barriers of omission must be eliminated so that persons with disabilities can come out of their homes or other residential situations to engage in recreation within community leisure settings and, if desired, alongside their nondisabled friends and neighbors.

Second, because the characteristics of a person's disability can limit his or her participation in regular programs (that is, those programs generally established for persons without disabilities), recreation professionals must develop a range, or a continuum of services (Figure 2.2) that are accessible to all persons with disabilities. This continuum of leisure service options for persons with disabilities ranges from segregated, special recreation programs focusing on skill development within homogeneous (i.e., handicap-specific) groups (e.g., craft activity for persons with developmental disabilities) to integrated programs.

Integrated programs incorporate the unique skills and abilities of each participant, disabled or nondisabled, into meaningful and functional leisure experiences. Ideally, accessible service options will become the norm for persons with disabilities who can identify and make use of preferred leisure settings and recreation programs with minimal assistance. Barriers of omission, negative attitudes, and various stigma threaten to keep persons with disabilities in the "basement of noninvolvement" unless recreation professionals and other key individuals take appropriate steps to facilitate movement of persons with disabilities along the continuum. Not only must access to community-based leisure environments be made available, but persons with disabilities must be provided with opportunities to learn new leisure and leisure-related skills (e.g., social, money management, transportation) and to practice these skills within settings that provide appropriate structure and staff support.

Utilizing a continuum approach to leisure service delivery for persons with disabilities is not a novel idea. In fact, many therapeutic recreation service systems in clinical, residential, and community-based agencies that serve persons with disabilities subscribe to

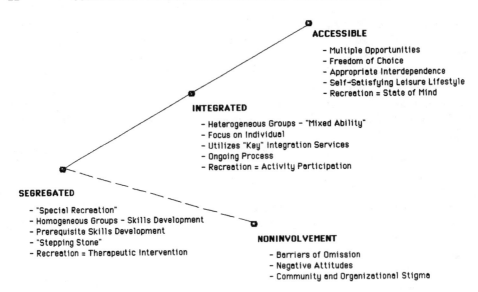

ACCESSIBLE

- Multiple Opportunities
- Freedom of Choice
- Appropriate Interdependence
- Self-Satisfying Leisure Lifestyle
- Recreation = State of Mind

INTEGRATED

- Heterogeneous Groups - "Mixed Ability"
- Focus on Individual
- Utilizes "Key" Integration Services
- Ongoing Process
- Recreation = Activity Participation

SEGREGATED

- "Special Recreation"
- Homogeneous Groups - Skills Development
- Prerequisite Skills Development
- "Stepping Stone"
- Recreation = Therapeutic Intervention

NONINVOLVEMENT

- Barriers of Omission
- Negative Attitudes
- Community and Organizational Stigma

FIGURE 2.2.   A continuum of leisure service options for persons with disabilities.

such a model. The National Therapeutic Recreation Society (NTRS) articulates this continuum approach in its philosophical position statement (NTRS, 1982). This model identifies three specific areas of professional service to the client with a disability, and is based on a design proposed by Gunn and Peterson (1978). Depending upon individually assessed needs and the service mandate, or mission, of the sponsoring agency, the client could receive recreational therapy, leisure education, or opportunities for voluntary recreation participation. The roles and responsibilities of therapeutic recreation staff vary depending upon the level of service. For example, if recreation is oriented to a more prescriptive approach, such as recreation therapy, the staff will be more intrusive using a variety of therapeutic approaches (Avedon, 1974) to facilitate development of functional abilities and behaviors as a prerequisite to more meaningful leisure experiences. Along with other members of the treatment team (including the client with disabilities), the recreation therapist can suggest optimal methods for ameliorating the effects of disabilities through the medium of recreation activity.

The level of intrusiveness diminishes in the leisure education and recreation participation service domains as clients with disabilities acquire leisure skills and values, and independently make decisions concerning when, and in what context, they wish to practice and develop these skills and values. As clients with disabilities visit community-based settings such as shopping malls and sports and health centers, they receive less specialized services, such as those found in therapeutic recreation programs utilizing highly adaptive equipment. Provision of these services helps to meet the intent of the normalization principle because therapeutic recreation personnel can facilitate client access to these less restrictive community leisure settings. In these settings, clients are expected to function appropriately and successfully.

The ultimate goal of providing leisure and recreation services is to enable the person to have as satisfying and as independent a leisure life-style as possible (Navar, 1981). The continuum model, also referred to as the "Leisure-Ability Model," serves as a guide for community recreation professionals to facilitate the movement of individuals with disabilities from more intrusive, specialized recreation services into integrated leisure environments that permit individuals to independently choose what they would like to do in their "free" or leisure time.

The leisure service option chosen as most appropriate for a particular individual will depend, in all cases, on the assessed needs of the potential participant who is disabled. As will be explained in more detail in Chapter 3, there are a variety of "key players" who can be consulted on specific strategies that can be used to determine what types of services in the model are the most appropriate for the participant. These key players will need to bear in mind that any decisions that are made should be based strictly on the needs and capabilities of the participant with disabilities, and that these needs and capabilities vary over time. This variation in needs necessitates constant reassessment of the leisure service to ensure that it is the most appropriate and least restrictive option for that individual. With this thought in mind, it is now appropriate to examine the three leisure service options and the unique features that characterize each.

Segregated Services

One must initially assume that barriers of omission have been overcome sufficiently to allow persons with disabilities to utilize community leisure environments, that is, they have been able to move from noninvolvement in community recreation programs to a segregated services setting. The first options likely to be encountered on the continuum are segregated, "handicapped-only" programs. Persons participating in these programs typically need special staff services, equipment, and environments in which to receive a positive and successful leisure experience. Specialized staff such as therapeutic recreation specialists, careproviders, or teachers are employed because they typically have a knowledge and understanding of the participant's skills, abilities, and behaviors. They can provide specialized services through appropriate interventions, such as speech interpretation or behavior management, to help ensure that the programs are conducted smoothly and that participants interact appropriately. Special adaptive equipment such as therapy balls or positioning cushions and facilities such as therapeutic swimming pools in hospitals, or activity rooms in institutional settings, can be scheduled to accommodate participants with disabilities. Persons utilizing segregated programs may be those individuals who prefer to associate with similarly disabled peers (in such activities as wheelchair basketball, or Friday night dances for persons with mental retardation), who are "placed" there by parents or careproviders, or who do not have opportunities to associate with nondisabled peers because any number of obstacles impede their ability to take advantage of integrated or "regular" recreation programs.

These specialized or segregated programs are typically developed by individuals who believe that service provision is most effective when persons with disabilities are grouped together. Therapeutic recreation specialists, community recreation personnel with backgrounds in serving special population groups, allied health professionals, advocacy agencies, or parent groups may believe that specialized services are developed and used more efficiently when participants with disabilities are congregated in one location. Special recreation programs can become extensions of therapeutic recreation programs and may border on being prescriptive and interventionist in approach. The goal of such programs is to habilitate or rehabilitate the participant with disabilities in order to prepare him or her for more normalized settings. A potential problem with this approach is that decisions about program content and process are left solely up to professionals who may believe they alone know what is best for the person with disabilities. The result is that often, persons with disabilities are not involved in program planning and implementation, because others are determining what is needed in terms of more "therapeutic recreation." This overreliance on professionals reinforces the stereotype that persons with disabilities do not know what is best for them. Overreliance also breeds dependency on professionals, who, without input from the participant or the participants' family, may not always know what is best for the participant.

While the main purpose of this text is to promote equal access and integration by persons with disabilities in community leisure service settings, the authors would be remiss if the more positive implications of special recreation services were not mentioned. If activities are age-appropriate and functional, and are offered in least restrictive or generic settings, that is, settings also used by nondisabled persons, segregated programs may provide individuals with disabilities with a safe, structured, and secure leisure experience. The participant must feel comfortable in new leisure environments if future integration efforts are to be successful. With the concentrated attention of staff, and the use of intervention strategies designed for each individual, participants with disabilities could acquire significant recreation and social skills in the context of an enjoyable leisure activity. Special or segregated recreation programs, therefore, can serve as stepping-stones to more integrated environments and experiences (Reynolds, 1981). It is critical, however, that specific "exit" criteria be delineated to ensure that participants in these programs can move through the continuum to less restrictive, integrated programs. Exit criteria include behavioral changes in the participant (e.g., in leisure and/or social skill acquisition, appropriate play behaviors), as well as a fixed amount of time (i.e., duration) for program implementation (e.g., an 8-week period). The latter criteria are typically determined by recreation professionals and activity leaders. Progress in other qualitative ways is jointly determined by recreational staff, careproviders, and participants with disabilities through specific evaluative methods (see Chapter 6). This does not imply that all supports for the disabled participant are immediately withdrawn. Rather, the participant will now have the opportunity to experience enjoyment and, possibly, disappointment in the same recreational contexts as his or her nondisabled peers. Participants with disabilities will no longer be insulated from the community by overprotective careproviders and professionals. Participants will be able to apply the skills they have acquired in the segregated recreation programs toward the multitude of leisure experiences available in the community.

There are many good community models illustrating special recreation services throughout the United States. The reader is encouraged to consult additional texts (e.g., Kennedy et al., 1987), for a detailed discussion of these types of services and the exemplary programs in existence throughout the country.

Integrated Services

The second leisure service option, integrated services, provides persons with disabilities the opportunity to be mainstreamed into regular community recreation programs and to participate alongside nondisabled participants. While specialized staff and services may still be used, little or no assumption is made beforehand that these considerations are appropriate or even necessary. The purpose of this text is to present a systematic process for ensuring the integration and accessibility of community recreation programs.

Whereas segregated programs comprise, by definition, more homogeneous "handicapped-only" groupings, integrated programs are more heterogeneous and bring together persons with "mixed abilities." The rationale of integrated programming is that participants bring into the recreation program intact skills and abilities, thus further contributing to the diversity typically found in such programs. This richness of experience creates a positive dynamic in the group that permits participants to learn from each other. If the primary mission of the public recreation agency is to contribute to the social, physical, educational, and cultural growth of the individual, what better forum is there than in an integrated program with participants of mixed abilities?

Because integrated recreation programs are viewed as a way for individuals to participate in and to enjoy their preferred leisure activities, the program focus moves from planning and implementing special recreation services for members of special populations to one of looking at the unique characteristics of individual participants. Recreation professionals in such programs will raise such questions as: Why did she or he register for this program? What are his or her expectations? What skills or experiences does he or she bring to the program? How will she or he interact with the other participants? How can I, as the recreation programmer, meet his or her needs? These questions require answers from the individual registering for the program. Since there are assumptions based on the characteristics of disability, these questions can be generally applied to any participant, whether or not the person has disabling conditions. Depending upon the answers to these and other pertinent questions (see Chapter 4, Environmental Analysis Inventory), community recreation professionals can begin to consider any combination of key strategies that will facilitate the physical and social integration of the participant with disabilities into the recreation program.

A final note must be made regarding integration. A chief corollary of the normalization principle (Reynolds, 1981; Wolfensberger, 1972) is that integration must be viewed as both a process and a goal. This means that successful integration will not be realized without the support and continual efforts of many individuals and agencies. Reynolds (1981) advised that integration will not occur if persons with disabilities are "dumped" into community leisure service settings. One should not make the assumption that the community leisure service system is ready and able to be accessible to persons with disabilities. Therefore, various leisure service personnel (e.g., therapeutic recreation specialists, or community recreators), advocacy agencies (e.g., the Association for Retarded Citizens), parents or careproviders, and potential participants with disabilities, must act together to ensure that integrated opportunities are possible.

These experiences must be successful and positive not only for the disabled participants, but also for the other (nondisabled) participants, the recreation staff, and the individuals who are involved in the process or who are directly affected by it. Taking a deliberate, systematic approach seems to be the best way to ensure that integrated services will, someday, become totally accessible. It also appears that this approach goes a long way toward helping to change the negative attitudes, stereotypes, stigma, and myths associated with persons with disabilities and the systems that serve them.

Accessible Services

The third leisure service option, accessible services, should be the ultimate goal of all recreation personnel and programs. Participants with disabilities should come to understand that independent access to community leisure settings and programs is possible. Persons with disabilities should be considered "participants," not "the handicapped." Therefore, they are entitled to the same respect and attention afforded any other member of the community when recreation programming is being planned and developed.

Accessible leisure services are so named in order to suggest that multiple leisure opportunities exist throughout the community. The individual who is disabled is able to select and access preferred recreation programs with no more effort than his or her counterpart who is nondisabled. Using appropriate levels of interdependence, the person with disabilities is able to call upon any number of necessary support systems to aid him or her in taking advantage of these recreation programs. The participant is able to realize his or her utlimate goal of achieving a satisfying leisure life-style, free of any significant individual (e.g., skill deficits, characteristics of disability) and external (e.g., transportation, barriers of a mission) constraints. While this may be an idealized or utopian view of leisure and recreation for the person with a disability, one must realize that most nondisabled people who utilize community recreation facilities are exercising their leisure needs in this very way. Persons without disabilities have come to expect and demand such variety and accessibility from public park and recreation systems.

In summary, it is apparent that there is a need for programs at all three levels of the leisure services continuum. Many persons with disabilities need the specialized training offered through segregated programs in order to participate in community leisure services. However, those persons with disabilities who have the potential to participate alongside peers within integrated programs, or who have the skills to independently choose and attend an accessible leisure setting, such as a park, should be given sufficient opportunities to do so. Segregated programs, therefore, become a means to an end: a stepping-stone to equal access and participation in community leisure settings. Decisions concerning at which level to start this process should be based upon a collective assessment of the skills and abilities of the potential consumer with disabilities. The continuum of leisure service options for persons with disabilities is represented, once again, in Figure 2.2. Key issues, such as freedom of choice or barriers of omission are listed under each option.

CURRENT PERSPECTIVE ON COMMUNITY LEISURE SERVICE SYSTEMS

If community recreation agencies and staff accept the continuum model of leisure service provision, use of this approach will be a positive step forward in meeting the individual leisure and recreation needs of persons with disabilities. It can be anticipated that greater numbers of individuals with disabilities will utilize the community leisure service system; the model proposes a strategy whereby these individuals will be given maximum opportunities to move through the full range of available leisure services. Regular participation in integrated and accessible programs will become the norm for individuals who had heretofore been relegated to special, segregated recreation programs or to the "basement of noninvolvement:" unseen, unwanted, and largely ignored.

However, for the continuum concept to work, community leisure service providers must closely examine their systems of service delivery. This would include making an objective appraisal of the mission or philosophical foundation of the agency and of the agency's procedures for selecting, implementing, and evaluating programs and management practices. If agency personnel or recreation personnel do not have a clear understanding of their purpose or methods of service delivery, there is the possibility that negative attitudes, organizational stigma, and other barriers of omission will continue to prevent or to inhibit persons with disabilities from taking advantage of leisure services.

Past studies have focused on the perceived or actual barriers encountered by recreation professionals and/or participants with disabilities that limit the latter's access to more generic and integrated community leisure environments. The most salient of these efforts is highlighted throughout Chapter 1 and will not be reiterated here. The authors of these studies have sought to identify both social and architectural barriers and to make suggestions on ways to overcome them. However, the studies appear to include an a priori assumption that it is the barriers themselves that prevent access to leisure services. The studies seem to suggest that if a specific barrier is eliminated, services will automatically be considered "accessible." This assumption is fallacious, because it does not address the broader issues related to the ongoing physical and social integration of people with disabilities into diverse leisure environments. Granted, overcoming isolated barriers may provide the participant with temporary access to services; unfortunately, the entire system of leisure service delivery is geared to an able-bodied population who are more adaptive or flexible in their ability to accept system inadequacies. If a service system fails to meet the needs of nondisabled individuals, for example, the individuals can either compromise standards and expectations, thus settling for less, or the individuals can choose to go somewhere else for leisure and recreation needs. If, more specifically, potential participants who are nondisabled do not like the services offered in a particular setting because the programs are not interesting, or because the program leadership is inadequate or incompetent, for example, they can choose to take advantage of a variety of alternative commercial or quasi-public leisure service settings, such as fraternal organizations or the YM/YWCA. For many people with disabilities, public recreation programs may be the only affordable alternative available to them for developing and practicing leisure skills and abilities. If the leisure service systems are inadequate or poorly administered, persons with disabilities may not have the necessary comprehension or ability to make appropriate choices among known opportunities.

In many ways, the practice of shopping around for services does a disservice to persons who have disabilities. For one thing, it hinders program improvement generated from constituent feedback. If low standards for leisure service delivery systems are maintained, there is little motivation or impetus to improve them so that they are more physically and programmatically accessible. If change occurs, it is probably due to the interest, enthusiasm, and tenacity of the people employed to administer the recreation and park programs and areas. Thus, any disappointment in service inadequacies should be expressed to the managers, superintendents, and service professionals, as they are the individuals empowered to make the necessary decisions that will result in positive system and program change. Similarly, it is important to reinforce those persons who have already made or are making these changes on behalf of everyone living in the community, including persons with disabilities.

Much of the effectiveness of service delivery for persons with disabilities is due, therefore, to the ability of the community leisure service professionals, parents, careproviders, and advocacy groups to react appropriately if and when specific barriers arise. Such responsiveness is important because if parents, careproviders, and individuals with disabilities perceive that a service system does not welcome them, they will stay away (West, 1984). If past attempts to utilize leisure services systems have failed due to the presence of any number of external or individual barriers (see Chapter 7), persons with disabilities, or those significant others facilitating decisions on behalf of these persons, will shy away from further attempts to utilize these systems. They will then create various segregated systems to meet the "special" needs of persons with disabilities.

By way of example: persons with mental retardation often depend upon the local Association for Retarded Citizens to provide opportunities for community leisure experiences. Although the 1964 Policy Statement of the National Association for Retarded Citizens (NARC) called upon local park and recreation agencies to assume responsibility for providing leisure services to persons with mental retardation, local ARCs continued to expand their own development and operation of community leisure services (Decker, 1980). These programs are almost always segregated, yet they meet the leisure needs of many persons who would otherwise be denied access to regular community recreation programs.

Community park and recreation agencies must take an active position regarding accessible leisure services. Community recreation agencies should fine-tune their own service delivery programs to maximize the ability of persons with disabilities to participate in leisure environments and recreation programs. Anticipating service needs is preferable to reacting to barriers that arise unexpectedly. The following provides a view of contemporary processes of community leisure service delivery systems. Also presented in the discussion is a proposal for making delivery systems more accessible.

THE DIAMOND ANALOGY

The use of graphic analogies and schematic drawings can be more useful than words alone to explain concepts and processes. Like acronyms (e.g., PIRC—Project for Integrated Recreation in the Community, or LIFE—Leisure is for Everyone), analogies can successfully play on words and images to clarify and illustrate ideas. When considering a useful way to present various processes of community leisure services, developing an analogy to a well-known item serves to get the point across readily to the readers. The author has selected the image of a diamond for the analogy in the following discussion.

Consider the diamond. As gemstones, they are highly valued and desirable investments. Owners who display their diamonds may be envied, revered or sought after. Diamonds can bespeak status, wealth, and at times, power. The cut and clarity of the diamond may dazzle and impress even the casual, uninitiated observer.

However, not all diamonds possess the same characteristics (See Figure 2.3). Diamonds are available in many shapes and sizes, and are appraised as having more or less value depending upon their weight, cut, clarity, and utility. Even imperfect diamonds are valuable. "Flawed" diamonds (Figure 2.3a), for instance, are used as abrasives to polish, grind, or cut other materials. These diamonds may not be pretty to look at, but they are useful. In this age of synthetics, it is possible to create realistic "diamonds" from cubic zirconia. These "fake" diamonds (Figure 2.3b) are manufactured through mass production for general consumption. However, because they are synthetic, they are not valued as highly as authentic diamonds. These fake diamonds give their owners a false sense of worth, with display, rather than investment, the chief concern. "Diamonds in the rough" (Figure 2.3c) are the next familiar diamond type. The facets, or sides, of such diamonds are incomplete or "rough." These diamonds lack polish, yet they have the potential for being refined by having their edges cut and polished by skilled lapidaries. The final, perfect diamond model is the "precious gem" (Figure 2.3d). Any discriminating person would prefer to invest in these, because these diamonds are of the highest quality. These diamonds are carefully cut and polished to bring out their greatest clarity and brilliance; these are considered to be the most valuable type of diamond.

Community leisure service delivery by municipal park and recreation agencies may be compared to the types of diamonds highlighted above. In the following discussion, four types of service delivery models are compared to the various grades of diamond mentioned above. Specific activities within each service model "diamond" are listed in the figures found throughout this chapter. The activities listed within each model represent the nature of the leisure service delivery process within individual municipal park and recreation agencies. In general, the service delivery process should follow the basic steps of the social systems planning process model illustrated in Figure 2.1. As each diamond analogy is presented, divergences from this model become apparent and are discussed. The activities identified in Figures 2.4 and 2.6 are similar to the idealized process listed in Figure 2.7 and described within this chapter and in Appendix A. The reader should refer to this process to further interpret the following discussions for Figures 2.4 and 2.6.

To begin with, segregated, "handicapped-only" models of service delivery may be compared to the "flawed" and fake diamonds in Figures 2.3a and 2.3b. Flawed diamonds (Figure 2.4) serve a utilitarian purpose, but are insufficient in several ways. Similarly, a

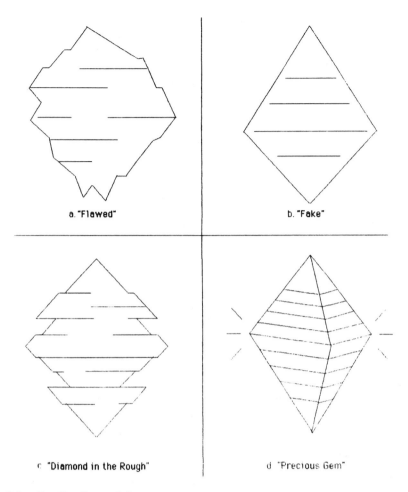

a. "Flawed"   b. "Fake"

c. "Diamond in the Rough"   d. "Precious Gem"

FIGURE 2.3.   Familiar diamond shapes.

segregated leisure service model is insufficient, because it does not provide for individual recreation needs or preferences. Additionally, segregated leisure service programs do not, in the authors' opinion, efficiently utilize available resources, promotional strategies, or program modification and improvement based upon feedback from staff, careproviders, or clients. Although there is service delivery in the segregated program, the lack of clarity (i.e., no clear purpose or mission), the presence of many rough, uneven edges (i.e., no systematic plan or approach), and the lack of "glamour" (i.e., no prestige associated with the agency), make this service system not worth owning or implementing. Such a flawed program, like a flawed diamond, is of diminished value.

The following scenario depicts a "flawed" program in action. Consider a municipal park and recreation agency in a suburban community. The program coordinator is aware that two of the more popular activities organized by the agency have been swimming at the community swimming pool and participation in the softball league. In response, the program coordinator increases staffing at the swimming pool and establishes a softball league. Participants purchase season passes to the pool and register teams and players for the league. By the Labor Day weekend, the program coordinator counts the number of participants and the amount of summer revenues and announces to her director that the summer

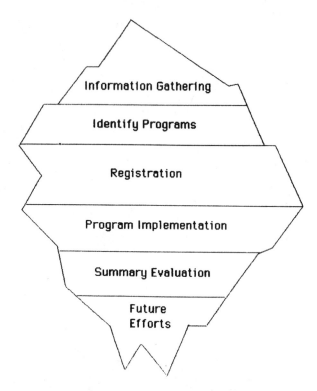

FIGURE 2.4.   Flawed diamond analogy: Inadequate service provision model.

recreation program has been a success. The director and the program coordinator decide to repeat the same program the following year.

What the program coordinator is failing to do is to consider the needs of the many other community residents who are not participating in her program. Examples of such residents are: the local teenagers who hang out at the shopping mall all day, nursing home residents who sit on their porches and play cards or just watch the world go by, and residents of large public facilities who have severe multiple disabilities and who stay indoors almost all the time. What do these people do all summer? They are not being served by the local recreation program. This "flawed" model of service is indeed unacceptable to the consumers who should be served within this community.

The next diamond model is the "fake" diamond (Figure 2.5). In this model, segregated leisure programs are compared to this synthetically produced gem. In this segregated program model, the agency assumes the chief decision-making role with little or no regard for input from potential participants or demographic information derived from needs assessments. Special population groups may be solicited by contacting advocacy agencies or special education classrooms, and may be provided activities that are stereotypical of such groups (e.g., bowling, arts and crafts, singing). Programs are terminated with essentially no evaluation or follow-up. Persons with disabilities must "wait" until recreation staff suggest a new program. The program and the gem are compared because outwardly, the park and recreation agency may appear to have a "gem" of a program: one that seems to be meeting the "special" needs of a "special" group of people. However, segregated service programs are poor investments, since they require the infusion of inordinate amounts of money and energy that go into constructing separate facilities, hiring specialized staff, pur-

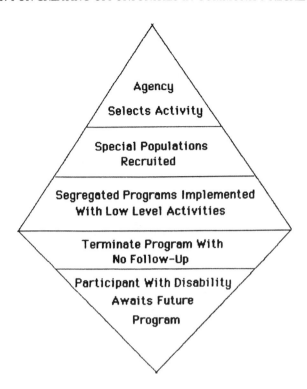

FIGURE 2.5.   Fake diamond analogy: Segregated leisure services model.

chasing adaptive equipment and materials. Examples of segregated services may include: Friday night dances for young adults with mental retardation, Sunday social groups for persons with autism, softball tournaments for persons with hearing impairments, or therapeutic swimming programs for persons with severe disabilities. Many of these activities are planned without regard to individuals' needs, preferences, skills, or abilities, particularly in relation to functional, community-based skills development, including social integration with nondisabled peers. Inattention to the needs of potential consumers with disabilities, coupled with the fact that most decisions are made on behalf of consumers by the recreation professional, distinguishes this segregated service from the "flawed" diamond model (Figure 2.4) described above. For example, the young adults with mental retardation who are attending the Friday night dances may also wish to socialize with nonretarded young adults. Yet, the activities in such programs may be advertised in such a way as to suggest to persons with disabilities that they are only permitted to participate in segregated, "handicapped-only" programs, because the community recreation professional has made a special effort to design these programs for them. In contrast to the high cost of segregated services, recent studies have demonstrated that integrated community leisure services are cost-effective (Voeltz, 1983) and need not be more expensive than other recreation programming efforts. As Sessoms (1984) noted, "society values and serves its 'normal' populations, those who can readily accept its resources and programs. Its 'special' populations deserve no less." (p. 212)

The third model, the "diamond in the rough" program (Figure 2.6), refers to service delivery programs that are almost—but not quite—"perfect." The areas in which such programs typically do not measure up include: lack of adequate information by the agency

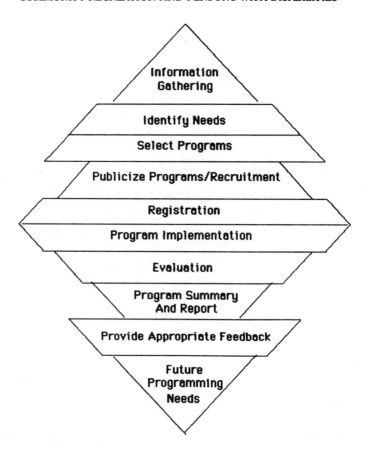

Information
Gathering

Identify Needs

Select Programs

Publicize Programs/Recruitment

Registration

Program Implementation

Evaluation

Program Summary
And Report

Provide Appropriate Feedback

Future
Programming
Needs

FIGURE 2.6.   Diamond-in-the-rough analogy.

regarding the community and those persons in the community who have disabilities, and insufficient publicity and recruitment activities to inform these persons that community recreation programs and services are available. Other program "rough spots" may be found in those service delivery programs where information needed to improve existing leisure services is either unavailable, or is not used appropriately to ensure that persons with disabilities are identified and successfully integrated into programs. Another rough spot may be found in recreation programs administered by unskilled recreation specialists. These specialists may be willing to include persons with disabilities in recreation activities, but may not understand how to do so effectively. Through systematic planning, staff training, and the use of community networks, these "diamond-in-the-rough" programs can reach full potential and can turn into "precious gem" programs. Until that time, these less-than-perfect programs continue to limit the full access of persons with disabilities to recreation and leisure services.

The fourth model (Figure 2.7), is the "precious gem" of community leisure service systems. Like the gem, these programs are multifaceted. In this program, the recreation professional carefully studies demographic data, leisure behaviors, and the recreation needs and preferences of his or her community. The recreation professional plans, implements, and improves programming with the understanding that he or she has ready access to this information through clear lines of communication. The element that makes this program superior to the "fake," "flawed," and "diamond-in-the-rough" programs is that the recreation professional is attempting to make recreation programs and services available to *every-*

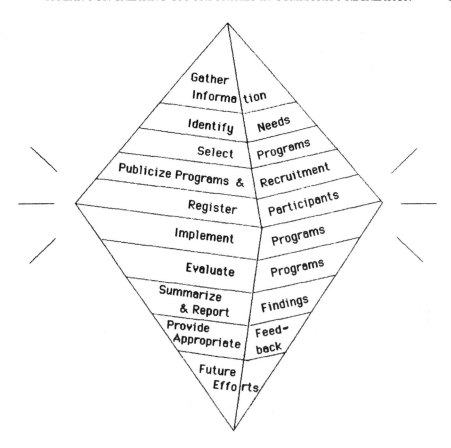

FIGURE 2.7.   Precious gem diamond analogy: An accessible leisure service model.

one in the community, including those persons with disabilities. Like a "precious gem," such a program becomes even more valuable over time, reflecting positively on the municipal park and recreation agency and staff.

A PROCESS ANALYSIS OF ACCESSIBLE LEISURE SERVICES

Because the recreation professional is trained not to be prejudiced against special population groups, he or she is likely to find accessibility to be an important feature in the provision of recreation services. Because the recreation professional has the resources, knowledge, and skills to provide accessible leisure services to everyone in the community, he or she is able to improve on the "diamond-in-the-rough" program model by incorporating various strategies for overcoming obstacles, thus making programs more accessible. Implementation of the "precious gem" recreation program model may have a profound effect on the provision of community leisure services to persons with disabilities.

At this point, it is appropriate to describe the accessible leisure service model (see Appendix A) and its components. All of the elements depicted in the "precious gem" analogy, Figure 2.7, are contained in this process. Readers should refer to this table for a list of specific tasks that can enhance physical and social accessibility of leisure services for persons with disabilities. Community leisure service professionals may wish to expand this process by identifying additional tasks and responsibilities to make services even more accessible.

Implementing Community Leisure Services: Preparation

Prior to the development of any plan to implement community leisure services, recreation personnel must be well-grounded in the philosophy of the municipal park and recreation agency, and knowledgeable about the provision of services to persons with disabilities. This knowledge gives the recreation professional guidelines with which to make program planning decisions and to practice his or her profession (Edginton et al., 1980). It is the municipal park and recreation agency that typically develops this philosophical mission around which individual community recreation professionals may design and implement programs. Specifically, the municipal park and recreation agency has the public interest at the center of its service philosophy. This philosophical mission is concerned with improvement in the quality of life in areas such as: health, well-being, self-concept, and happiness, and with the affirmation that recreation and leisure experiences are important in achieving this improved quality of life, however it may be defined. Thus, a sound program philosophy is composed of a successful blending of personal, professional, and community beliefs and values into clear operational methods.

Before starting out, recreation professionals may wish to bear in mind several key tenets that may guide them in the provision of community leisure services:

1. People have a right to recreation that is personally satisfying.
2. The essence of leisure is freedom: freedom to choose between a variety of leisure options and experiences.
3. The leisure experience differs between individuals; therefore, programs should be designed to address various needs, interests, and abilities.
4. People have a right to have access to quality leisure environments.
5. Leisure opportunities should be provided in a consistent manner to all potential participants without regard to sex, religion, age, socioeconomic status, or physical or mental ability.

When considering his or her responsibility to provide accessible leisure services for persons with disabilities, the community recreation professional must first ensure that the philosophical position of the agency is nondiscriminatory in practice, policy, and in attitudes. Second, the professional should make certain that programs and services are: physically accessible, chronologically age-appropriate, and flexible enough to allow participants to enter the continuum of leisure service options at the most appropriate, least restrictive level. Additionally, programs and services should adequately address the personal needs and preferences of potential participants with disabilities, and should be affordable and conveniently reached by participants. The following is a list of steps for implementing community leisure services.

A. Gather Information   An absolute necessity for effective recreation service provision is the possession of a comprehensive knowledge of neighborhood residents, the potential users of community leisure services. The community recreation professional must have a sense of the diverse leisure attitudes and preferences of the residents. Knowledge of community demography has also been demonstrated to be critical when considering the "variety, emphasis, and type of recreation activities enjoyed by people" (Russell, 1982, p. 70). Demographic factors that influence such preferences include: ethnic heritage, residence, age, educational level, occupation, social status, family life-styles, and religious affiliation. Metropolitan and regional planning agencies can generally provide recreation staff with this information and are easily approached via telephone.

A third component of the information gathering phase of the Accessible Community Leisure Service Process concerns available resources. Knowledge of available resources helps to avoid costly duplication of services. Also, it helps to maximize coordination of resources to ensure efficient and effective programming (Edginton et al., 1980). Resources of interest to recreation staff include facilities, settings, materials and equipment, staff, budget, neighborhood support, and alternative leisure service systems (e.g., voluntary/ youth-serving, private, or commercial).

A final component concerns the leisure behavior of neighborhood constituencies. Information regarding community participation patterns and motivations gives the recreation planner additional bases for decision-making. However, recreation staff must be careful not to assume that past recreation behavior is a sole predictor of future preferences and needs (Russell, 1982). Instead, recreation planners must rely on preference assessments, as described next.

B. Identify Needs Closely related to the fact-finding process highlighted in *Section A* is the identification of individual needs and preferences of potential participants. The most effective way of determining such preferences is to couch activities in "plain English" rather than in professional terms. For example, potential participants may express interest in health and fitness through aerobic dancing rather than by saying they have a "desire for enhanced socialization," "improved cognitive ability," or "increased gross motor coordination." Community recreation professionals, program leaders, and other recreation professionals are most likely aware of these types of therapeutic activity goals. Recognizing that individuals relate differently to activities and experiences, the recreation professional endeavoring to survey his or her community usually begins by developing a list of diverse activities which community residents are asked to rank according to preference or interest (example in Appendix B). The recreation professional might also take a less formal approach and simply ask persons in the community what types of activities they would like to see offered at the community recreation site. The community recreation professional can then begin to identify programs and activities based upon these expressed preferences, and to construct a program that will more effectively meet individual participant needs within preferred activities.

The recreation professional utilizes similar techniques for determining the activity preferences of persons with disabilities. Parents, careproviders, teachers, or therapeutic recreation specialists may assist with the assessment of preferences. These people are in a position to offer the community recreation professional information concerning the lifestyles, interests, and leisure behaviors of persons with disabilities. An additional means of gaining knowledge about the leisure needs and preferences of persons with disabilities is to contact advocacy agencies. These agencies typically have a sense of the general needs of persons with a particular disability type. For example, the local Association of Retarded Citizens might recommend that the community recreation professional offer teens with mental retardation more opportunities to socialize with nonhandicapped peers. The recreation professional could then suggest programs that are social and integrated in nature such as teen dances, team athletics, and cooperative art projects.

C. Identify Programs The community recreation professional must use the demographic information and the recreation preferences indicated in the community to develop a number of program alternatives. The challenge for the professional is to address as many of these diverse community preferences as possible, while bearing in mind the available resources and anticipated rate of participation. It is not surprising that preferred programs have a greater chance of being attended than those that were developed based on the preferences of the community recreation professional. Also, the recreation professional should endeavor to offer a range of programs that permit potential participants to choose between active (e.g., athletic) or passive (e.g., crafts) activities. Additionally, the recreation professional can expect participants to have a varying range of abilities, skills, and familiarity with any given activity. Programs must be designed in such a way as to allow participants opportunities for personal growth and socialization, as well as for having fun in a stimulating, yet comfortable, environment. Instructors can maximize participants' potential for meeting these needs through empathy with participants, clear articulation of program objectives, nonjudgmental attitudes, and recognition of individual potential. Of course, programs should be offered for every age group represented in the community, and should anticipate expanding should the need arise. For example, if a greater percentage of participants are adults rather than children, then more adult programs should be offered.

Community recreation professionals should demonstrate extreme caution when identifying segregated programs for persons with disabilities. Using nomenclature such as "handicapped programs" or "special needs programs" has a tendency to stigmatize persons with disabilities and could send a clear message that persons with disabilities are not welcomed in regular programs. By being characterized as "handicapped," persons with disabilities are denied their right to be persons first and to participate in programs developed for other, nondisabled, persons of the same age group. The community recreation professional must make it clear that programs and services are accessible to everyone. If segregated programs are offered, consumers should be made aware that these programs are designed for persons with disabilities as stepping stones to more integrated and accessible experiences.

D. Publicize Programs/Conduct Recruitment   It is essential, at this point, that the community recreation professional consider various means to advertise program offerings. A variety of print media (e.g., flyers, brochures, newspapers, posters) can be utilized for this purpose. However, the professional must consider the audience to whom leisure services are to be marketed and sold. Having determined what type of print media will be used, a marketing plan must be devised by the recreation professional to address issues related to user recruitment. A comprehensive marketing plan takes into consideration all known resources. Included in this plan is a knowledge of individuals and agencies that provide all types of social and health services to persons with disabilities (e.g., advocacy groups, allied health professionals), as well as a list of the names and addresses of potential consumers, including persons with disabilities. The community recreation professional collaborates with others (see Networking Matrix, Chapter 3) to implement this marketing plan.

As Russell (1982) advises, "turning potential users into actual ones . . . entails communication, persuasion, and timing" (p. 247). Communication occurs, initially, in the information gathering and needs identification stage. If the message between the community recreation professional and the constituency is clear, appropriate leisure programs and services can be identified. At this point, the recreation professional attempts to persuade potential users to register and to be active participants in proposed programs. When considering potential users who have cognitive impairments, the recreation professional must communicate with parents and other careproviders. As the recreation professional discusses the individual merits or benefits of participation in community leisure programs, he or she may need to explain how modifications and adaptations to programs and settings to suit the individual needs of the participant will take place (see Chapter 4). The recreation professional, when in the persuasion phase, may wish to refer back to *Section B, Identify Needs*, for further support. Finally, the promotional effort must take place early enough to ensure that potential participants are not informed about programs after registration has taken place. As noted by Russell (1982) "ideal timing takes experimentation with local media deadlines, the scope of the program (i.e., duration, frequency), and the life style of the constituency" (p. 248).

A common method of advertising programs is through a published program brochure that identifies the program, meeting time, dates and duration, restrictions (e.g., fees, age, personal equipment needs), locations, and instructor. Also essential for inclusion in this brochure and necessary for integration and accessibility purposes, is a statement of nondiscrimination that openly invites the active participation of persons with special needs, particularly persons with disabilities. Sample nondiscrimination statements are included in Appendix C. Community recreation professionals should avoid using generic nondiscrimination statements in the brochure that sound like "legalese." In the authors' opinion, from working with various parent groups, it is necessary for brochure statements to sound friendly, sensitive, and inviting in order to make a person feel welcomed to the leisure setting.

E.   Conduct Registration   If program offerings have been identified and designed according to the preferences and needs of potential users, and if the community recreation professional has implemented a successful publicity campaign, the result should be programs that are filled to capacity. However, programs cannot be implemented until specific characteristics of the participants are identified. The program instructor will want to know facts about the participants such as: age, gender, past experiences in similar activities, how participants learned of the program, their motivations for registering, their personal goals or expectations, and so forth. A comprehensive registration process will ensure that this information is obtained.

Conducting a comprehensive registration becomes critical when a person with disabilities desires to participate in the program. It is at this stage of the Accessible Community Leisure Service Process that special considerations are identified. These special considerations may include, but are not limited to: extent and level of physical and/or mental disability, presence of adaptive behaviors (i.e., ability to understand and to participate in recreation experiences with minimal assistance), past experiences in integrated environments, medical concerns, behavioral approaches, and so forth. The Environmental Analysis Inventory (Chapter 4), provides the community recreation specialist with a specific format to explore specific individual and program considerations.

Once these special considerations are identified, the community recreation professional may determine if, and what, program modifications must be made to successfully accommodate the participant with disabilities. Decision rules governing program modification and strategies to achieve the goals of accessible and integrated programs are further detailed in Chapters 4 and 5.

F.   Implement Programs   While clearly not the most important phase of the Accessible Community Leisure Service Process, program implementation translates preparation and planning into action. The participant may or may not understand the comprehensive organization conducted prior to participation in the program. However, depending upon how the program is implemented and the positive or negative reactions of other participants, the community recreation professional should be able to ascertain the efficacy of his or her program planning approach. The entire purpose of moving systematically through this process is to avoid potential pitfalls (such as program objectives not being met) that may affect future program efforts. Specifically, one objective to be met is of particular importance to participants with disabilities: that of overcoming barriers to successful access and participation in community leisure programs. The next section addresses methods to evaluate client outcomes, program efficacy, and planning procedures in order to determine the success of the program. An entire chapter in this text has been devoted to program evaluation (see Chapter 6). Therefore, discussion on evaluation at this time will be brief.

G.   Evaluate Programs   Evaluation, in itself, is a process. The community recreation professional may be interested in using this process in order to determine whether the programs met the leisure and social skill needs of individual participants. Program evaluation may also yield information concerning utilization of resources, needs assessment, program identification and planning, and program implementation. Evaluation aids in program and administrative accountability from an individual, an organizational, and a community perspective. Recreation staff and activity instructors demonstrate accountability to participants of leisure services at specific recreation centers and programs by ensuring that programs and facilities are open to everyone, and that special considerations can be made to those participants who need them. Additionally, the municipal park and recreation agency demonstrates its commitment to comprehensive and accessible leisure service provision as mandated by its service mission and the law. In short, information gleaned from evaluation efforts assists the recreation professional to improve the overall delivery of community leisure services.

H. Summarize Findings and Report Without a concise analysis of the evaluation data and a clear mechanism for reporting these data, appropriate modifications to improve implementation of the Accessible Community Leisure Service Process cannot be made. Conducting such an analysis permits the recreation professional to identify and act upon program or administrative strengths and weaknesses prior to planning and implementing new programs. The evaluation findings must be succinctly written in narrative form and in language easily understood by administrative personnel within the municipal park and recreation or local government agency, and by parents and careproviders. These findings, when reported to key individuals, or "key players," can be useful to recreation personnel and to persons with disabilities who are current or potential customers. Presentation of findings (particularly regarding successful programs!) are also useful to recreation planners for public relations and promotion of future programs. Such presentations demonstrate to the public that programs are becoming more accessible, that successful community integration is possible, and that the municipal park and recreation agency has the personnel, organization, and motivation to ensure community leisure services will be open and accessible to *all* community members.

I. Provide Appropriate Feedback Criticism is valuable, particularly when it is constructive. Recreation personnel are likely to share criticisms and suggestions for program modification throughout implementation of the leisure service process. Further support for changes in the process should come from individuals and agencies who are involved with community leisure services. Soliciting feedback from others is an essential link to successfully implementing this process. It also strengthens the bond developed by individuals and agencies through networking. This, in turn, provides continued support for the provision of accessible leisure services by the community recreation professional. As the process is refined and reworked, accessible community leisure services will become less of a novelty. The planning and implementation of recreation programs and leisure services for persons wtih disabilities will be a common occurrence with broad community acceptance and support.

J. Determine Future Programs and Interventions Implementation of this part of the Accessible Community Leisure Service Process is critical if year-round accessible community leisure services are to be provided. The entire process should be scrutinized by community recreation personnel and by the community as a whole. The philosophy and mission of the municipal park and recreation agency may be modified during this time to reflect improved approaches to delivery of leisure services based upon evaluative findings and feedback from colleagues and participants. Through their efforts to improve service provision, community recreation professionals and the agencies they represent assume an advocacy role. Their position is "proactive" versus reactive. These professionals will continue to employ systematic, organizational tactics and appropriate service methodology in order to bring about accessible community leisure services.

SUMMARY

This chapter has considered the nature of municipal park and recreation agencies, and the various leisure service delivery models that may exist within these agencies. A continuum of leisure services for persons with disabilities was discussed, and a schematic drawing of this model was presented in Figure 2.2. This model proposes utilizing segregated, "handicapped-only" programs with the condition that persons with disabilities are not restricted from achieving independent access to other leisure services. Segregated programs, therefore, are to serve as stepping stones to integrated and accessible recreation opportunities and experiences.

Also, a "diamond" analogy was presented to give the reader a sense of service delivery models within community settings. The "flawed diamond" is so-called because its service provision is grossly inadequate or incomplete. The "fake diamond" model represents segregated services; it appears valuable, but is a poor investment in time and money. The "diamond-in-the-rough" program has great potential, but possesses service gaps that diminish its value. Finally, the exemplary model program is the "precious gem diamond." In this program, service gaps are eliminated and various integration strategies are implemented. This model is nondiscriminatory and allows equal and appropriate access for persons with disabilities.

The following three chapters describe various methods of achieving accessible community leisure services. Strategies such as networking, conducting architectural accessibility surveys, and staff training and development, are discussed. These approaches are best employed during the phase described in **Section J, Determine Future Programs and Interventions,** highlighted earlier in this chapter. Also discussed at length are specific strategies to overcome the barriers to community recreation integration that are identified through the Environmental Analysis Inventory. Careful reading of these chapters, plus attention to the suggested strategies, should ensure successful implementation of the Accessible Community Leisure Service Process.

Chapter 3

Setting the Stage for Integrated Recreation
Preparing People and Environments

It should be clear by now that developing a specific process to systematically plan for the integration of community leisure services by persons with disabilities is both appropriate and necessary. However, community recreation professionals must generate momentum to set the community leisure service process in motion. Implementing this process may be a difficult task for personnel who lack the training to do so. This chapter presents various strategies that are essential for achieving accessible and integrated community leisure services. These strategies include: development of networks or communication linkages between persons and agencies concerned about community leisure services, surveys of architectural accessibility of leisure service settings, and provision of comprehensive staff inservice training. All of these steps are precursors to the systematic integration of persons with disabilities into recreation activities or settings. Obstacles formerly thought to be insurmountable by parents, consumers, and the community recreation professional, will be dissipated as information is obtained about community support systems and the accessibility of current facilities and programs. Additional strategies for meeting individual participant's unique needs will be covered in depth in subsequent chapters.

GENERAL PROGRAM STRATEGIES

Effective Networking

While it is expected that the community recreation professional has the requisite skills and knowledge to plan and implement appropriate recreation programs and services for the neighborhood constituency, seldom does she or he operate alone in this process. The key to successful integration of persons with disabilities into community leisure service settings depends greatly on the amount and quality of networking that is done. Networking involves making connections with professionals from various disciplines, with community members, and with parents and consumers—all persons who share common interests and concerns regarding leisure opportunities in the community for persons with disabilities. Networking is a process. As such, it involves the establishment of ongoing and productive working relationships by the recreation specialist with others who are striving to meet similar ends. Networking can begin with a telephone conversation, a personal meeting, or a workshop that one attends. The astute recreation professional will determine the strengths of these social contacts and will solicit the assistance of others in planning and delivering community leisure services.

An effective way to identify significant and worthwhile contacts is to develop a "Networking Matrix" (Figure 3.1). This matrix lists key players who can aid in the implementation and delivery of community leisure services. The matrix also identifies their roles and responsibilities within this process (Appendix D). This matrix and the responsibilities involved may vary from community to community. The community recreation professional is encouraged to use the matrix as a guide and to adapt it to his or her agency's and community's needs. Additionally, one may find that certain key players, in fact, play a more significant role in the community leisure service process than is listed in this matrix. For example, one may find that parents have to assist with program implementation, a task normally reserved for the recreation professional. The community recreation specialist may wish to further personalize each category by identifying individuals and agencies by: contact person, agency or category affiliation, address, and telephone number. A sample form called the Networking Referral List is found in Appendix E. This list provides a ready-

Community leisure service process / **Key players**

Community leisure service process	Community rec. professionals	Parents and care providers	Consumers	Advocacy groups	School/Day program personnel	Allied health professionals	Private rec. services	Quasi-Public rec. services	Professional/Educational resources
1. Information	X	X	X	X	X	X	X	X	X
2. Identifying needs	X	X	X	X	X	X		X	X
3. Selecting programs	X	X	X	X	X		X	X	X
4. Publicizing programs and recruitment	X	X	X	X	X	X	X	X	X
5. Registering participants	X	X	X		X	X			
6. Implementing integration strategies	X	X	X	X	X	X	X	X	X
7. Implementing programs	X			X			X	X	
8. Evaluating programs	X						X	X	X
9. Summarizing findings and reporting	X								X
10. Providing appropriate feedback	X	X	X	X	X	X	X	X	X
11. Determining future program efforts	X	X	X	X	X	X	X	X	X

FIGURE 3.1.   Networking Matrix for identifying responsibilities of "key players" in the community leisure service process. (Circumstances related to community, participants, and/or agency may require additions, deletions, or other changes in these recommendations.)

reference of community service professionals for the individual who is planning or administering services.

The Networking Matrix process is a simple one. For example, assume that the community recreation planner is beginning to plan for the agency's summer programs, the busiest season of the year. The planner would first ensure that all information regarding potential participants and available resources is obtained and evaluated. First, refer to the Accessible Community Leisure Service Process described in Chapter 2 and Appendix A to identify the steps one would take to achieve these objectives. Next, consider those key players who could assist in each step of the process. At this time, the community recreation planner could refer to or add other individuals to the list of the key players in the Networking Referral List. The recreation planner can then contact individuals and agencies by telephone, through the mail, or face-to-face in order to solicit such information as special needs considerations, referrals of potential participants, and leisure preferences. Proceed through each step of the process, working collaboratively with the various key players identified within the matrix. Not only will the task of planning and implementing the summer season programs be completed more efficiently, but chances are that participation rates will increase and successful integration of services will be achieved. Furthermore, consumers with disabilities, parents, careproviders, and advocates will be satisfied by these efforts. This networking process affirms that the cooperation of the various individuals and agencies concerned with the needs of persons with disabilities is critical to the success of accessible community leisure services. This proactive approach assures the community that tax dollars are being spent appropriately and that capable recreation professionals are administering these programs.

Establishing a Community Advisory Board

Two important components of the Accessible Community Leisure Service Process are communication and service planning. Community recreation professionals need assurance that their efforts in planning and implementing accessible leisure services are appropriate for meeting the leisure needs of persons with disabilities. They also need to know that these efforts are supported by the general community and that the services could be continued throughout the year. One method to communicate feedback about such issues is through the establishment and maintenance of a Community Advisory Board that specifically addresses the leisure needs and services of persons with disabilities. This advisory board could be made up of a number of representatives from each category of key players (e.g., advisory groups, parents or careproviders, persons with disabilities). The community recreation professional is the logical person to establish the advisory board, as he or she represents the agency responsible for meeting the recreation and leisure needs of all citizens of a given locale. Representatives from advocacy groups such as ARC may express a willingness to assist in the coordination of the advisory board. However, ARC's primary concern, as mandated by its organizational mission, is with service provision for persons with mental retardation. Thus, ARC is not in the best position to advocate for all citizens with and without mental or physical disabilities. For this reason, and because the purpose of this advisory board is to address leisure and recreation issues related to persons with disabilities, 30%–50% of the board should be made up of individuals with disabilities (Wolfensberger, 1972). This would ensure that the board's decisions truly represent the wishes of the persons the advisory board has been founded to serve.

The objectives of this Community Advisory Board should include the following:

1. To bring together individuals and agencies to facilitate community recreation opportunities for members of special populations through networking, advocacy, and action;

2. To serve as a resource to individuals with and without disabilities, and to advise leisure service providers on methods to achieve integration within community settings;
3. To promote public awareness about the value and availability of recreation opportunities in community settings through dissemination of information;
4. To develop a working relationship with a variety of community leisure service agencies to effect greater opportunities for community recreation participation;
5. To develop and maintain an advisory board that actively promotes community recreation opportunities and is representative of consumers with disabilities and other interested persons and agencies.

The advisory board can focus on broad, general issues relating to leisure services such as integration and community-wide accessibility, or on specific neighborhood concerns such as obtaining volunteer advocates for a particular program serving individuals with special needs. Decisions on how to achieve accessible leisure services is generally done by consensus. The combined efforts of all participants in the networking process, including the members of the Community Advisory Board, should ensure that persons with disabilities have equal opportunities to participate in integrated and accessible community leisure services.

ARCHITECTURAL ACCESSIBILITY SURVEY

Disabled citizens in all communities are in need of facilities and programs that allow them to meet the daily living needs that contribute to their welfare and growth. These needs include recreation and leisure. Many persons with disabilities have special requirements that must be met in order for them to participate in recreation activities in community environments. It is the recreation professional's responsibility to understand accessibility issues, and all relevant disabilities and their attendant special requirements, and to plan programs and facilities accordingly. For example, specific adaptations may need to be made in order to eliminate architectural and attitudinal barriers in parks and recreation facilities. One way to analyze what specific adaptations or modifications may be needed is through an architectural accessibility survey.

The National Policy for a Barrier-Free Environment has estimated that 1 in 10 persons in the United States has limited mobility due to a temporary or permanent physical disability. The number of these individuals will continue to expand as improved medical techniques continue to make mobility possible for an increasing number of individuals. Also, as the overall population ages, an ever-increasing number of older persons, many with mobility problems, will make up much of the constituency served by community leisure organizations.

Although the federal government and individual states have recognized the necessity of providing legislation to make facilities accessible for persons with disabilities in such measures as Section 502 of the Rehabilitation Act of 1973, which created the Architectural and Transportation Barriers Compliance Board to enforce the Architectural Barriers Act of 1968 (PL 90-480), the physical environment of our communities continues to be designed to accommodate the able-bodied only. Lack of enforcement of such laws and the preponderance of waiver claims combine to restrain architectural accessibility in the environment. Also, most guidelines on barrier-free design focus solely on accessibility for the wheelchair user. Such guidelines assume that persons with all types of disabilities will be able to use a facility that is accessible to people who use wheelchairs. This assumption is faulty, since a few barrier-free features designed for wheelchair users only, such as the elimination of curbs, may actually be dangerous to blind individuals who rely on curbs for guidance.

It is necessary that recreation planners recognize the inherent rights of all citizens, regardless of their disability, and that they mobilize their planning resources to successfully integrate persons with disabilities into barrier-free environments. A necessary first step toward achieving barrier-free facilities is through an architectural accessibility study. This study provides a comprehensive review of architectural and environmental barriers that limit participation of individuals with disabilities in community recreation programs and activities. A careful analysis of the survey data could provide an understanding of how architectural barriers could limit participation of individuals with special needs. It might also give planners useful information about standards and criteria for designing and modifying facilities in order for them to be used by all citizens of a given locale.

In order to obtain a comprehenesive, in-depth analysis of the physical accessibility of municipal park and recreation facilities by persons with disabilities, a detailed survey instrument would have to be developed and implemented. Many "homemade" survey instruments are of limited use to recreation planners who need specific dimensions and requirements in order to modify facility structures so that they are physically accessible. Structures need to be accessible not only for persons who use wheelchairs, but also for others who have limitations due to visual or hearing impairments or other physical disabilities, such as arthritis or cerebral palsy. A comprehensive and detailed survey instrument that sets forth federal and state mandated design characteristics would provide individual surveyors with a thorough and systematic method for examining the accessibility of all essential features of public facilities. Attention should be given, at a minimum, to the following features[1]:

1. **Parking**—This category includes information on the location, dimensions, and visibility of accessible parking spaces. For example, the surveyor would be directed to record how many handicapped parking spaces were allocated per total number of existing off-street spaces (e.g., 1 per 50), how they were so designated (i.e., type and number of signs displayed), parking space width (e.g., 12' minimum), and their proximity to accessible building entrances.
2. **Exterior Path**—This category includes information concerning the transition of the pathway to the street level (i.e., are curb cuts needed?), to the texture of the ramps (e.g., coarse aggregate preferred), the width of the path (e.g., 4' minimum), and the need for handrails, if the slope is too great.
3. **Entrance**—The entrance must be level with little (i.e., less than ½″) or no threshold. The width of the entry door must be useable (i.e., 31″ required; 34″ recommended) with the height (42″ maximum) and the type of door latch hardware (lever handle) operable by persons using wheelchairs and/or with limited manual dexterity. Also, it is desirable to have the International Symbol of Accessibility displayed on the doorway.
4. **Interiors**—When evaluating building interiors one must consider accessibility of various building levels (i.e., presence of ramps or elevators), passages or aisle space between rooms, doorways and door latch hardware (i.e., same as exterior), flooring (i.e., not plush carpet and slick flooring), and seating accommodation (i.e., number of spaces reserved for persons in wheelchairs). Other considerations include accessibility of public telephones, and of various controls such as manual fire alarm pulls, thermostats, light switches, outlets, and intercoms. Controls should also be indicated in

---

[1]The accessibility features described are based on a survey instrument developed by the Minnesota State Council for the Handicapped, St. Paul, MN. This "Building Access Survey" (1984) is based on Minnesota Building Code Chapter 55 and establishes minimum requirements of accessibility for all new construction and structural renovation after November, 1975. A complete copy of this survey is found in Appendix F.

braille or raised letters so that they are identifiable by persons with visual impairments; visual cues should be available for hearing impaired persons.

5. **Sanitation Facilities**—Public sanitation facilities (e.g., toilets, urinals, sinks, soap dispensers, hand towels or dryers, and bathroom shelves), and doorways and entryways must be accessible to persons using wheelchairs and labeled as such. Use of grab bars, openings under sinks, lowered dispensers or controls (i.e., 40" maximum height), and adequate manuevering space, are all methods to assure compliance with requirements or recommendations in this survey category.

6. **Bathing Facilities**—Entry to and accessibility of showers or tubs is related to requirements noted in Section 5 above. Shower heads and water controls must accommodate persons with disabilities. Use of grab bars and alternative seating arrangements are also required to ensure complete accessibility.

7. **Kitchen Facilities**—Adequate knee space (i.e., 29" minimum) must be available under the kitchen sink and countertops to accommodate persons using wheelchairs. Water control valves (lever action preferred) and front or side controls for the stove or oven must also be considered.

The survey instrument should be arranged in a readable manner that allows the surveyor to move through the building or facility in a systematic way. A sample of questions concerning parking, interior, and sanitation facilities has been provided in Figure 3.2 to illustrate the survey format. A complete copy of an architectural accessibility survey is found in Appendix F; this form may be reproduced for use in the reader's community.

Parking

1. How many off-street parking spaces are provided?

| current status | requirement | recommendation |

2. How many of these parking spaces are provided for use by disabled persons?

1 per 50 or fraction of 50

| current status | requirement | recommendation |

Interior

1. What is the working height of the following?:

			current status	requirement	recommendation
a.	fire alarm pulls			60" maximum	36"–48"
b.	electrical outlets			60" maximum	24"–48"
c.	light switches			60" maximum	36"–48"

Sanitation Facilities

1. Are there any public toilet facilities equipped for disabled persons?

Yes

| current status | requirement | recommendations |

2. Is the door or entry identified as accessible?

Yes — Use International Symbol of Accessibility

| current status | requirement | recommendations |

3. What are the working heights from the floor of the following?

		current status	requirement	recommendations
a.	soap dispenser		40" maximum	
b.	towel dispenser		40" maximum	
c.	mirror's lowest edge		40" maximum	

FIGURE 3.2.   Architectural Accessibility Survey Sample Questions (Minnesota State Council for the Handicapped, 1986.)

Community recreation professionals or facility planning staff within the leisure service agency should take primary responsibility for surveying all relevant community or neighborhood recreation settings. The authors have successfully utilized university students to assist with data collection. Students received preservice training on how to conduct surveys of 42 recreation centers within a major Midwest metropolitan area. This training consisted of the following:

1. Philosophical and legislative rationale for architectural accessibility of community leisure settings
2. Purpose of the survey, including intended outcomes, current status of facility accessibility, and the utilization of the findings by the leisure service agency recreation staff
3. Methods to conduct the survey, deadline for completion of the survey and for reporting the data

Recreation sites were divided among pairs of students working together to analyze each category within the survey instrument. Tape measures or yardsticks, and one survey instrument per recreation center, were provided to each student dyad. To enhance communication and understanding between the investigators, recreation staff, and student surveyors, a memorandum describing the proposed architectural accessibility survey and listing survey procedures was sent to each recreation center director prior to data collection. (An informational meeting at a central location could also be scheduled.) Drawing from this memorandum, students were then given a standard "telephone protocol" for initial contact; this served as a means of introduction, and allowed students and recreation center staff to arrange a time to conduct the survey. The recreation center director was given the option to participate in the survey; it was anticipated that the survey would take 90 minutes or less to complete. The investigators continued to facilitate implementation of the survey and to serve as a resource to the student surveyors during data collection. (Smaller communities with fewer park and recreation facilities may not need to utilize this many volunteers.)

Upon completion of the surveys and return of the data accumulated about each recreation center, the name of the center and the total number of code violations per category were recorded on a simple matrix. This matrix listed the municipal park and recreation facilities surveyed and the features of each (e.g., parking, sanitation). Areas of noncompliance, including total violations within that area, were then noted. This summary information was then submitted to the recreation agency for further analysis by personnel in the recreation and planning divisions. Recommendations for elimination of specific architectural barriers cited in the surveys could then be examined by municipal park and recreation administrators, planners, and recreation program and facility staff.

Upon receipt of the survey data, the recreation agency followed the procedures below to aid in the interpretation of the data. Aspects of this particular system of analysis are generalizable to other recreation agencies.

1. The survey data were entered into the agency computer corresponding with the agency's five geographic districts.
2. Spread sheets were created that allow survey questions and data to be correlated with each recreation center within that district.
3. All noncompliance information was identified for correction.
4. Information from the survey was disseminated to recreation staff and agency administrative personnel.
5. Staff reviewed the data and verified or updated information. New data were entered into the computer.

6. Correction activities were cataloged under one of two major headings: Maintenance or Capital Improvement.
    a. Maintenance catalog activities could include: replacing or adding grab bars at the correct height and distance; placing strips and signs in parking stalls to permit handicapped accessibility; placing tactile identification on doors.
    b. Capital Improvement catalog activities could include: doorway enlargement; restroom remodeling; major building renovations.
7. Recreation, Planning, and Maintenance staff reviewed the catalog and established a method of merging requests for maintenance with identified access deficiencies.
8. Center personnel request use of maintenance catalog.
9. Repairs and changes would be made in accordance with the survey requirements or recommendations under state and federal statutes.

Architectural accessibility issues, once raised, must be approached jointly with other personnel within the municipal park and recreation agency. Certainly, funding priorities must be considered when anticipating changes or renovations to bring facilities "up-to-code." More importantly, one should become aware of the capacity of recreation settings to become physically accessible for persons with disabilities. If accessibility features are known, one can make informed decisions during program planning and implementation to ensure accessibility. For example, instead of denying access to a person with a physical disability because the facility is not wheelchair accessible, the community recreation planner may want to develop a reciprocal agreement with another organization such as a church, synagogue, school, or rehabilitation hospital to use their facilities if these are more accessible than the recreation agency's facilities. These arrangements are best made before the need becomes apparent. Having completed an architectural survey, one knows the capacity of the facility to be architecturally accessible. Effective networking offers the community recreation planner opportunities to make alternative facilities available in case they are needed.

Staff Training and Development

Inservice training is an integral component of ongoing professional training and development, and it is typically offered within organized municipal park and recreation agencies. Training topics vary according to the current or anticipated needs of the staff, and may cover issues such as program planning and implementation, activity analysis, fiscal responsibility, personnel concerns, and leisure trends. Staff are expected to attend these inservice training programs as part of their professional responsibilities.

An important element that should be present in any comprehensive inservice training plan is a segment devoted to delivery of leisure services to members of special populations. Topics of importance that should be presented during these inservice programs are presented below. In fact, the content of this inservice training program may be an abbreviated form of this text.

—Characteristics of persons with disabilities
—Rationale for integrated services
—Benefits to integrated leisure services
—Methods to achieve successful integrated programs
—Identifying and overcoming obstacles to integration
—Evaluating programs
—Effective and ongoing networking

Because of the vast amount of information available in the literature concerning the characteristics of different disability types, the authors have elected not to include that information in this text. However, persons coordinating inservice training programs are encouraged to write to nationally recognized organizations (See Appendix G) to receive information on disabilities represented in their community. Furthermore, it is recommended that an individual from the recreation agency contact his or her state or local chapter of these organizations to establish a contact for future networking and participant referral. Often, representatives from these agencies will come to the recreation agency to speak and to share information about their particular constituency group. Also, individuals with disabilities from the immediate community should be invited to participate in the inservice training sessions as speakers or as resource persons. Having a person discuss his or her disability is a useful way of educating audiences and dispelling negative attitudes. Additionally, a resource file on characteristics of disability groups, updated annually, could be created and made available for reference by recreation staff. Pamphlets from advocacy groups, informational brochures from sports and recreation associations for persons with disabilities, and comprehensive mailing lists of national, state, and local agencies serving persons with disabilities could be included in this resource file.

In an effort to strengthen the linkage between various key players in the recreation and leisure network, inservice training coordinators and/or community recreation professionals should contact individuals within each category or advocacy group to invite them to participate in some aspect of the inservice program. It is useful for recreation staff to be exposed to the experiences of others who have either had contact with potential consumers of community leisure services or who are themselves disabled. This approach lends credibility to the inservice program and legitimizes the process used to achieve accessible and integrated leisure services. This outreach approach demonstrates to the community that the municipal park and recreation agency is interested and concerned about the services it offers. The approach also demonstrates the agency's desire to interact as an advocate with the community to increase the chances that appropriate programs serving the needs of all citizens are considered and made possible. These public relation efforts are practical and useful and could result in increased recreation participation by persons with disabilities. They may also generate interest among persons without disabilities to serve as volunteer advocates by becoming role models or "Special Friends" to participants with disabilities.

There are several manuals created for the purpose of aiding recreation personnel in achieving accessible community leisure services. Examples of these manuals include:

Integrating Persons with Disabilities into Community Leisure Services
(Project for Integrated Recreation in the Community [PIRC])

Editors: Stuart J. Schleien, Director
           M. Tipton Ray, Project Coordinator
School of Physical Education and Recreation, University of Minnesota
   Minneapolis, MN, 1986

The PIRC manual provides a field-tested guide for planning, implementing, and evaluating integrated leisure programs. Specific case studies illustrate practical application of theoretical concepts and principles. Sample forms are included to enable community recreators to immediately begin integrated leisure programming. This manual served as the guide for this text.

Mainstreaming: A Total Perspective

Authors: Laura Wetherald
           Joy Peters
Montgomery County Department of Recreation-Therapeutic Section
   Silver Spring, MD, 1986

Developed as a guide for recreation staff to integrate or mainstream public recreation services in Montgomery County, Maryland, this manual can serve as a useful resource to other municipal and county park and recreation agencies. It provides a comprehensive overview of and rationale for mainstreaming community recreation programs. Implementation of the mainstreaming process is extensively covered. Useful appendices include a glossary of terms and information on specific disability groups. Sensitivity training exercises about common disability types are included.

LIFE Resource and Training Manual
(Project LIFE [Leisure is for Everyone])

Editors: Charles C. Bullock, Project Director
            Rayal E. Wohl
            Tracy E. Webreck
            Angela M. Crawford
University of North Carolina-Chapel Hill
    Chapel Hill, NC, 1982

The LIFE inservice training manual is practically-oriented. It is designed to provide concrete and specific information to human service professionals, paraprofessionals, and volunteers who are providing recreation services to persons with disabilities in both integrated and segregated programs. The manual is intended as a resource and training guide. Contents include: a discussion of the concepts of normalization and mainstreaming; characteristics of persons who have disabilities; attitudes of human service workers toward persons with disabilities; physical accessibility issues; administrative concerns; leadership and programming; resources. LIFE-EXTENDED, a 3-year continuation of the original grant that produced the LIFE inservice training model, is currently underway. The LIFE-EXTENDED program intends to develop additional inservice training tools by using audiovisual media.

WE CAN DO IT! A Training Manual for Integrating Disabled People Into Recreation Programs

Editor: Ann Fitzgerald
Bay Area Outreach Recreation Program, Inc. (BORP)
    Berkeley, CA, 1982

The We Can Do It training program is designed to instruct recreation and school personnel on procedures for integrating persons with physical disabilities into existing recreation programs. This inservice training guide introduces concepts of integration, stimulates disability awareness, teaches adaptive programming skills, promotes professional development, and presents a process for establishing integrated recreation programs. We Can Do It incorporates diagrams, photographs, forms, checklists, and curricula to illustrate these areas.

Therapeutic Recreation Inservice Training Manual

Editors: Richard Dlugas, Project Director
            Jean R. Tague, Project Director
            Cynthia Stanley, Project Coordinator
Denton Parks and Recreation Department
Texas Woman's University
    Denton, TX, 1985

This training manual was developed collaboratively by several community recreation, university, and advocacy agency personnel. It presents to community recreation planners a conceptualization of the therapeutic aspects of leisure, as well as various methods of addressing the recreational needs of persons with disabilities. These methods include: accessibility, equipment and activity adaptations, and behavior modification. An extensive overview of disability characteristics is presented. Also, several activities in the categories of arts and crafts, outdoor activities, creative arts, fitness, and sports and games are presented. Goals, adaptations, and special considerations are highlighted for each. Finally, the appendix gives the recreation planner a variety of resources for additional reading.

Community Recreation for Handicapped Persons: Inservice Education Program

Editor: Jacquelyn Stanley, Director
Office on Community Recreation for Handicapped Persons
Division of Community Resources, Bureau of Recreation
New Jersey Department of Community Affairs
    Trenton, NJ, 1980

The Office on Community Recreation for Handicapped Persons was created to provide inservice training and education to community and state agency personnel to develop, implement, and improve community recreation services for persons with disabilities. A variety of inservice training materials were developed to address the leisure needs of persons with physical disabilities, sensory impairments, emotional disorders, autism, learning disabilities, and mental retardation. The first section outlines clearly and comprehensively the characteristics of particular disability types. The second section details specific methods on how to develop and implement integrated recreational programs for persons with disabilities. Numerous resources are cited within each monograph to allow community recreation personnel to pursue additional information.

SUMMARY

This chapter has proposed a variety of general strategies to ensure that community recreation services and settings are integrated and accessible for persons with disabilities. The creation of a networking matrix of local key players in the community leisure service delivery process is a necessary first step to ensuring that agencies and individuals work together on accessibility issues. The chapter also suggests that an active and viable Community Advisory Board should be established to address community leisure services issues concerning persons with disabilities. The community recreation professional should also implement a comprehensive architectural accessibility survey of existing municipal park and recreation facilities and settings. Recommendations to upgrade physical accessibility of leisure settings would then be forwarded to park planning personnel. Additionally, continuing education and training of community recreation professionals, part-time staff, and volunteers regarding development, implementation, and evaluation of community leisure programs and services for persons with disabilities must be provided on an ongoing basis. The processes outlined for each of these areas of concern have been articulated in order for the community recreation professional to have the means to develop a solid foundation for accessible community leisure services.

These processes are not setting- or community-specific. That is, even though urban and rural communities exhibit differences in population distribution, availability of resources, convenience of services, and leisure life-styles (e.g., limited leisure options in certain areas), each strategy highlighted above can be implemented to a greater or lesser extent and can remain functional for that community setting. In fact, planners in isolated rural communities that do not have community leisure service agencies or advocacy groups may need to emphasize implementation of these basic strategies to optimize leisure service delivery to persons with disabilities.

One should feel free to use these approaches as a guide for implementation of these strategies, and to adapt them to the unique circumstances of the particular community or leisure setting. This text could also serve as an effective training tool for staff and volunteers. These individuals are reminded to invite the assistance of the Community Advisory Board in program planning and strategy development for achieving accessible and integrated community leisure services. The community recreation professional must acquire the necessary skills, knowledge, and experience to provide leisure services; he or she should then be in the best position to detect those areas in greatest need of integration, and to solicit the support of other persons or agencies to see that accessible community leisure services are realized.

Chapter 4

An Ecological Approach to Community Recreation Integration

Within the last few years, human service professionals have attempted to provide services to individuals with disabilities in community and other noninstitutional settings. The term "least restrictive environment" (LRE) is commonly used to describe this noninstitutional service approach. Leisure and discretionary time use in the LRE refers to the acquisition and performance of leisure skills by persons with disabilities in normalized community environments. The use of the adjective *normalized* is critical to distinguishing these two service approaches, since many human service providers conduct programs in the community, but in segregated—that is, nonnormalized—settings.

The acquisition of functional leisure skills (i.e., skills that are naturally occurring, frequently demanded, and have a specific purpose), that are age-appropriate (i.e., activities typically performed by persons in a particular age group), and comparable to nondisabled peer skill performance presents a powerful tool to integrate disabled persons into normalized community environments. The selection of leisure skills for individuals with disabilities should reflect this potential benefit. Only those skills or activities that have the potential of being performed in the presence of, or in interaction with, nondisabled peers should be selected for instruction. Anything short of this goal will do little to mitigate the unnecessary, long-term segregation of disabled persons, and could result in the acquisition of leisure skills that meet only the substandard performance demands of protective segregated settings.

The purpose of this chapter is to detail the process of community recreation integration. Additionally, a strategy adapted from an approach to analyze vocational tasks (Belmore & Brown, 1976), is presented as a guide to developing leisure skill instructional content that is based on the skill performance of nondisabled individuals.

This inventory identifies specific needs of individuals with disabilities and provides an excellent starting point from which to consider necessary program modifications to enhance successful participation. A discussion of the principle of partial participation will follow the presentation of the Environmental Analysis Inventory. Individualized program and activity adaptations, which are related to the principle of partial participation, are considered and illustrated next. Finally, descriptions of additional integration strategies, including volunteer advocacy and cooperative grouping arrangements, are provided.

The Environmental Analysis Inventory provides the human service professional with a systematic approach to facilitating the leisure involvement of persons with disabilities in community recreation settings (Certo & Schleien, 1982; Certo et al., 1983). Use of the inventory helps to heighten public awareness and to increase the level of sensitivity of all persons involved in the process of integrating community leisure services. This approach can be applied in the home, in schools, in vocational and community settings, and in a variety of recreation or leisure settings. The Environmental Analysis Inventory is beneficial in a variety of ways:

1. It provides a *step-by-step procedure* to integrate persons with disabilities into community leisure services;
2. It offers an *individualized approach* to community recreation participation by persons with disabilities;
3. It provides helpful *information* to careproviders (e.g., how to plan and prepare for the leisure experience) and community recreation personnel (e.g., guidance and direction in the planning and delivery of leisure services for current and future program instructors).
4. It identifies basic and vital skills and other useful information for participation in the targeted leisure activity, and is *compared to nondisabled peer performance*. This data can be used repeatedly. For example, whenever a person with a disability is identified as a potential participant, the inventory data from previously completed inventories can be used again.

It appears that most consumers follow a particular step-by-step procedure when using community recreation settings. This procedure, in its simplest version, consists of the following four steps:

1. Identifying a community leisure setting or recreation activity that is of interest
2. Making the necessary arrangements to arrive at the setting or activity
3. Participating in the setting/activity
4. Determining if a return to the recreation setting for future participation is desired

A more comprehensive examination of each element of this procedure is detailed below.

PROCESS FOR PARTICIPATING IN A COMMUNITY RECREATION ACTIVITY

Procedures for the Consumer

A. Identify the Preferred Leisure Setting/Recreation Activity

1. Become aware of a community recreation setting/activity by reading about it in a newspaper or program brochure, or hearing about programs on the radio or T.V.
2. Express interest in going to community recreation setting/activity.
3. If needed, request more information about location and directions to facility; re-

quest program brochure for specific information on activity, dates, time, and activity fees.

B. Make Arrangements to Attend Leisure Setting

1. Determine tasks to be completed before participating. Tasks should include the following:
    a. Completing registration procedure (Potential participant may need to determine an ideal time to travel to the setting to complete registration procedures.)
    b. Obtaining guardian permission (if under a certain age restriction)
    c. Determining program costs
    d. Arranging transportation for future visits to agency
    e. Determining appropriate attire for activity
    f. Obtaining necessary material/equipment (e.g., for tennis, one would need a tennis racquet and balls, tennis shoes, headband)
    g. Optional: Inviting a friend or sibling to participate with you
2. At the appropriate time, gather necessary material and equipment such as clothing, money, and tennis racquet, appropriate to the recreation setting or activity.

C. Travel To Recreation Program

1. Travel to the selected recreation setting using previously arranged transportation.

D. Arrive and Enter the Recreation Setting

1. Exit vehicle and safely cross streets and/or parking lot. (Participant may first locate entrance from vehicle.)
2. Locate main entrance.
3. Proceed in direction of facility's entrance.
4. Enter facility and locate activity or program area.

E. Participate in Targeted Recreation Activity

1. Procedure
    a. Request information about selected activity from information desk.
    b. Complete equipment/material checkout procedures.
    c. Locate appropriate area to engage in activity.
    d. Engage in activity; demonstrate appropriate behaviors.
    e. Return equipment/materials following termination of activity.
    f. Leave program area.

F. Leave Community Leisure Setting

1. Exit community recreation facility.
2. Cross streets and/or parking lot safely and enter vehicle.
3. Return to place of residency or other prearranged location.

G. Consider Future Involvement (Optional)

1. Return to community recreation facility for future participation.

When participating in a community recreation setting, the nondisabled individual can perform many of the steps of this process without extensive planning. To illustrate this process in action, two scenarios have been presented below.

1.   **Participation in Community Recreation by Nondisabled Persons**

Joe Brown, a nondisabled computer programmer, while on his way home from work, hears an advertisement on his car radio for a new physical exercise class at the neighborhood recreation center. The advertisement states that new members who register and pay for 20 sessions will also receive five free bonus sessions. This is an activity that Joe has been interested in pursuing for quite some time. From the directions given on the radio broadcast, he knows the recreation center is in proximity to his home. Joe also makes a mental note of the activity schedule, program costs, and registration procedures.

After relaxing at home and "psyching" himself up to enroll in the exercise class, Joe decides to call his friend and let her know about this exciting offer. Joe's friend expresses an interest in the program, and decides to meet Joe in one-half hour. Joe understands the appropriate attire needed for participation in the program and the amount of time required to get to the recreation agency. After changing into his exercise clothes, Joe grabs his billfold and coat. He leaves, excited in anticipation of this new experience. Joe and his friend arrive at the community recreation center 15 minutes early, with ample time to request assistance with the registration procedure. They are directed to the multi-purpose room where the exercise instructor can answer their questions. They are informed that the first class, to be held that evening, is a general orientation, and that they can attend for only one dollar. Additionally, a medical liability release form has to be read and signed. Following the orientation class, participants can register for the 20–session exercise program and can take advantage of the new member bonus offer.

Joe and his friend enjoy the exercise orientation class. They learn about exercise, health, and fitness, and meet others their own age. Before leaving, they register for the 20–session class. For three evenings per week, they enjoy participating in this healthy, educational, and meaningful community leisure experience. Additionally, Joe and his friend discover other activities, such as the pottery workshop, the holiday dances, and the neighborhood picnic, that are also conducted at the recreation center throughout the year.

Joe's continued involvement in these activities has facilitated his personal growth and development, and has greatly improved his quality of life and leisure life-style. The program has helped him become an active participant in the community. Joe has invited other friends and family members to share in his leisure and social experiences at the community recreation center.

Now one might ask: "If a person with a disability has an interest in participating in the same recreation activity/setting as Joe and his friend, would the procedures for participation be the same?" The second scenario describes a situation wherein the participant has developmental disabilities.

2.   **Participation in Community Recreation by Persons with Disabilities**

While listening to the radio in her bedroom at the group home, Sue Winters hears the same advertisement for the physical exercise program. She believes that this activity would be healthy and fun. Sue understands that the exercise class meets several days a week and requires money to participate.

Sue is a 22-year-old developmentally disabled woman living in a group home with five other individuals also diagnosed as being developmentally disabled. The group home residents (ages 22–37) are functioning in the moderate to severe range of mental retardation. Sue is moderately mentally retarded with an I.Q. of 48. She has limited expressive language (e.g., uses simple words and phrases) and frequently exhibits inappropriate social behaviors (such as vocalizing loudly at inappropriate times, touching others inappropriately, and forgetting to attend to personal hygiene). Sue is ambulatory, but has an unsteady gait and a noticeable limp. At times, she requires assistance with dressing skills such as putting on her coat, buttoning her blouse, tying her shoe laces, due to the limited use of her disabled, yet dominant, right arm. Sue attends a sheltered workshop during the day and independently commutes there on a public bus. The only consistently planned leisure activity in which Sue participates is a Tuesday evening Bible study class sponsored by the local church and conducted solely for persons with mental retardation. Occasionally, she participates in large group recreational field trips that are planned by the group home staff (e.g., movies, Association for Retarded Citizens' monthly dances, trips to the local diner for coffee). At other times, Sue and the other residents are left with a great deal of unstructured leisure or discretionary time.

How does Sue inform her careproviders of her interest in the exercise class? For the last 5 years she has resided in a supported living environment; much of the decision-making and planning in her life is conducted by paid professional staff on her behalf. Unlike Joe Brown, Sue is not allowed to decide on her own that she will participate in the exercise class. She must undergo a completely different process in order to become involved in the community recreation center program.

Each time Sue hears the radio advertisement for the exercise class, she becomes excited at the thought of participating. One evening, Sue expresses her desire to participate in the class. She does this by pointing to the radio, nodding her head, and laughing in the presence of a careprovider as the advertisement is being broadcast over the radio. Her careprovider acknowledges her attempt to communicate by stating that she has already received information about the exercise class in a community recreation center brochure. The careprovider explains to Sue that she will contact the recreation center director later in the week to receive more information. However, she will first discuss Sue's potential participation in a class with the group home's director and the other staff.

During a staff meeting shortly after, the information about Sue's interest in the program is shared with the other staff members. The group home director and staff identify several problems or potential barriers that could prevent Sue from participating in the program. The current insufficient staffing situation, the lack of personal and agency finances, and the unavailability of transportation appear to be major obstacles to participation that cannot be overcome at this time. The decision not to allow Sue to participate is shared with her, although she is not certain what the reasons are behind this decision. Sue continues to be excited about the program and seeks staff attention each time an exercise class broadcast is heard on the radio. Staff members continued to respond: "Sue, we're looking into it for you!" Sue remains hopeful, but as time progresses, she becomes frustrated and begins to experience feelings of helplessness. Group home staff begin to have difficulty controlling her inappropriate behaviors, for example, she throws a tantrum every time the exercise class advertisement is heard. The group home staff find they are not able to motivate her to participate in other recreation and social activities.

During the next staff meeting, it is decided that action will be taken to effect Sue's involvement in the exercise program. A group home careprovider telephones the community recreation center to solicit additional information regarding the program, and to notify the agency of Sue's participation. Having been informed that Sue is a potential participant with special needs due to her mental and physical disabilities, the recreation center director responds:

> Since we attempt to meet the leisure needs of all persons in our community, including those with disabilities, I am pleased that you called our center. Let's discuss Sue's needs, and then, the exercise class. I must ask you several questions to determine if this class is an appropriate and feasible leisure option for Sue. If it is, then we will want to discuss the best ways to involve Sue so that she and the other participants will benefit from the program. I could ask you these questions over the telephone or in person, whichever is most convenient for you. We look forward to having Sue in our program. Thank you for calling.

COMPLETING THE ENVIRONMENTAL ANALYSIS INVENTORY

The community recreation center director will use the Environmental Analysis Inventory to facilitate Sue's participation in the integrated community recreation program. The Environmental Analysis Inventory is a 4-part tool to be used during the initial steps of program planning. This planning process includes identifying an appropriate activity/setting and addressing preplanning issues and tasks such as program dates and times, activity costs, and transportation needs. The Inventory includes a general analysis of the program and a discrepancy analysis to determine how well the participant's current abilities match the skills necessary to participate in the activity. This analysis includes the identification of possible program modifications, if such are needed, to enhance participation.

The application of the Environmental Analysis Inventory to Sue's participation in a community recreation program will be presented next. Each section of the Environmental Analysis Inventory will be accompanied by a discussion of its implementation and useful-

ENVIRONMENTAL ANALYSIS INVENTORY
FIGURE 4.1

PART I: (A) APPROPRIATENESS OF RECREATION ACTIVITY/SETTING

When an activity or setting is being examined for recreation involvement, there are key areas that should be addressed prior to implementation of the program. These areas relate to the *appropriateness* of the activity or setting under investigation to an individual's needs, preferences, and skill level.

With such a wide variety of leisure-related activities and settings available to individuals with disabilities, the information gained from the following questions will assist the person with a disability, their care providers, and recreation staff in determining the appropriateness of the activity and setting for participation. In situations where a decision between two or more activities must be made, this information may assist in determining the best activity to meet the individual's needs and skill level.

Please record the participant's name, activity, setting, and date and check the correct response to the following seven questions. If the responses to the questions are affirmative (i.e., yes), proceed to the next step of the Environmental Analysis Inventory (PART II: ACTIVITY/DISCREPANCY ANALYSIS). If the responses to these questions fail to show positive results, an alternative recreation activity or setting should be selected for analysis and potential participation.

Name of Participant: __Sue Winters__   Date: __3-1-87__

Name of Activity/Skill: __Exercise Class__

Community Leisure Setting: __Hiawatha Recreation Center__

1. Is the activity or setting selected appropriate for nonhandicapped persons of the same chronological age? __X__ yes ____ no

2. Does the individual demonstrate a preference for this activity or could he/she benefit (i.e., individual has related goals/objectives stated in program plan, IEP, IHP, etc.) from participation in this particular activity or setting? __X__ yes ____ no

3. Can the individual financially afford/receive financial assistance to access this specific activity/setting? __X__ yes ____ no

4. If materials or equipment are necessary for participation in the activity or setting, does the individual own or have access to the necessary materials/equipment (i.e., borrow from recreation center, family, friend, etc.) __X__ yes ____ no

5. If necessary, are material and/or procedural adaptations available for the individual with physical disabilities? __X__ yes ____ no

6. Does the individual have access to some form of transportation to get to the leisure setting? __X__ yes ____ no

7. If physical accessibility is a special consideration for participation, does the setting provide easy access (i.e., handicapped parking, curb cuts, ramp to entrance, etc.)? __X__ yes ____ no

---

ness, including completion of all necessary forms. A flow chart depicting the use of the inventory follows the implementation example.

The completion of the ENVIRONMENTAL ANALYSIS INVENTORY, PART I: (A) APPROPRIATENESS OF RECREATION ACTIVITY/SETTING (Figure 4.1) and PART I: (B) GENERAL PROGRAM AND PARTICIPANT INFORMATION (Figure 4.2) is conducted during a second telephone conversation between the careprovider and center director.

The completion of PART I: Sections A and B are viewed as an initial assessment or screening technique. The seven questions in Section A and general information in Section B address critical areas of concern that could help determine whether the leisure experience under consideration for this particular disabled individual will be a successful one.

For Sue, it is determined that the exercise class at the community recreation center is a *chronologically age-appropriate* activity (Question 1). The appropriateness of this activity is determined by the observation of nonhandicapped peers participating in the identical activity.

It is apparent that Sue has demonstrated a *preference* for this activity by continuously seeking staff attention and by smiling each time the exercise class advertisement is heard on the radio. In the past, Sue exhibited these same behaviors when she enjoyed herself

FIGURE 4.2

ENVIRONMENTAL ANALYSIS INVENTORY

PART I: (B) GENERAL PROGRAM AND PARTICIPANT INFORMATION

General Information

Recreation Program Experience: **Exercise Class**

Directions: Check or write in the requested information on the following items. If necessary, use space on back.

1. Dates: from **3-16-87** to **5-11-87**
   Days/times: **M,W,F 5 to 6 p.m.**
   Number of sessions: **20 plus 5 free sessions**
   Total: 25 (Approx. 9 weeks)

2. Registration required: **X** yes ___ no
   Procedure: **X** in person ___ mail ___ phone
   Deadline date: **none** *
   This class is ongoing. One can register at any time.

3. Guardian permission required:
   ___ no **X** yes Comment: **Medical release form must be signed.**

4. Fee charged or money required: **X** yes ___ no
   Amount: $ **1.00** Payment procedure: **Pay instructor each session — maximum $20.**
   Are memberships available for free or reduced entrance fee?
   X no ___ yes; Cost: ___ Good for how long? ___

5. Transportation provided: ___ yes **X** no
   If yes, is it handicapped accessible (e.g., wheelchair lift?) ___ yes
   ___ no
   Other comments: ___

6. Comment on type of dress worn: **Exercise clothes; tennis shoes required**

7. List required equipment and materials:
   a. Facility owned: **Exercise mats**
   b. Participant owned: **None**
   Optional: Exercise weights

8. Special rules related to this activity (e.g., appropriate dress): **No eating during class; work at your own pace.**

Participant Information

Name: **Sue Winters** Date: **3-1-87**

Directions: Refer to item in left hand column. Check correct response for participant. Add comments when appropriate.

1. **X** Can participate
   ___ Any conflicts (i.e., arrive late, leave early?); Comment: ___

2. ___ Registration not required
   ___ Can register independently
   X Needs assistance; Comment: **Staff from group home will assist as needed**

3. ___ Permission not needed
   X Permission granted (consent form attached?)

4. **X** Participant can afford financial costs.
   ___ Other arrangements; Comment: ___

5. Participant's transportation choice(s):
   ___ Walk ___ Drive **X** Bus ___ Bike
   ___ Dropped off ___ Other: ___
   Assistance needed: **X** yes ___ no
   Initial bus training required

6. **X** Participant has appropriate attire.
   ___ Other; Comment: ___

7. **X** Equipment/materials are supplied
   ___ Participant has equipment
   ___ Equipment/materials need to be purchased
   ___ Other; Comment: ___

8. **X** Participant can meet requirement
   ___ Other; Comment: ___

in highly preferred activities. Upon further investigation, it is determined that Sue's participation in the exercise class is consistent with the *goals and objectives* in her program plan (Question 2).

It is confirmed that, with careful budgeting, Sue can *financially afford* to participate in the exercise class (Question 3). If the leisure option selected does cost money, one must be able to afford the costs to participate in the activity, either through personal resources or through the receipt of financial assistance. The recreation agency informs the group home staff that it can apply a sliding fee schedule for persons in financial need.

Sue possesses the necessary *materials and equipment*, in this case, exercise clothing and tennis shoes, for participation in the exercise class (Question 4). Owning or having access to the required materials/equipment is necessary if complete and functional participation in the recreation environment is to transpire.

Sue's minimal physical limitations do not present a problem for participation; therefore, material and/or procedural *adaptations* were not, at least initially, necessary (Question 5). However, for individuals with more severe physical impairments who require additional assistance to participate, it would be necessary to implement material and/or procedural adaptations to promote successful participation, success, and enjoyment in at least a partial manner.

Sue demonstrates independent *transportation* skills (i.e., riding the city bus to and from the sheltered workshop). With additional training, Sue could learn to ride the city bus that makes stops at the recreation center and one block from her home (Question 6). Incorporating additional transportation skill training into Sue's program could be of value in her attempts to utilize community recreation environments in the future.

Physical accessibility is not a special consideration that could hinder Sue's participation in this setting (Question 7). Further investigation reveals that the recreation center is physically accessible; there are, for example, handicapped parking spaces, curb cuts, no steps to contend with, and lowered drinking fountains with push plates. These factors will probably assist Sue in her independent, functional, and successful participation in this setting.

The exercise instructor and careprovider then complete PART I: (B): GENERAL PROGRAM AND PARTICIPANT INFORMATION (Figure 4.2) to identify preplanning tasks.

Based on the information above, the exercise class is deemed appropriate for Sue's participation. Following the directions stated in PART I, a meeting is arranged in order for the center director, a group home careprovider, and the exercise class instructor to complete PART II: ACTIVITY/DISCREPANCY ANALYSIS, of the Environmental Analysis Inventory.

The completion of PART II: ACTIVITY/DISCREPANCY ANALYSIS (Figure 4.3) provides the careprovider, exercise class instructor, and center director with an overall inventory of the basic and vital skills necessary for participation in the activity.

Following the completion and review of the ACTIVITY/DISCREPANCY ANALYSIS, PART III: SPECIFIC ACTIVITY REQUIREMENTS (Figure 4.4) is filled out. The social/emotional demands of the exercise class that would be placed on Sue are still areas of concern (See PART IV, (C): SOCIAL/EMOTIONAL CONSIDERATIONS in Appendix H) (implementation example found in Figure 4.5).

PART IV, (C): SOCIAL/EMOTIONAL CONSIDERATIONS of the inventory is then completed to analyze further the social and emotional skill requirements of the exercise class that would need to be addressed. In this manner, social and emotional concerns can be alleviated with additional training and activity modifications. Strategies to enhance Sue's participation are developed by group home staff and the exercise class instructor. The use of a volunteer advocate, additional skill training in social skills, and peer social reinforcement and modeling are identified as strategies to facilitate a successful leisure experience for Sue. If Sue had additional skill deficits relative to the exercise class demands in the physical and/

Leisure Skill Inventory

Inventory for Participant with Disability

Activity/Skill: __Exercise Class__

Name: __Sue Winters__

Leisure Setting: __Hiawatha Recreation Center__

Directions: Below, give a step-by-step breakdown of those *basic* and *vital* skills a nonhandicapped person would need in order to participate in the activity. Include all components (i.e., breaks, using restrooms, drinking fountain, telephone, etc.)

Directions: Read the step(s) in left column. If participants can perform the step, mark a plus (+) in the center column. If the participant cannot perform the step, make a minus (−) in the center column. If the participant's performance is marked (−), identify a teaching procedure or adaptation/modification for that step in the right column. Upon completion, go to Part III: SPECIFIC ACTIVITY REQUIRE-MENTS.

STEPS (Activity Analysis):	+	−	Teaching Procedure, Adaptation/Modification, Strategy for Partial Participation
1. Enter the recreation center.	+		1.
2. Acknowledge recreation staff and others, if appropriate.		−	2. Initially, group home staff will appropriately model interactions with rec. staff and others. (Staff may not be available.)
3. Locate and proceed to the multipurpose center.		−	3. Group home staff will teach Sue to ask for assistance in locating the room. After a few classes, Sue will know where the room is.
4. Locate coat rack along the wall and proceed in that direction.		−	4. Initially, group home staff will model and assist Sue in this step.
5. Take coat off, hang on coat rack or place it with other belongings (i.e., sport bag, purse) along the wall.	+		5.
6. Find a space on the exercise mat and proceed in that direction.		−	6. Initially, group home staff will model and assist Sue in this step.

(continued)

61

FIGURE 4.3 (continued)

7. Wait for class to begin.	7.	
8. Optional: Appropriately speak with others and stretch out.	8. + / −	Appropriate role modeling needed
9. When class starts, listen to and follow instructor's directions.	9.	
10. Do warm-up exercises.	10. +	
11. Do strength training exercises.	11. / −	Sue may have difficulty with some of these exercises. The instructor will provide modified exer. or assistance as needed.
12. When instructor offers a break, use drinking fountain if necessary.	12. +	
13. Do aerobic exercises.	13. / −	Assistance/modification, as needed.
14. Check heart rate (3 x).	14. / −	Assistance/modification, as needed.
15. Do cool-down exercises.	15. +	
16. Upon completion of class, help put mats away.	16. / −	Appropriate role modeling/ teaching may be needed.

(continued)

(continued)

PART II: *(continued)*

STEPS (Activity Analysis):	+	−	Teaching Procedure, Adaptation/Modification, Strategy for Partial Participation
17. Optional: Talk to other participants		−	17. Group home staff will appropriately model interactions with others.
18. Optional: use drinking fountain/ restroom, if necessary.	+		18.
19. Collect personal belongings.	+		19.
20. Put on coat.	+		20.
21. Exit recreation center.	+		21.
22.			22.
23.			23.
24.			24.
25.			25.

(If needed, use additional space on back)

63

ENVIRONMENTAL ANALYSIS INVENTORY
PART III: SPECIFIC ACTIVITY REQUIREMENTS

FIGURE 4.4

Name: __Sue Winters__   Date: __3-8-87__

Question: After completing and reviewing the ACTIVITY/DISCREPANCY ANALYSIS, if particular responses would be difficult for the participant to perform, would special material/procedural adaptations or teaching procedures be readily available to enable at least partial participation?

     ____ yes   __X__ no

If yes, participate in the program.

If no, please check the area(s) of concern listed below. This allows for an in-depth analysis of the specific requirements needed for this activity in the identified area of concern (i.e., physical, cognitive/academic, social/emotional).

____ Physical Skill Requirements: refer to ENVIRONMENTAL ANALYSIS INVENTORY PART IV (A).

____ Cognitive/Academic Skill Requirements: refer to ENVIRONMENTAL ANALYSIS INVENTORY PART IV (B).

__X__ Social/Emotional Skill Requirements: refer to ENVIRONMENTAL ANALYSIS INVENTORY PART IV (C).

---

or cognitive/academic areas, SECTIONS A and B (i.e., PHYSICAL SKILL REQUIREMENTS and COGNITIVE/ACADEMIC SKILL REQUIREMENTS), respectively, would have been provided. Copies of these sections are found in Appendix H.

Use of the 4-part Environmental Analysis Inventory allows for an individualized and systematic approach to integrating persons with disabilities into community leisure settings. To follow the Environmental Analysis Inventory process in its entirety, refer to the flow chart illustrated in Figure 4.6. Blank forms from the Environmental Analysis Inventory are presented in their entirety in Appendix H and may be reproduced for use.

Inventory Summary

The first part of this chapter delineated the components of the Environmental Analysis Inventory that was organized to secure relevant community recreation instructional information. This recreation skill and facility inventory was designed to modify or eliminate the various obstacles that are often encountered by persons with disabilities. Following the four-part process in this inventory might allow one to overcome obstacles that interfere with the selection and implementation of functional, age-appropriate leisure skills in community recreation environments. Overcoming such obstacles would permit interactions between persons with and without disabilities in integrated community leisure contexts.

As used here, the inventory outlines a systematic method of conducting an observation of an event as it occurs in a natural setting under typical conditions. Utilizing an inventory approach to the development of instructional sequences and related information provides recreation professionals, educators, and parents with an accurate, detailed description of a recreation activity. Since such a description is generated from the observation of nondisabled individuals, it can be compared to performance criteria exhibited by nondisabled persons. As a result, important, yet subtle, component responses such as finding an unoccupied space on the exercise mat, or qualitative response characteristics such as performing warm up exercises for the appropriate amount of time that might be easily ignored, are highlighted for instruction. Incorporating such subtle component or qualitative responses can minimize unnecessary performance discrepancies between the participants with and without disabilities who are using a recreation facility or who are simply performing the

FIGURE 4.5

ENVIRONMENTAL ANALYSIS INVENTORY

PART IV: FURTHER ACTIVITY CONSIDERATIONS—(C) SOCIAL/EMOTIONAL CONSIDERATIONS

Activity: _Exercise Class_

Name: _Sue Winters_   Date: _3-5-87_

Directions: Check, circle, or write in the correct information.

Directions: Refer to information in left-hand column. Answer yes or no as to whether the participant can participate at the level requested. If the answer is "no," comment on the assistance that is required.*

1. a. Does this activity occur: ____ alone ____ with 2 ____ in small
      group (3–8) _X_ in large group (8 or more)
   b. This activity is structured:
      _X_ class structure ____ no structure ____ combination
   c. Comment on the type and amount of supervision:
      One exercise instructor leading the group.

2. This activity involves: _X_ females _X_ males
   Age range: ____ preschool (under 5)
   ____ children (5–12)   ____ teens (13–19)
   _X_ adults (20–64)   ____ senior citizens (65 +)

3. a. Check the social interactions listed below that pertain to this activity.
      _X_ Share materials ____ Take turns ____ Compete
      _X_ Communicate with other participants
      ____ Have physical contact with other participants
   b. Noise level: ____ quiet ____ medium ____ loud ____ mixed

4. List words or common phrases associated with or used during this
   activity (e.g., nice shot)
   Stretching out counting 1-2-3, work it jog
   bend to the left right down on the mats,
   arms in front, legs out, etc.

1. a. _X_ yes ____ no
      Comments:

   b. _X_ yes ____ no
   c. _X_ yes ____ no
      Comments:

2. _X_ yes ____ no
   Comments:

3. a. ____ yes _X_ no → Sue displays inappropriate
      Comments: social skills (e.g., vocalizes loudly).
      If a group home staff person cannot assist
      ____ no w/ approp. role modeling and ver-
   b. ____ yes ____ bal correction, it may be necessary to
      Comments: solicit a class participant (volunteer)
      advocate) to assist, as needed.

4. ____ yes _X_ no
   Comments: Sue will require additional
   training and peer social reinforcement
   and modeling to respond to
   instructors directions.

*If social/emotional considerations have been met, proceed as planned. If not, an alternative activity or setting should be considered for investigation and potential participation.

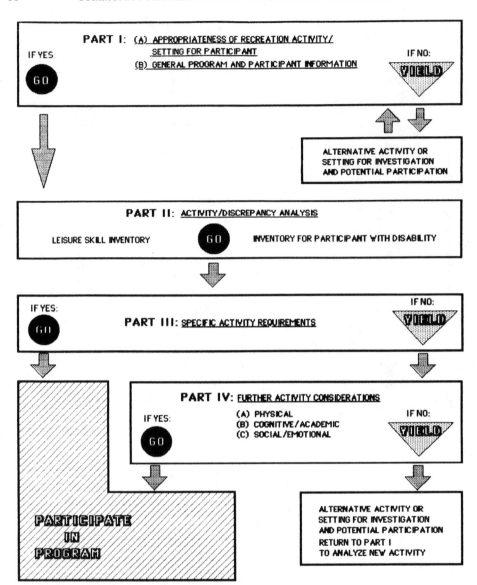

FIGURE 4.6   Environmental analysis inventory flow chart.

same leisure skill. In addition, using an observational inventory requires recreation professionals and educators to leave residential facilities and school buildings, and parents to leave homes, in order to develop instructional content. A visit to the recreation facility by parents or group home staff to determine its appropriateness for recreation instruction can be useful. For example, such a visit would reveal the variety of support elements needed by the participant, such as available transportation, or the number and complexity of location cues within the facility, or the types of activities available to the student as part of his or her leisure skill instruction. Completion of the Environmental Analysis Inventory can provide a broader and more complete view of an activity or skill.

PARTIAL PARTICIPATION AND INDIVIDUALIZED ADAPTATIONS

Depending upon the extent and level of their physical and/or mental disability, individuals with disabilities often lack the full range of motor, cognitive, or social skills needed to fully and successfully participate in a variety of leisure experiences. Community recreation professionals typically organize leisure services and programs to meet the needs of nondisabled persons. Because community recreation professionals often lack awareness of how to address the leisure needs of potential participants who have disabilities, programs and services traditionally organized and implemented have generally been unnecessarily restrictive and closed to persons with disabilities. As a result, segregated or special recreation programs are offered to persons with disabilities as substitutes for regular programs. The worst possible scenario would be a situation where no leisure programs are planned, and there are no options available for persons with disabilities. Persons with disabilities would then be relegated to the "basement of noninvolvement" due to the barriers of omission described in Chapter 2.

The case of Sue Winters, the hypothetical situation presented earlier, illustrates that use of the Environmental Analysis Inventory is an important strategy to ensure equal program access for persons with disabilities. Another strategy, that of partial participation (Baumgart et al., 1982; Ford et al., 1984), affirms this right to participate alongside nondisabled peers in a variety of recreational programs that are advertised to the general public. The principle of partial participation affirms, among other things, that persons with disabilities should be allowed to participate in environments and activities (e.g., recreational pursuits) at least partially, without regard to degree of dependence or level of functioning (Baumgart, et al., 1982). Furthermore, this principle assumes that participation in these environments and activities is advantageous to the person with a disability. Participation is particularly beneficial when it is approached systematically and with an awareness of not only the inherent skills and abilities of the participant but also the individualized adaptations necessary to enhance participation. The community recreation professional who spoke with Sue's group home careprovider was able to determine, by way of a comprehensive and systematic process, Sue's appropriateness to participate in the exercise class, her current skills and abilities related to the activity, and the physical and social needs that might require individualized attention prior to participation. An important step to be taken next by the community recreation professional, along with Sue, the careproviders, and, if necessary, other key players, is the identification of specific modifications or adaptations needed to facilitate Sue's involvement in the recreation program.

Suggested Program Modifications

The following principles must be considered by key players, that is persons responsible for adapting community recreation activities (Wehman & Schleien, 1981; Wehman, Schleien, & Kiernan, 1980).

Adapt Enough to Increase Participation, Success, and Enjoyment. Only Adapt When Necessary.   In Sue's situation, the Environmental Analysis Inventory and, in particular, the discrepancy analysis sections, identified Sue's need for assistance for successful and enjoyable participation.

View Any Changes or Adaptations as Temporary. Work Toward Engagement in Original, Nonmodified Activity.   Unless the adaptation is always necessary (e.g., prosthetic adaptation such as a built-up tennis shoe for persons with a shorter leg, or a sighted guide for a blind cross-country skier), program modifications must be designed as temporary changes so the person requiring the changes can learn the necessary skills and can eventually participate in a standard fashion like his or her nondisabled peers. For example, initial volunteer advocates assisting Sue may be close acquaintances, such as careproviders; later, the advocates may be other class participants, such as new friends. Finally, the need for a volunteer advocate is discontinued as Sue independently participates in community recreation programs.

Make Adaptations on an Individual Basis Meeting Individual Needs.   When the community recreation professional discovered Sue's needs for specific program adaptations, he based his findings on the information he gathered from the Environmental Analysis Inventory. He did not have any preconceived notion that people "like Sue", that is, persons with mental retardation, are "special" and should automatically require one-to-one attention during participation in recreational programs. However, the analysis by the community recreation professional determined that Sue would initially require some type of one-to-one arrangement, in her case, a volunteer advocate, to increase Sue's chance for successful and enjoyable participation in the exercise class. Other modifications were noted in Part II: ACTIVITY/DISCREPANCY ANALYSIS (Figure 4.3).

After making certain that all of the above principles are thoroughly considered and deemed necessary, the community recreation professional, in collaboration with key others, considers what types of adaptations must be made in recreational activities prior to Sue's participation. The recreation professional identifies five areas of the program that need to be modified: activity materials or equipment, the rules of the game, skill sequence, facility and environment, and lead-up activities. The following is a list of modifications that can be made in these five program areas. Modifications specific to Sue's participation in the exercise class are followed by a more general list of modifications that can be made to accommodate other persons with disabilities in a variety of recreation activities offered at a community leisure setting.

1. **Activity Materials or Equipment:** Leisure materials or equipment are modified to facilitate participation of persons with disabilities.
    Modifications for Sue: uses built-up tennis shoes or orthotic insert
    Other Activity Modifications: tubular steel bowling ramp
    lowered basketball backboard and rim
    built-up handles on paint brushes
    sport versus standard wheelchair
    Braille reading materials
    close-captioned video tapes
    soft versus hard rubber balls
    picture card of recreation center activities to make activity selection easier
    handicapped-accessible playground equipment
    tee-ball versus pitched baseball

2. **Rules of the Game:** Change the original rules to simplify activity.
    Modifications for Sue: Due to limited income, makes partial rather than lump sum payments for lessons
    Other Activity Modifications: stand closer to horeshoe pit to ensure greater accuracy
    allow two-handed basketball dribble
    require one- versus two-handed play on fooseball table

allow table tennis ball to hit same side before going over net

use personal item versus driver's license as collateral to borrow games in recreation center

3. **Skill Sequence:** Rearranging component steps of an activity to enhance safety and efficiency

Modifications for Sue: dresses in exercise clothing at home

does not perform activity until instructor verbalizes, then demonstrates exercises

does one-half of the normally required exercise repetitions

Other Activity Modifications: place finger on camera's shutter release button before raising camera to eye level

enter classroom earlier than other participants

place food item in oven, before turning oven on

4. **Facility and Environmental:** Renovating or constructing facilities and outdoor environments that are physically accessible.

Modifications for Sue: none

Other Facility Modifications: ramp curbs and steps

handrails from building to ice skating rink

installation of accessible toilets, sinks, water fountains

asphalt versus sand or dirt walking paths

tree branches trimmed so they cannot injure visually impaired persons

5. **Lead-Up Activities:** Simplified version of traditional activity allowing practice in component skill of the game leading to full participation in the future.

Lead-Up Skills for Sue: uses a chair when necessary to aid balance

practices exercises at home

works with a volunteer advocate

Other Lead-Up Activities: kickball leads to baseball

tricycle leads to bicycle

using only low numbers on dart board as scoring numbers in Cricket dart game

boot hockey leads to skate hockey

game of "catch" over a net leads to volleyball

volunteer advocate leads to participation with friend or independent access

VOLUNTEER ADVOCACY

A critical component in the integration of persons with disabilities into community leisure services is the recruitment, training, evaluation, and recognition of volunteers. Because it is determined that some individuals with disabilities (based on the Environmental Analysis Inventory) need personal assistance to participate successfully in a recreation program, volunteers become essential. This need was illustrated in the example of Sue Winters. Program leaders must necessarily focus their attention on all participants, both disabled and nondisabled, in a program. Therefore, the addition of a volunteer advocate, who could individually assist the participant with disabilities, when and if necessary, is helpful to the leader. The tasks of the volunteer advocate might include:

1. Assisting the participant during registration
2. Explaining to nondisabled peers the nature of the participant's disability, if the participant is not able to do so him or herself
3. Managing problem behaviors, if they occur
4. Facilitating interpersonal relationships with classmates
5. Physically prompting the participant to perform a task (e.g., helping a person with poor balance to bend over to touch toes in an exercise class)
6. Task analyzing and teaching leisure skills to the participant
7. Evaluating participant involvement in the recreation program
8. Providing transportation assistance to and from the recreation program site
9. Assisting during toileting, dressing, grooming
10. Assisting mobility throughout program length (e.g., pushing wheelchair, walking beside and providing needed support)
11. Other assistance needed as determined by the Environmental Analysis Inventory and joint recommendations of key players

Recruitment

It is the primary responsibility of the participant with disabilities and/or their parents or careproviders to provide a volunteer advocate, if needed. However, it is sometimes difficult to identify individuals to assume this role. A major task of the Community Advisory Board should be to assist in volunteer advocate recruitment. Parents, siblings, friends, school classmates, and neighbors of persons with disabilities should be contacted as potential volunteer advocates. Additionally, agencies providing youth services such as Boy and Girl Scouts, 4-H clubs, or YM/YWCAs often look for service projects for their membership. Volunteer advocacy is an excellent way to involve these groups. Corporations have also been known to provide volunteer resources for recreational programs and special events where persons with disabilities are expected to participate.

One role of the community recreation professional is to assist in identifying volunteer advocates, if an individual needs one. There are two important steps one might take to recruit and retain volunteers in case the need for volunteer advocates arises:

1. Develop a Volunteer Advocate Job Description format that outlines specific responsibilities and expectations (sample form Appendix I). Include:

Basic Information Needed	Where to Find Information
a. Title	(e.g., Volunteer Advocate, Special Friend)
b. Job description	(based on individual participant needs)
c. Days needed	(consult program brochure)
d. Hours needed	(consult program brochure)
e. Length of program	(consult program brochure)
f. Location of program	(facility; classroom)
g. Immediate supervisor	(program leader's name)
h. Special skills needed	(based on individual participant needs)
i. Description of participant with disabilities and his or her needs	(from registration form)
j. Other considerations	(e.g., transportation needs, self-care)

2. Recruit potential volunteer advocates from the community, local schools, youth service agencies, businesses, etc. Appropriate methods to solicit involvement include:

   a. Advertising in municipal park and recreation program brochures
   b. Distributing news releases to the media
   c. Writing public service announcements for local radio, TV, and cable network stations
   d. Creating a speaker's bureau made up of parents, consumers, and advocates to speak to agencies and organizations such as schools, parent groups, advocacy groups, and senior centers
   e. Registering the municipal park and recreation department and/or individual community centers with the local volunteer clearinghouse

The following list suggests ways to follow-up volunteer advocate recruitment:

1. Conduct a media saturation campaign calling for volunteers.
2. Send out a Volunteer Application (Appendix I) and job descriptions to interested persons who respond by phone call. (Note: Be sure to include a stamped, addressed return envelope with the application. The easier it is for a prospective volunteer to respond to the agency, the greater the likelihood of successfully recruiting him or her). Complete the Volunteer Advocate Call Sheet (Appendix I).
3. Follow-up with a phone call to the individual asking if he or she has received the application and has any questions. At this point, it is a good idea to ask the volunteer candidate if he or she could identify a specific task of interest.
4. Once the written application is returned by the volunteer candidate, review the application and call the applicant to set up a personal interview.
5. During the interview, discuss the volunteer's goals, specific talents and preferences, and hours during which he or she can volunteer his or her time.
6. Match volunteer advocate with a program and a disabled participant. Fill out a Volunteer Advocate = Participant Match Form (Appendix I). Complete the job description and give a copy to the volunteer.
7. Arrange for the volunteer to meet the program leader or disabled participant before the program begins. Be sure the community recreation professional or another representative from the agency is present at the first meeting. Once the volunteer has made a commitment, it is the recreation professional's responsibility to provide comprehensive inservice training and information to the volunteer advocate.

Other key players may be involved in this training; the training covers many of the same topics as the staff training program described in Chapter 3. Other inservice training topics could include: site orientation, goals and objectives of the program, and policies and procedures of the agency, including emergency procedures. Depending upon how many volunteers have been recruited, it could be easier and more efficient to provide volunteer orientation concurrently with staff orientation. However, if there is a large number of volunteers, orientation should be provided separately.

In order to assess whether the individual volunteer's needs and the needs of the agency have been met, it is essential to conduct program and volunteer evaluations upon completion of the program. The program staff should evaluate the volunteer not only to assess the volunteer's personal competencies, but also to determine if the volunteer was actually needed and, if so, did he or she enhance the program and the recreation experience of the participant with a disability. The volunteer should assess his or her own experience by evaluating whether the training and supervision were adequate, and whether the volunteer received respect from other staff. Evaluation formats are presented in Appendix I.

Volunteers need to feel important about their own work. Many programs and tasks could not be accomplished without them. Because the recreation agency has invested time and energy in training a volunteer, it is important to the agency that the volunteer continue his or her involvement with the agency. Volunteer recognition is the best way to ensure that trained volunteers return and provide the necessary program continuity and support for persons with disabilities. Recognition can be handled in a number of ways. Regular and sincere praise are the most natural ways to reinforce volunteers. Awarding certificates of recognition, and organizing small social events such as pizza parties and picnics, as well as full-scale annual recognition dinners with awards are additional methods to honor and reward volunteers. Each agency must decide how much it will commit to volunteer advocate recognition in terms of staff time and dollars.

"Special Friends" Training

The "Special Friends" program, which is operated by volunteer advocates within community recreation programs, is a direct outgrowth of the "Special Friends" concept (Voeltz, 1980; Voeltz, 1982; Voeltz et al., 1983) that was initiated in the early 1980s by special educators and university faculty in the Hawaii public schools. The intent of this school-based training program was to prepare children, with and without severe handicaps, for social interactions with each other within classroom settings. Because nondisabled students had little or no personal contact with severely handicapped peers, the "Special Friends" training program was devised to increase their awareness of persons with severely handicapping conditions. Students also had opportunities to ask questions and to participate in discussions regarding ongoing interactions with their peers who were disabled. Teachers and program coordinators used this time to introduce preferred strategies and methods to aid students in these interactions and to encourage the students to accept roles as volunteer advocates in the future.

The "Special Friends" concept has demonstrated its effectiveness in several of the exemplary programs PIRC has established as part of its grant project efforts (Schleien, Krotee, Mustonen, Kelterborn, & Schermer, 1986; Schleien, Ray, Soderman-Olson, & McMahon, in press). The use of a slide presentation illustrating interactions between participants with and without disabilities can help "Special Friends" volunteers to become familiar with and confident in their new roles as advocates. In addition, the program encourages questions and discussions to help increase volunteer awareness and sensitivity to the needs of persons with disabilities. During these discussions, adequate time is provided for volunteer advocates to express their concerns about socializing and engaging in recreational activities with disabled persons.

The recreation agency can develop their own "Special Friends" program simply by developing an orientation package suitable for presentation at volunteer advocacy recruitment programs. Basic elements of a "Special Friends" orientation include:

1. A 5-minute overview of accessible leisure services within the community
2. A 5–15 minute slide presentation with script illustrating successful integration efforts
3. A 10–15 minute question/discussion time

The 20–35 minutes spent on the "Special Friends" orientation represents a sound investment of time, effort, and money, as it may allay fears and apprehensions of persons who may wish to become future volunteer advocates.

COOPERATIVE GROUPING ARRANGEMENTS

An effective way to maximize participation by persons with disabilities in integrated community recreation programs is to use the technique of cooperative grouping arrangements. Based on the concept of cooperative goal structuring (Rynders, Johnson, Johnson, & Schmidt, 1980), cooperative grouping arrangements could enhance social interaction among participants with and without disabilities, augment positive attitudes of nondisabled persons toward their peers with disabilities, and increase the possibility that activity skills will be learned by participants with disabilities. This strategy can be applied to the many recreation programs that commonly offer isolated activities designed to meet individual needs (e.g., crafts, woodworking, photography, cross-country skiing), and competitive games and team sports, such as bowling, volleyball, floor hockey, or softball.

During Steps A and B on the Accessible Community Leisure Service Process (see Chapter 2 and Appendix A), the community recreation professional will have identified the need for a diverse range of programs and leisure services as defined by the expressed needs of persons with disabilities who register as participants. The recreation professional must also realize that, in many cases, activities may need to be modified somewhat to allow, at a minimum, the partial participation of persons with disabilities in that activity. In other words, there is a likelihood that a disabled person's mental or physical impairment will limit the extent to which he or she can participate independently in a recreational activity. Therefore, in SELECTING PROGRAMS, STEP C of the Accessible Community Leisure Service Process, one must carefully consider the functioning level of potential participants and then propose programs that can be modified so that persons with disabilities can be successfully integrated with nondisabled persons. By restructuring activities to make them less individualized or competitive, that is, by having participants work toward a common goal rather than playing alone or against one another, the recreation professional can encourage social integration. This strategy has been demonstrated to be effective in integrated art education programs (Schleien et al., in press).

A diagram representing cooperative grouping arrangements is presented in Figure 4.7. In this figure, three leisure activities—art project, cross-country skiing, bowling— that may be typically considered as either individual or competitive activities are used to illustrate this integration strategy. Individual participants of each activity are distinguished as O (nondisabled persons) and X (persons with disabilities). Each activity illustrates the interaction patterns of participants before and after the cooperative grouping arrangement program modification is implemented. The following are specific scenarios demonstrating this strategy to enhance social integration and positive, enjoyable leisure experiences. The reader should note that, in each case, the principle of partial participation as described earlier, applies in these scenarios. If performed carefully and effectively, the original program objectives are not compromised. Rule changes and other activity modifications are made prior to program implementation. As a result, positive client outcomes associated with cooperative activities (e.g., peer acceptance, equal participation) can be realized.

Activity #1: Art Project

This program is designed to provide nine children with opportunities to create a collage using a variety of art materials, including: scissors, paste, poster board, sawdust, sand, confetti, crayons, and colored paper and markers. The children are told to use these materials to make a picture of a farm. After receiving their assignment from the instructor, the students are told to collect the appropriate materials and to spread out around the room, either by sitting on the floor or at a table.

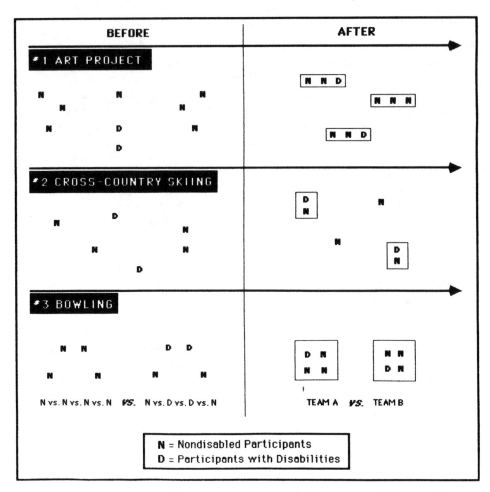

FIGURE 4.7.   Cooperative grouping arrangement strategy to enhance integrated leisure activity participation by persons with disabilities.

However, there are two students who are disabled. One child is mentally retarded and has difficulty understanding what a farm is, or what it may look like. The other child has cerebral palsy, uses a wheelchair, and has difficulty with her fine motor skills. Realizing that it may be difficult or unrealistic for these two students to produce the collage independently, the instructor assigns three teams of students to work collaboratively on the project, and includes the students on two of the teams. The two children with disabilities are assigned to different teams to encourage social integration. The instructor begins to apply the integration strategy of a cooperative grouping arrangement with each of the three teams responsible for producing a collage.

Once the groups are formed, students must answer the following questions as teams: Who in the team should draw the farm? What subjects (animals, buildings, equipment, people) should be drawn? What materials should be used in the picture (e.g., sand for the driveway, colored paper for the barn, confetti for fields)? Who in the team should apply the materials? Team members then work together to complete the collage. If the child with mental retardation cannot conceptualize a farm, then he or she can apply materials, such as glue or sand, to the picture while another child on the team draws the farm. If the child with mobility impairments cannot draw the picture or cut paper, then she can share ideas about the content or the materials used to make the collage. Additionally, she might be able to apply sand or confetti to glued areas, even if her fine motor skills are limited. At the completion of the art project, each group receives positive verbal reinforcement from the instructor. The instructor seeks to encourage the students, and is thus careful to avoid making any negative value judgments about individual works of art. Additionally, social integration and appropriate group work skills are enhanced.

Activity #2: Cross-Country Skiing

Cross-country (X-C) skiing is a popular leisure activity in northern climates, even in areas that have only a few inches of snow. It is believed by many that "if you can walk, you can X-C ski." Unfortunately, the activity itself requires that the participant have sufficient visual acuity to discern variations in the terrain, in snow conditions, and in ski trail markings in order to enjoy a safe and pleasurable ski outing. Because of the need for sight, most individuals with visual impairments are unable to X-C ski independently.

The BEFORE aspect of this activity, illustrated in Figure 4.7, shows a clear absence of persons with visual impairments in the ski area. However, through the use of the cooperative grouping arrangement strategy, sighted X-C skiers can be teamed-up with X-C skiers with visual impairments, serving as their guides on snow.

Norbie (1983) and others (Opel, 1982) have articulated techniques for training sighted individuals to be X-C ski guides, and have also presented successful ways of integrating persons with disabilities into X-C skiing. An exemplary program detailing a method that enhances volunteer advocacy, for example, by developing a X-C ski guide network, and that utilizes the cooperative grouping arrangement strategy, may be found in Chapter 8. These techniques have been used successfully for over 2 decades in Scandinavian countries. In the United States, the techniques have been systematically used since 1975 by the Ski-for-Light organization based in Minneapolis, Minnesota (Rostad, 1985).

Activity #3: Bowling

Bowling is a popular leisure activity for persons of all ages. Using the cooperative grouping arrangement strategy in a bowling activity that includes persons with disabilities has been demonstrated to be an effective means of enhancing positive attitudes and social interaction between youth with and without disabilities (Rynders et al., 1980). Specific modifications and adaptations to enhance the bowling skills of persons with developmental disabilities has also been presented in the literature (Certo et al., 1983).

In this scenario, two persons with disabilities are bowling with six other non-disabled friends. Both disabled individuals are mobility-impaired; one person is using a wheelchair and the other person, although not using a wheelchair, is having severe motor (ambulation) difficulties. Each of the eight players is striving to produce his or her best combined score, based on the three games they will bowl this day. Since they are not regular bowlers, point handicaps (i.e., adjustments in the individual's score to help equalize chances to win) are not computed. The bowlers with disabilities seem to be at a disadvantage due to their inability to adjust their bowling techniques to accommodate their disabilities. These two persons consistently have the lowest scores of the group.

To make bowling more competitive, teams of four persons each are formed. Team A has one of the individuals with disabilities as a member. The other disabled person is on Team B. The winning team is the team with the highest combined score (i.e., each person's three-game score added together for a team total score) declared the winner. The outcome of the tournament between Team A and Team B now depends on team members supporting each other.

To summarize, many of the programs offered by communities are oriented toward team athletics, which are competitive, or toward individual, independent activities, as in arts and crafts classes, self-help groups, and technical skills classes such as auto mechanics and knitting. It has been demonstrated that both competitive group activities (Rynders et al., 1980) and individually performed activities (Schleien et al., 1985) can be modified in ways that create better opportunities for truly integrated recreation experiences. Following are examples of how other common community programs can be adapted so that they are accessible for persons with disabilities.

1. A designated runner can be used for the baseball batter who is a double amputee.
2. Cumulative team scores are the only basis for winning a recreation league bowling tournament. A person in a wheelchair can be a member of the bowling team and can compete by using a tubular steel bowling ramp.
3. Participants in the photography class are told to work in two-person teams to complete their class project. One person in the class happens to be mentally retarded.
4. Participants in a woodworking class work in groups of four to complete a shelving unit. Three of the participants are not disabled and do the cutting and joining of the parts. The fourth member, who happens to be severely disabled with cerebral palsy, does the varnishing.
5. Children are gathered in groups of three to explore the "Haunted House" at the recreation center. One child holds the flashlight, while another hides effectively behind the third friend's wheelchair, which she helps to push.
6. Players at a frisbee "golf" tournament in a park are awarded individual stroke handicaps similar to those awarded in a regular golf game. The person who earns second place is severely mentally retarded.

SUMMARY

This chapter has presented a conceptual framework for community recreation programming and leisure skill instruction for persons with disabilities. The authors' position is that persons with disabilities should be taught functional, age-appropriate leisure skills that are comparable to those used by nondisabled individuals and that lead to successful performance in integrated community recreation settings. Through the selection of such leisure skills, maximum gains in independent community performance may be expected, over time, to accrue.

In order to facilitate this transition to more functional recreation and leisure skill instruction for individuals with disabilities, a multiple component inventory strategy was presented. The Environmental Analysis Inventory was designed to provide the community recreation professional, educator, or parent with relevant instructional content and the information needed to make viable recreation instructional decisions. The inventory provides useful information about the potential participant with disabilities, the skills and abilities of the potential participant, and the program modifications needed to complement these skills and abilities. The authors acknowledge that the inventory process is long and initially tedious. However, the inventory helps develop functional, age-appropriate, integrative recreation skills in individuals with disabilities; skill development is a benefit that far outweighs the inconvenience of completing the inventory.

The chapter concludes with specific methods to facilitate successful participation in community leisure settings by persons with disabilities. Several approaches, including strategies for partial participation, individualized adaptations, volunteer advocacy and special friends training, and cooperative grouping arrangements, are described, and examples are provided. The implementation of one or a combination of these key integration strategies is often necessary if persons with disabilities are to appropriately participate alongside their nondisabled peers in community leisure settings and activities. In the next chapter, a practical approach to the use of behavioral methods in community recreation settings is presented. The combination of behavioral principles and the integration strategies discussed in this chapter can provide the community recreation professional with a potent arsenal of techniques to make community leisure settings accessible to all individuals.

Chapter 5

Behavioral Principles in Community Recreation Integration

Richard S. Amado

This chapter continues discussion and presentation of specific methods or strategies to integrate existing community leisure services and to overcome common barriers that may be encountered by persons with disabilities. The Environmental Analysis Inventory, described earlier, provides the basis for selection of one or more of these key strategies. The reader should find this information immediately useful. However, this survey is no substitute for the information and approaches one might gain by communicating with the many key players identified earlier. The following are guidelines for decision-making; these should be adapted or expanded to serve individual, agency, or community needs.

BEHAVIORAL STRATEGIES

A key strategy that is essential and must be addressed for integration to take place is behavioral programming. A comprehensive review of this strategy is provided in this chapter. The management of problem behaviors of persons with disabilities is an issue that many community recreation professionals hold in common. Specifically, persons organizing and leading recreational activities are concerned about a number of program-specific behaviors. Such behaviors include: interpersonal relationships between disabled and nondisabled participants, and the presence (or absence) of antisocial behaviors (e.g., screaming, hitting, spitting, or self-injurious behaviors). Recreation planners are also concerned with specific management techniques that may be employed without detracting from the objectives of the recreational program or the enjoyment of the other participants. These professionals are also interested in the current abilities and skills of the participant with disabilities to per-

Dr. Richard Amado is with the Human Sciences Support Network, in St. Paul, Minnesota.

form program tasks in the "normal" manner, and in the best ways to motivate the person with disabilities to participate in the activity.

The reader will want to determine to what extent inappropriate behaviors become a problem for any particular individual who becomes a participant in the community recreation program. To determine general behavioral characteristics associated with specific disability types, one should contact local or national advocacy organizations (See Appendix G). For example, persons with autism often need consistent routines to enhance successful participation in programs. Another method for identifying problem behaviors is to discuss individual characteristics of potential participants with parents and careproviders. These key individuals can identify any potential problem areas that may arise (e.g., sudden, loud noises may trigger tantrum or self-abuse behaviors in certain individuals). Parents and careproviders can also advise as to the most effective ways to direct and motivate participants, and can encourage appropriate participation, thus increasing the chance for successful integration. A third approach to behavioral programming, which will be discussed in this chapter, involves use of task-analytic procedures.

There are many ways to modify behaviors (e.g., contingency management, reinforcement schedules, and stimulus control), to increase chances that participants with disabilities will participate appropriately and socially within the context of a particular recreation program. It is not within the scope of this book to address all of these techniques. For the most part, community recreation professionals, program leaders, and volunteer advocates must rely on positive reinforcement procedures to manage participant behaviors. The activity itself should be a strong enough reinforcer to persons with disabilities that they will find involvement in a community-based program motivating and personally rewarding. More powerful reinforcers come from staff, volunteer advocates, and peer participants who provide constant positive attention through social interactions such as conversation, praise, smiles, appropriate touching (e.g., hugs, pats on the back, handshakes), and cooperative assistance in specific tasks within the activity. Nondisabled persons, particularly other participants, are excellent role models from whom persons with disabilities can learn by observing. The community recreation planner should observe participants with disabilities and to see what is naturally motivating, and should seek ways to nurture friendships that could promote and enhance enjoyable and accessible recreation programs.

Solving the Problem of Undesirable Behaviors

Behavior problems are not a significant barrier to integrating recreation programs in community settings. Most people with disabilities do not have behavior problems; those who do can usually be served very easily with simple interventions. The number of intense behavior problems will be few and far between. Even intense behavior problems can be addressed in integrated settings with appropriate professional input and adequate supports. In short, behavior problems are a barrier to participation only to the extent that individuals allow them to be so.

Behavior Occurs in a Context

It is common knowledge that behavior is affected by environment. In fact, it is popularly believed that moods and behaviors are affected by the weather, the time of day, whether or not one is hungry, and so forth. Some of those incidents that affect behavior are like cues, that is, they precede certain behaviors. Common cues and their associated behaviors include:

Cue	Behavior
A red traffic light	Stepping on the brake pedal
Someone saying "hello"	Responding with "How are you?"
The doorbell ringing	Asking, "Who's there?"
The firing of a starting gun	Runners leaving the starting line

In fact, cues precede almost every action a person makes. That cue is referred to as an *antecedent* because it comes before behavior. Antecedents tell individuals when to do a particular behavior. The red traffic light tells drivers it is time to step on the brakes; the green light tells drivers it is time to step on the gas; the referee's whistle tells players to begin the basketball game; the horn tells them to stop the game.

Those actions that follow certain behaviors are referred to as *consequences*. Examples of familiar consequences include:

Behavior	Consequence
Doing a job for someone	The worker is paid money
Putting on sunglasses	The bright light dims—relief!
Stubbing one's toe	It hurts—ouch!
Arguing with the sports official	The player is "thrown out" of the game

Consequences are very important because they influence how often a certain behavior is likely to occur. Behaviors that produce money and stop painful light in the eyes, for example, are likely to be repeated; behavior that results in stubbing a toe is not likely to be repeated.

The antecedents and consequences for any behavior can usually be identified, although this is sometimes a difficult task. There are times when the antecedent or consequence is very subtle; there are times when the consequences follow only certain instances of a behavior; there are times when the antecedent is invisible without special observation equipment. Nonetheless, most of the time, the antecedents and consequences of any action can be identified, and the relationship between the antecedents, behaviors, and consequences can be revealed by making a simple model:

Antecedent	Behavior	Consequence
Red light	Step on brake	Car slows and stops
Gun fires	Start to run	Compete in race

This model is often referred to as the "A-B-C" model, and through this model the problem behaviors that make it difficult for some learners to participate in recreational settings can be understood, and often changed.

Identifying the Problem

The first step to fixing a problem is identifying the problem. Rather than simply saying, "John is aggressive," or, "Mary does not pay attention," it is important to clearly state the problem in precise terms. Rather than calling John aggressive, identify the aggressive behaviors he displays and specify how often he displays that behavior: "John hits other participants in the tumbling class an average of 8 times per 40-minute class session." Similarly, rather than calling Mary inattentive (which could be noncompliance or daydreaming, etc.), describe the behavior that Mary displays: "Mary follows about 4 out of every 5 of the instructor's directions in all of her classes."

When identifying problem behaviors, it also helps to identify why the targeted behavior is a problem. Behaviors are usually a problem when they (1) occur too often in a particular setting, (2) occur at the wrong time or in the wrong place, or (3) do not occur as often as one would like in a particular setting. For the authors' purposes, it is more than adequate to identify behavior that occurs too often as a behavioral excess, behavior that occurs at the wrong time or place as misplaced behavior, and behavior that occurs too infrequently as a behavioral deficit.

Putting it Together

After identifying the problem, the next step is to identify the antecedents (As) and the consequences (Cs) of the target behavior. To find the As and Cs, make a record each time the target behavior occurs. The record should include a description of what action took place immediately before and after the behavior. After recording 10 instances of the target behavior, scan the records for common elements in the antecedents and common elements in the consequences. Look for similar events changing in similar ways. For example, a consequence might be correction from an instructor, escape from the activity, laughing from peers, or self-stimulation.

If there is not enough information to identify the A's and C's, simply collect the information for 10 more episodes. Continue collecting data in this fashion until conclusions can be drawn about the antecedents and consequences, then fit the information into an A-B-C model. Following are examples of this process.

Example I

Antecedent: Children are working on crafts projects.
Behavior: Child will not sit still and is going around the room disturbing others.
Consequence: Instructor tells child to sit down and work on the project.

Example II

Antecedent: Children are instructed to choose an activity.
Behavior: Child does not comply but instead climbs on furniture and railing.
Consequence: Instructor talks with child about his behavior and redirects his activities.

The next step is to find similarities among the antecedents, and then to find similarities among the consequences. In the first situation above, the children have a task, a crafts project, on which they are to be working. In the second incident the children are given an instruction to choose an activity. Being given an instruction creates a "task available" situation in which there is something that the child is expected to do, just like the crafts project situation. In both situations, the child has been provided a task that he or she is expected to do.

Similarities in the consequences can be identified in the same way. In the first situation, the instructor directs the child back to the task; in the second situation, the instructor talks with the child. The common element in both consequences is attention from the instructor. Often, there is more than one consequence for a behavior. In both of the immediate situations, the second consequence of not doing the assigned task is escape from, or avoidance of, the task. Getting out of doing something undesirable is a very potent and prevalent motivation. So, two of the possible consequences for climbing on furniture and roaming around the room are: 1) attention from the instructor, and 2) avoiding a nonpreferred activity. The craft project and furniture-climbing incidents can be reduced to the A-B-C model in the following manner:

Antecedent	Behavior	Consequence
Child is provided a task	Child leaves assigned task	Child receives instructor's attention and avoids the assigned task

By putting these situations into an A-B-C model, one can readily see that the child is getting attention for doing what he or she should not be doing. The child's behavior demonstrates that being noncompliant has significant rewards or payoffs: receiving attention from the instructor and escaping a task.

PROBLEM BEHAVIOR AND THE ENVIRONMENT

By now, it should be fairly obvious that the environment plays an important role in the existence and nature of undesirable behaviors. In fact, the environment can support problem behavior, as can be seen in the following situations:

Antecedents and Problems

Antecedents for Appropriate Behavior are Unclear, Unavailable, or Obscured by Other Cues.   For example, a driver pulls up to an intersection with a stop-and-go light that just changed to yellow—first he lightly touches the brakes, then he slams the gas pedal. Another example: during a basketball game the coach is shouting out instructions to his players faster than they can respond; the players miss some of the moves the coach requests because of the speed of his instructions and the background noise from the fans. A third example: when a student in swimming class gets out of the pool after swimming laps, another student says, "You made great time," and the swimmer hits him in the mouth because through the water in his ears he heard the student say, "You'd make great slime." Consequences also support or generate problem behaviors.

Consequences and Problems

Consequences of Problem Behavior Act as Reinforcers to Strengthen that Behavior.   Every time the class clown does something humorous, the whole class laughs at her. In another situation: several times a week after doing things he is told not to do, a young troublemaker gets large amounts of individual attention from the instructor who attempts to "get to the hidden causes of the participant's behavior". Or: a youngster who has fallen off the parallel bars several times creates a disturbance whenever his physical education class has gymnastics because he is then sent to the principal's office and thus successfully avoids the parallel bars.

Consequences for the Appropriate Alternative to the Target Behavior are Punishing Consequences.   Doing the required activity ineptly in front of the entire class produces ridicule; practicing swimming with the face in the water results in swallowing water; sewing can include pricking one's finger with a pin or needle.

Consequences for the Appropriate Behavior are Inadequate Reinforcers that Cannot Strengthen the Behavior.   At the end of each session the instructor tells all the participants, "you all did a great job today!", but there is no other consequence for behaving well and performing as the instructor desires. Similarly, after playing very hard during a contact sport (and being physically battered), members of the losing team are likely to play with less interest and intensity the next time out.

In the following situation, behavior itself can facilitate the development of problem behaviors:

Problem Behavior

Emotional Arousal Interferes with Acceptable Behavior.   When a participant who is playing basketball is upset over missing a basket, angry about a referee's bad call, or distracted by physical pain, the likelihood of acting out in response to minor annoyances is increased. At times like this one, a little teasing or an instruction to do a nonpreferred task can result in verbal and/or physical aggression.

Appropriate Behavior May Be Unavailable; The Person May Never Have Learned the Right Way to Behave.   One often expects people to behave a certain way because "it is the right thing to do." In reality, people need to learn the subtle, and sometimes not so subtle, social amenities and rules for dealing with other people effectively. Each sport and organized activity has its written and unwritten rules. These rules are often learned inadvertently by participants through participation in an activity. Other learners do not learn by accident, and for these participants, recreation planners must arrange specific opportunities for the participant to learn the rules, so that he or she may actively take part in recreation.

Summary

In summary, before attempting to change a problem behavior there are several things that must be done. First, one should identify the *antecedents* and *consequences* of the targeted problem behavior. Second, one should determine precisely what the problem is: a behavioral excess, a behavioral deficit, a misplaced behavior, or some combination of the three. Third, one should identify the reason why the problem exists in terms of the A-B-C model. That is, one should describe how the *antecedents, behaviors,* or *consequences* are supporting the problem behavior and interfering with the desired adaptive behavior.

EXAMPLES

The following examples are provided to illustrate the process of selecting a behavior-changing intervention after completing the antecedents, behaviors, and consequences analysis.

Example I

Antecedent: Children are playing in a gymnasium program.
Behavior: Child leaves the gymnasium.
Consequence: Instructor brings child back into the gymnasium; child leaves again.

Two things occur when the child in this example leaves the activity: first, the child escapes from the activity, and second, the child receives individual attention from the instructor. It is not possible to tell from the existing information if one or both consequences are supporting the behavior, but it is evident that the consequences for staying in the activity are not as strong as the consequences for leaving. Therefore, one possible solution to this problem is to provide the youngster with a positive reinforcer for being in the gymnasium, for remaining there, and for participating in the activity. Because it is possible that youngsters might also be leaving the room because this act produces individual attention from the instructor, it makes sense for the instructor to use frequent, individual attention as the reinforcer for encouraging the children to remain in the gymnasium.

At the same time, if attention is what the child is seeking, the instructor will want to be certain that the youngster receives little or no attention for leaving the gymnasium. Therefore, the instructor should monitor the child who leaves the gymnasium as unobtrusively as possible, in order to ensure his or her welfare. If unobtrusive monitoring cannot be used, a staff member can wait outside the gymnasium door to turn the youngster around if he or she tries leaving the environment.

Example II

Antecedent: The group of children were asked to begin an art project.

Behavior: The participant becomes withdrawn and will not approach the group.

Consequence: After verbal prompts, the participant becomes more determined not to join the group. The participant is given the art project and proceeds to work on the project away from the rest of the participants.

It is very important to scrutinize the relationship between the participant's behavior and the instructor's behavior in this example. While the instructor's behavior is described in the *consequences* component as "verbal prompts", the result of the instructor's behavior was an increase in the participant's resistance. Because the prompting strengthened the behavior it followed, it is reasonable to assume the prompting was actually reinforcement. Given this analysis, there is an immediately available solution: withhold attention for non-participation and provide much more attention for participation. Because the participant engaged in the activity when away from the rest of the group, there is also a second possible solution: slowly bring the participant and the group into closer physical proximity over a period of time by arranging the seating in a tighter pattern before each class period.

Example III

Antecedent: The participant is involved in an integrated arts and crafts class.

Behavior: The participant attempts self-abuse with a pair of scissors.

Consequence: Teacher removes the utensil; the participant finds another item with which to continue the self-abuse behavior.

Self-abuse is a special behavior only because the result of doing things that are self-abusive can be permanently disfiguring and debilitating. Otherwise, it is important to re-member self-abusive behaviors just like other behaviors: they occur within an environment that supports them. Adding to the difficulty of trying to change self-abusive behaviors is the problem of preventing the participant from doing damage to him or herself; other-wise, the same process used above for modifying other problem behaviors is applied.

Because the behavior continues after the scissors is withdrawn, one can assume the behavior is not specific to the scissors. A fair assumption here is that the participant does not know what to do with the scissors. Additional observations indicate the participant goes on to use other materials for self-abuse. Because there is no apparent lengthy or repeated inter-action between the instructor and the participant following or during the participant's self-abuse, one can further assume the instructor's attention is not significant to the child's be-havior. What is left? Escape from boredom!

Many children with disabilities have not been taught to participate in group instruc-tion, to use arts and crafts materials, nor to enjoy crafts activities; however, they may have learned to entertain themselves by stimulating their senses in ways that also result in damage to their bodies. This behavior of the disabled learner is not very different from the fingernail biting or hair-twisting behavior displayed by nondisabled persons. The likely so-lution to managing the self-abuse behavior is to teach the participant the correct way to use the materials and to enjoy the activity. This teaching will require the use of small steps with substantial prompting for the participant, as well as the use of strong reinforcers delivered for participating in the learning experience (see the information on "Effectively Teaching New Skills" in this chapter).

Example IV

Antecedent: The instructor directs the group to run laps around the recreation room; the instructor then steps out of the room.

Behavior: The nondisabled participants initiate horseplay, including inappropriate use of equipment and name calling.

Consequence: Upon returning to the room, the instructor reprimands all the class members and has them sit with their heads down on the gym floor.

Most young recreation class members are not enthralled with running laps in a gymnasium. It is likely that the instruction to do so cues the participants to engage in a behavior that avoids running laps. The instructor's response in this instance is exactly the wrong one if the participants are trying to avoid the activity. Rather, the instructor should have had the class run the laps so the class members would not have succeeded in avoiding that exercise.

Another way to eliminate the problem of avoidance behavior is to create group activities in which the participants have a stake in the outcome of their performances. Having the students agree to work toward a desirable goal (e.g., the students select a game in which teams compete to run the most laps in a period of time, or they run to raise funds for a charity), can motivate the student to participate rather than avoid the undesirable activity.

This final example introduces a method to influence the behavior of individuals in groups; this method can, in fact, be very effective and efficient behavior management. There is sufficient data available from group management methods to discuss them at length.

BEHAVIOR MANAGEMENT METHODS FOR PEOPLE IN GROUPS

In this section, the antecedents and consequences of the behaviors of individuals will once again be examined. Even though the techniques are applied to groups of people, the antecedents and consequences do not operate on this group, but act instead on the individuals within the group. In fact, the underlying premise of this section is that groups do not behave, but people do.

Now, bearing this background information in mind, the reader can review some procedures for influencing groups effectively and efficiently. These procedures complement the discussion in Chapter 4 on cooperative grouping arrangements as an effective integration strategy.

Consequences and the Group

The Consequence for a Group is Dependent on the Performance of One of its Members.   When one member of the group is provided the opportunity to earn something desired by the entire group, the group's members tend to support the individual, to rally behind his or her efforts to earn the consequence, and to dissuade the individual from acting in ways that are inconsistent with earning the consequence. Therefore, this procedure is particularly effective for creating social relationships for an individual who has few or no relationships, and for improving the quality of existing relationships when they are not constructive.

Example I

Antecedent: The physical education class has been assigned to do sit-ups.

Behavior: John, who is overweight, tries a few sit-ups and then begins to clown around, drawing others off-task.

Consequence: John avoids the discomfort of doing sit-ups and produces "agreement" from his peers by entertaining them.

A group consequence procedure, in which John earns something for the group by doing sit-ups, would be particularly effective in this situation. For example, permitting John to earn 10 minutes of a preferred activity daily, or, through participating for a week, to earn the opportunity for the entire group to select its preferred sport on Friday, or some other readily available event, would be more effective. The rest of the students in the class will be more inclined to cheer for him when he does sit-ups, and to ignore him when he clowns around. This intervention is likely to produce appropriate participation and to create constructive peer relationships.

A Desired Consequence for the Group is Dependent Upon the Performance of All the Members of the Group. This procedure is similar to the way in which team sports already work. When the team scores high, every individual on the team wins. While this procedure will support the development of constructive social relationships, it does not single out any particular individual as in the last procedure.

Example II

Antecedent: The class is given a list of words to learn for a spelling test 1 week before the test. Just before the test, they are given 15 minutes to review the words.

Behavior: The class members study individually and in pairs for varying amounts of time and with varying amounts of effort.

Consequence: The students produce a range of scores; some scores are marginally acceptable and some are not acceptable at all.

If there was a preferred activity or event contingent upon the total group score, there would be adequate reason for the students to help one another study in order to raise the scores of all the individual students. A situation in which this procedure is in place will produce cooperative efforts to raise every score and may possibly produce new relationships and friendships.

Special Concern

There is one special concern to be addressed when using any group management procedure. While the procedures can, and usually do, foster constructive relationships, there is potential for a particular undesirable side effect. In any of the group consequence procedures, it is possible for the group members to be unkind and vindictive toward anyone who does not contribute to earning the desired outcome. In fact, to minimize the likelihood of this side effect, the instructor should present information to participants regarding the benefits of working together, supporting others, etc. In addition, the instructor should observe the participants for any indication of retribution, and should intervene at the earliest moment to discourage such behaviors.

Summary

Behavior occurs in a context of antecedents and consequences. The easiest way to effect long-term change when someone displays a problem behavior is to identify the antecedents and consequences that support that behavior and then to change one or both of them. This approach to managing problem behaviors is referred to as "Behavior Analysis" because the emphasis is placed on analyzing the context in which behaviors occur. Several examples of behavior analysis have already been provided to illustrate the application of this methodology. One must develop solutions to these problems by conducting analyses of the unique environments in which those behaviors occur.

EFFECTIVELY TEACHING NEW SKILLS

Four behavioral techniques for enhancing teaching effectiveness are: activity and task analysis, shaping, prompting, and error correction. While the procedures can be used independently, powerful learning could result from their combination during instructional activities.

ACTIVITY AND TASK ANALYSIS

Activity and task analyses are useful strategies that break down programs or skills into component parts and aid facilitation of leisure participation by persons with disabilities. Each type of analysis is illustrated within this manual. Activity analysis procedures may be found in Part II: Activity/Discrepancy Analysis of the Environmental Analysis Inventory. Task analysis, as a method to evaluate participants' progress toward acquiring specific leisure skills, is explained and illustrated in Chapter 6. A further examination of task analysis, or skill sequencing, should be helpful to the recreation professional in planning and implementing recreational programs for participants with disabilities.

Task-analytic procedures are particularly useful for assessing and teaching skills to persons who are developmentally disabled (e.g., persons with severe/profound mental retardation, or with severe physical disabilities) (Knapcyzk, 1975; Nietupski, Hamre-Nietupski, & Ayres, 1984; Wehman & Schleien, 1981). Breaking down social and recreation behaviors and motor skills through use of task analyses may seem anathema to traditional recreation programming which is intended to offer fun and enjoyment to the participants. Also, persons responsible for developing recreation programs may not use task-analytic procedures if they, themselves, have not been exposed to the efficacy of this approach (Wehman, 1977).

Activity and task analysis procedures could enable many persons, who traditionally have been excluded from integrated community leisure services, to participate successfully in recreation activities. A complete task analysis will break down specific activities, such as playing a board game, into distinct behavioral components, such as picking up a die, rolling the die, determining the value of the die, or picking up a playing piece, or moving the playing piece on a game board according to the value of the die, etc. Instructors or volunteer advocates will be able to determine, through a discrepancy analysis, the skills the participant currently possesses and those he or she needs in order to successfully perform the targeted recreational activity. Persons with disabilities could begin to acquire appropriate skills that lead to successful participation in future recreation programs. Further, as a result of task analysis, the community recreation professional could develop increased self-confidence in his or her professional abilities, thus leading to the development and implementation of more accessible recreation programs in the future.

Shaping

Shaping is a very simple procedure that is characterized by gradually changing the requirement for reinforcement to change some dimension of a behavior. Dimensions of behavior that are typically modified using shaping include intensity, duration, form, and frequency. If participants in an aerobics class, for example, do not seem to be able to keep up a high pace early in the program, slower music could be used initially and gradually replaced with faster music. A tennis player's ability to return fast or hard serves can be improved by gradually increasing the speed of the serves that are hit to him or her. Shaping is one of the most flexible and useful of the behavioral teaching procedures. The community recreation planner will find many uses for it.

Prompting

Before the consequences of a particular behavior can be examined, the behavior first has to occur. This dilemma is referred to as the problem of the first response, and it repeatedly confronts every teacher and instructor. Prompting procedures have been designed to address this problem. Initially, the prompt is used with the normally occurring antecedent to supplement it. In this way, the prompt clarifies the antecedent. As the behavior occurs more readily, the prompt is phased out until the behavior is no longer present, leaving the normally occurring antecedent to precede the behavior.

There are many forms of prompts; only the most common forms are included here. Further information about prompting procedures may be found in B. F. Skinner's *The Technology of Teaching* (1968).

Gesture Prompts   Many people use their hands as they talk. It is not unusual to see hands waving in the air as a speaker gets more and more excited while speaking. When speaking to someone over loud background noise, the speaker might beckon wtih his or her hand as well as speaking the request: "Come here!" At another time, a speaker might point at a particular cabinet while speaking, "Put it in there!" In these instances the gesture is not simply a prompt, it is an integral part of the instruction from the speaker. However, in the process of teaching someone to put, for example, the field hockey equipment in the correct locker, the speaker might point to the locker next to the door and say, "That equipment goes in the locker by the door." Eventually this pointing will be eliminated as the learner becomes familiar with the location of the equipment locker.

Verbal Prompts   Verbal prompts can be thought of as extra instructions. After telling the participants in exercise class to reach up as high as they can, the instructor might then add, "Higher, that's it! Higher, keep reaching!" When asking where the bathroom is, a new participant in a program might be told, "Go to the far corner, the red door." In this example, "the red door" is a prompt because it supplements the necessary instruction, "Go to the far corner . . ."

Model Prompts   This type of prompt is one of the more familiar. Instructors are used to explaining how to do a particular task to a neophyte, following instructions with, "Like this, watch me!", and then proceeding to act out the performance just described to facilitate faster learning. As with other forms of prompts, these prompts should be phased out as quickly as possible without disrupting the teaching that is dependent on the prompts.

Physical Prompts   Physical prompts are often used absent-mindedly. An instructor might take a child's hand as the instructor starts to walk off, saying, "Let's go!" When teaching a youngster to put on a coat independently, the instructor may guide the child's hands into the arm holes on the child's coat. These physical contacts are supportive and can guide voluntary participation in the training. Such contacts are not to be confused with guidance procedures designed to produce compliance with instructions when the learner is resisting. *Never* force a participant to do anything against resistance as a prompting procedure. Force against resistance is not prompting, it can be dangerous to the learner, and it must be done with appropriate professional supervision. A correct application of physical prompting in a recreation setting occurs, for instance, when the coach wraps his arms around the batter from the back and guides the participant through an even, level swing of the baseball bat. Similarly, the trainer might assist a learner in mastering the swing of a tennis racket or a volleyball serve.

SELECTING AND USING PROMPTS

Effective prompts can only be identified as effective after they have demonstrated their effectiveness in use. While this logic may seem absurdly obvious, it is presented to remind the reader that there is nothing wrong with the participant who does not respond to specific prompt forms; rather, the prompt should be changed. However, instructors may automatically tend to react as if there were something wrong with the participant.

There are two rules of thumb the instructor should use when selecting prompts. First, the instructor should identify the distinctions the participant already makes. That is, can he or she readily imitate a model? Or, can he or she understand verbal instructions, or respond to gestures? Select a form of prompt that the participant can already distinguish, not one that requires even more learning. Second, the instructor should choose a prompt that, as it is phased out, draws the participant's attention to the new distinction you are trying to teach.

For example, the instructor might draw a bright red square on the basketball backboard behind the net to mark the appropriate area to hit with the ball in order to make a basket. After the ball players routinely hit the area in the square, the red lines that define the box could be faded in intensity and width slowly until they no longer exist at all. In a second example, the seams on a baseball could be painted bright orange so that the batters-in-training can see the seams more readily. The paint could be faded as the participants demonstrate sufficient hitting ability.

ERROR CORRECTION

No matter how well instructors teach, it seems they will never do so well that students make no errors at all. Therefore, it is imperative that instructors have an error correction procedure (ECP) ready for these situations. There are several characteristics of an effective ECP:

1. The correct response is necessary before moving on to additional training or training trials.
2. There is no reinforcement for the error.
3. Prompts are provided following an error to the degree necessary to assure the participant exhibits the correct behavior.
4. Reinforcement is provided following the correct response, but it is of lesser quality or quantity than the reinforcement for performing without error.

If errors occur repeatedly, it is a good idea to evaluate them for patterns. It could be that the reinforcers are too weak to maintain consistent performance, the prompts are not strong enough for the participant, or the steps in the task analysis are too large. When a pattern of errors exists, discovering the source of the errors and incorporating necessary changes in teaching procedures can reduce the error rate significantly.

SUMMARY

Proper use of activity and task analysis, shaping, prompting, and error correction procedures will have a significant effect on the instructor's success at teaching new skills to others. Although simply reading this chapter will not give instructors the necessary skills, using this material could serve as a practice guide to enhance proficiency.

There are many introductory books that contain useful information about the application of behavior principles. Two series of introductory workbooks are: the 1) *How to teach series,* which consists of 16 booklets, each covering a different behavioral technique, and 2) the *Managing behavior series,* which includes three workbooks on different areas of behavior analysis.

Chapter 6

Evaluating Community Recreation Programs

Individuals with disabilities can be physically and socially integrated into recreation activities and environments. Physical integration, that is, placing individuals with disabilities alongside nondisabled persons, has been shown to have positive effects on the participants (Matthews, 1977). The physical integration of community recreation programs has been typically evaluated by simply counting the number of persons with disabilities participating in the setting. This method of evaluation provides *quantitative* information.

PROGRAM EVALUATION: QUANTITATIVE AND QUALITATIVE ANALYSIS

Quantitative information may allow a program evaluator to determine whether there are increasing or decreasing numbers of disabled and nondisabled persons participating in the program. Furthermore, such information may reveal frequency of participation. However, this method of evaluation may not provide any information on the *quality* of the participants' recreation experiences.

Qualitative information could be gained by evaluating the social aspects of the integrated community recreation program. The successful (or unsuccessful) social integration of participants may be determined by observing certain behaviors between participants with and without disabilities. These behaviors may include initiating social interactions, eye contact between peers, physical proximity, appropriate physical contact, sharing or offering equipment or materials, appropriately participating in a cooperative activity, friendship development, and changing attitudes toward other participants, to name a few. These participant behavioral outcomes or dependent variables must be evaluated in order to better understand the impact and effectiveness of the recreation program on its participants.

Why must the recreation professional evaluate the qualitative aspects of the program? The most salient benefits may be that it could:

1. Provide valuable information to the instructor for objective program decisions and revisions
2. Enhance accountability to administrators
3. Help the recreation center staff gain support for the program from administrators, professional colleagues, parents, and consumers
4. Enable one to better understand how the program is improving the participants' quality of life
5. Provide information that could be used to promote funding for future programs
6. Assist in the recruitment of volunteers
7. Increase community awareness of the recreation program by providing concise information concerning the impact it is having on participants
8. Assist in the determination of whether program goals and participant learning objectives are being met

Several questions are typically raised when an agency attempts to socially integrate participants with and without disabilities into a recreation program. These questions include:

1. Are the participants acquiring the recreation and leisure skills that are targeted for instruction?
2. Are the participants interacting appropriately or inappropriately with their peers?
3. Can individuals or groups of clients be identified so that they could be used to increase participation and socialization within the group?
4. Are nondisabled participants interacting, sharing conversation, and making friends with their peers who are disabled, and vice-versa?
5. Are attitudes of the nondisabled participants changing toward their disabled peers?
6. Are participants' levels of self-concept increasing due to their participation in the program?

Qualitative program evaluation and the strategies and tools to be used for this purpose are presented in this chapter and may assist the community recreation professional in answering many of these questions.

The process of recreation program evaluation (see Figure 6.1) must be a systematic procedure that is formative or ongoing in nature. This process may include the following 11 components. The process commences by:

1. Determining the need for the recreation program
2. Determining program goals and instructional procedures
3. Selecting evaluation tool(s) that will determine whether the program goals are being met
4. Implementing the recreation program
5. Gathering data on the performance of participants
6. Analyzing the data
7. Incorporating necessary revisions into the program
8. Concluding the program
9. Summarizing the data following the conclusion of the program
10. Making program revisions and recommendations and disseminating these to administrators, participants, and other interested persons
11. As the program evaluation process commences once again, a new program may be implemented with revised goals and instructional procedures.

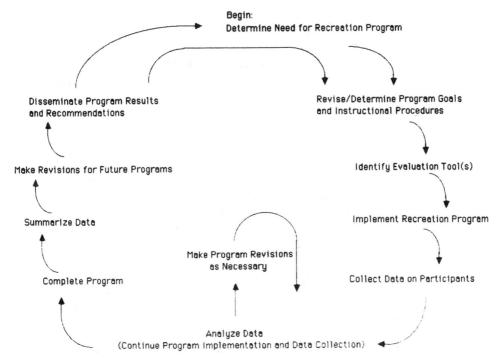

FIGURE 6.1. Process of recreation program evaluation.

The process of program evaluation is a dynamic one. The program evaluator must continue to seek ways to improve the program to benefit the participants. To provide optimal recreation services, evaluation must be viewed as a helpful process that allows the professional to gain important insights, feedback, and information concerning the impact of the program. It is only through systematic and ongoing evaluation that the community recreation program will continue to be beneficial to all of its participants.

As one may have realized by now, evaluation is crucial to planning and implementing community recreation programs for individuals with disabilities. Two major forms of evaluation influence the success of an individual's program. The first is baseline assessment, an initial observation of the participant's ability level before actual implementation of a program. A second form of evaluation is ongoing or formative evaluation of the progress that the participant is making throughout the program.

Both forms of evaluation are essential to an integrated recreation program because: 1) without baseline assessment, it will be impossible to determine the individual's skill level on the activities or skills that are to be taught, and 2) without ongoing evaluation, it may be difficult to verify the progress made by the participants.

Recent special education legislation (PL 94-142 and its amendments) have also created a heightened awareness of the importance of program evaluation by mandating that evaluation data must be provided in the student's individualized education program (IEP) or adult participant's individualized habilitation or treatment plan (IHP, ITP), and periodically updated.

The purpose of this chapter is to discuss relevant program evaluation in the context of designing and implementing an integrated community recreation program. The relationship of program evaluation to an IEP or IHP, frequency, reliability, and validity of evaluation, and an overview of six evaluation tools are discussed.

Relationship of the IEP or IHP to Evaluation of Participants with Disabilities

Each client's individualized education/habilitation plan calls for an annual evaluation of short-term instructional objectives. The individual's program also must be completely re-evaluated once every 3 years by the interdisciplinary team of which a therapeutic recreation specialist is often a member. These are minimal standards for evaluation and they are, in the authors' opinion, far too limited.

For a client's IEP or IHP to be properly developed, it is necessary that the therapeutic recreation specialist and teacher or careprovider make evaluation a continuous, ongoing process as opposed to following time periods that have been set arbitrarily. For instance, the recreation professional must regularly communicate the participant's current level of performance to others. Evaluation of skill mastery will confirm the individual's strengths and weaknesses in different activity areas (e.g., sports, games) throughout the year.

There are other reasons why ongoing evaluation is a critical aspect of the IEP or IHP. Following the initial assessment of the client's present performance levels, frequent follow-up assessments provide for tracking overall progress in each activity area. Daily or weekly evaluation of recreation objectives can indicate the effectiveness of training programs.

The dynamic process of regular evaluation of instructional procedures, as well as short-term learning objectives, will make the IEP or IHP a more vital blueprint of the disabled individual's educational progress and not simply a piece of paper to be shuffled into one corner of the desk. The progress of each participant should be followed systematically throughout the year and reported periodically to careproviders.

Considerations in Evaluating Progress

Frequency of Evaluation   A decision that must be made, usually by the teacher or recreation professional, is to determine exactly how often short-term instructional objectives will be evaluated. Objectives may be evaluated at the end of each day, or they may be evaluated weekly, bi-weekly, or once a month. As a general rule, the individual's progress on a specific skill should be monitored often enough for the instructor to:

1. Receive feedback on the progress of the participant. The more frequently the participant's skill level is evaluated, the easier it is to assess problem areas.
2. Make necessary modifications in methods or materials and ascertain whether the instructional sequence is effective or not.
3. Verify that the participant has attained the learning objective. Once the participant has acquired the skill, the next skill in the instructional sequence can be taught with the newly acquired skill being reviewed periodically.

It is advisable, however, to evaluate measures continuously; for example, one should evaluate the progress of persons who do not display clear-cut gains in their programs at each session. Keeping a chart or plotting a graph of the participant's performance will reveal the rate of the individual's mastery of the skill. If the program is working, there will be an ascending rate of progress. For those who work with persons with severe disabilities, charting and continuous evaluation are critical for determining if any progress in skill acquisition is occurring.

Reliability of Evaluation.   The reliability, or accuracy of data, is dependent upon a number of factors, including the method by which data is collected. The process of monitoring the participant's progress can be influenced by a number of factors. If the participant or specialist is ill, for example, or if the same person does not always do the evaluating, or if there is confusion or inconsistency about the method of evaluation, the data collected will be suspect.

One means of increasing the reliability of observations is to have a second trained person collect data independent of the primary observer. For example, in order to achieve a reliability of agreement that the target behavior is actually occurring at a given rate, two or more independent observers must simultaneously view the response. In this way, an index of the consistency of agreement may be established. Reliable recording of behavior is the foundation of a good evaluation. Inconsistent agreement between observers casts serious doubt on the credibility of evaluation data.

Validity of Assessment   The validity of the evaluation technique addresses the question, "Does the instrument that is used to assess the participant's progress measure what it purports to?" In order for data to be valid, participants must be evaluated with instruments that provide a true picture of the individual's performance level.

One way to ensure validity of evaluation measures is to employ different types of techniques. For example, if a community recreation planner is interested in improving a participant's basketball shooting accuracy, then an observational assessment of percentage of successful field goals obtained by the participant might be computed and recorded daily. This would be an example of criterion-referenced evaluation.

As an initial evaluation, however, the participant's basketball shooting accuracy could be compared to the scores of other individuals of the same chronological age. This procedure is norm-referenced, that is, performance levels are computed on the basis of how well a large number of other respondents have performed on the same task.

By utilizing two types of evaluation, student performance can be cross-checked. Although improvement on one measure, observational assessment, might not be mirrored by similar advances in the norm-referenced standardized tests, the use of these measures allows for two independent methods for tracking an individual's progress. However, only criterion-referenced evaluation tools are described in this chapter. For a more comprehensive review of criterion-referenced and norm-referenced evaluations in therapeutic recreation, refer to Wehman and Schleien (1980).

Evaluation Tool #1-SKILL ACQUISITION
EVALUATION TOOL: TASK-ANALYTIC ASSESSMENT

Although there are a number of areas that can be assessed in a recreation environment, an initial question that must be answered to determine the first area of study is whether the individual knows how to interact appropriately with the recreation materials. Also, can the individual use the facility independently? Stated another way, when placed in a leisure skill environment and supplied with recreation materials, can the participant use them appropriately? If not, then systematic instruction is required.

What is required for evaluating leisure skill proficiency is task-analytic assessment (Knapczyk, 1975; Nietupski et al., 1984). An instructional objective must be written for a given material or environment. The objective should reflect the specific skill that the instructor wants the participant to learn.

There are multiple advantages to this type of observational assessment. First, the information collected about the participant performing a particular leisure skill or playing in a specific recreation environment helps the instructor to pinpoint the exact point where instruction should begin. Therefore, the participant does not receive instruction on skills in which he or she is already proficient. Another advantage is that step-by-step individualized instruction is facilitated. Evaluation of the participant's proficiency with different materials or in different environments over an extended period of time will also be more objective and precise, and will be less subject to instructor bias.

The *Skill Acquisition Evaluation Form* (Figure 6.2) could be used to determine which parts of a larger leisure skill or recreational activity has been acquired by the participant. A task-analytic assessment will provide instructors with information on where to begin teaching the skill in each session, and at what rate the participant is acquiring the skill. To conduct the assessment, the evaluator must familiarize him or herself with the completed Skill Acquisition Evaluation form that follows. (Blank copies of this form and all other evaluation tools that are discussed in this chapter appear in Appendix H.)

The process begins when the instructor identifies and lists on the evaluation form each step that is required to independently complete the selected skill. The steps should be listed sequentially. In each session, following the completion of instruction on the selected skill, a verbal cue can be provided to the participant that instructs him or her to begin the activity. Without offering any reinforcement to the participant, such as giving positive feedback to the participant for his or her performance, the instructor observes the participant attempting to complete the task or skill. During observation and recording, the instructor records a plus (+) by each step of the task analysis the participant completed independently, and a minus (−) by those steps not performed independently. The recorded plus signs reveal which steps of the skill the participant has mastered. The beginning of consecutive minuses determines where instruction should begin during the following session. By totalling the number of pluses, the instructor can identify the participant's progress in learning the skill and the rate of skill acquisition.

Skill acquisition evaluation enables the instructor to provide individualized instruction on a specific step of the skill that has not been mastered by the participant. It also gives the instructor immediate feedback about the progress each participant is making on the targeted skill in the program.

The benefits of utilizing a Skill Acquisition Evaluation Tool could include:

1. A participant's current level of mastery of a specific leisure skill is determined.
2. The specific step of a task analysis at which to begin instruction of the selected leisure skill is identified.
3. The rate of increase (or decrease) of the participant's level of mastery of the selected leisure skill is documented.

DIRECTIONS FOR SKILL ACQUISITION EVALUATION FORM

Before the Program Begins:

1. Write the participant's name on line "A".
2. Determine a skill relevant to the program that the participant needs to acquire. Write the skill on line "J".
3. Write the goal statement on line "B".
4. Determine a phrase (verbal cue) that you will consistently use to instruct the participant to begin the task. Write this verbal cue on line "C".
5. Write the name of the program, the days it meets, and the time the sessions are held on line "D".
6. Observe an individual who has already mastered the skill and perform this skill by yourself so that you may write each step necessary to independently complete the skill

FIGURE 6.2

SKILL ACQUISITION EVALUATION

Date: 4-22-87

A. Name: Sue Winters

D. Program: Exercise Class

B. Goal Statement: To independently participate in an exercise class. M + W: 5-6 p.m.

C. Verbal Cue: "Sue, we're here for your exercise class."

F.

	Task Analysis Steps	a	b	1	2	3	4	5	6	7	8	9	10	11	12	13	14	15	16	17	18	19	20	21
25																								
24																								
23																								
22																								
21	Exit the recreation center	-	-	+	+	+	+	+	+	+	+	+	+	+	+	+	+	+						
20	Put coat on	-	-	+	+	+	+	+	+	+	+	+	+	+	+	+	+	+						
19	Collect personal belongings	-	-	-	-	-	-	+	+	-	+	+	+	+	+	+	+	(+)						
18	Optional: use drinking fountain/restroom	-	-	-	+	+	+	+	+	+	+	+	+	+	+	+	+	+						
17	optional: talk to other participants	-	-	-	+	+	+	+	+	+	+	+	+	+	(+)	+	(+)	+						
16	At the end of class, help put mats away.	-	-	-	-	-	-	-	-	-	-	+	(+)	(+)	+	-	+	+						
15	Do cool-down exercises.	-	-	-	-	-	-	-	-	-	-	+	+	+	+	(-)	-	-						
14	Check heart rate (3 x).	-	-	-	-	-	-	-	-	-	-	(-)	-	-	-	-	-	-						
13	Do aerobic exercises	-	-	-	-	-	-	-	(-)	-	-	-	-	-	-	-	-	+						
12	When instructor offers break, use drinking fountain	-	-	-	-	-	-	-	-	-	(-)	-	-	-	-	-	-	+						
11	Do strength training exercises.	-	-	-	-	-	-	(-)	-	-	-	-	-	-	-	-	+	+						
10	Do warm-up exercises.	-	-	-	-	-	-	-	-	(-)	-	-	-	+	+	+	+	+						
9	When class starts, listen to and follow instructor	-	-	-	-	-	-	-	-	+	+	+	+	-	+	+	+	+						
8	Optional: approp. speak w/others + stretch out.	-	-	-	-	(-)	(-)	-	+	-	-	-	+	+	+	+	+	+						
7	Wait for class to begin.	-	-	-	(-)	-	-	-	+	-	-	-	+	+	+	+	+	+						
6	Find a space on the mats + go in that direction	-	-	+	+	+	+	+	+	+	+	+	+	+	+	+	+	+						
5	Take off coat, hang it on coat rack	-	-	(-)	-	-	-	+	+	+	+	+	+	+	+	+	+	+						
4	Locate coat rack along wall + walk in that direction	-	-	-	-	-	-	+	-	+	+	+	+	+	+	+	+	+						
3	Locate + proceed to the multipurpose room.	-	-	+	+	+	+	+	+	+	+	+	+	+	+	+	+	+						
2	Acknowledge rec. staff + others, if approp.	-	-	-	-	+	+	+	+	+	+	+	+	+	+	+	+	+						
E. 1	Enter the recreation center.	-	-	+	+	+	+	+	+	+	+	+	+	+	+	+	+	+						

Sessions

	a	b	1	2	3	4	5	6	7	8	9	10	11	12	13	14	15	16	17	18	19	20	21
G. Total # of +'s	0	0	5	7	8	8	11	12	11	12	14	16	16	17	15	17	19						
H. Your initials	ab	ab	ab	ab	ab	ab	ab	ab	ab	ab	ab	ab	ab	ab	ab	ab	ab						
I. Date	3/16	3/18	3/20	3/23	3/25	3/27	3/30	4/1	4/3	4/6	4/8	4/10	4/13	4/15	4/17	4/20	4/22						

J. Partic. in comm. rec. program

Skill

in the "Task Analysis Steps" column. Write step #1 on line "E.1", step #2 above it on line 2, and so forth.

Note: Your targeted skill may require more or less than the 25 rows provided; modify the form as necessary.

To Evaluate the Initial Sessions:

1. Before you begin instruction on the targeted skill, give the participant the general verbal cue; record each step of the task analysis that the participant performs independently with a plus (+) and those not performed independently with a minus (−). Record your observation under "F" in column "a". Repeat the procedure during each session and record your observation under "F" in column "b", etc.
2. A plus (+) or minus (−) should appear after each step listed in the task analysis in column "F", in both the "a" and "b" columns, by the end of the first two evaluation periods.
3. The information gathered during the first two sessions is referred to as the "baseline assessment." This baseline assessment identifies the participant's current level of mastery of the task before instruction begins. At least two assessment probes on different days should be conducted to establish a true baseline rate. When the baseline rate appears stable (i.e., forms a horizontal line) instruction on the targeted skill should commence. A stable baseline followed by an increase of steps mastered in the task analysis documents the effectiveness of the recreation program.
4. To complete the remainder of the form, refer to the directions on "Evaluating All Other Sessions During Instruction."
5. Refer to the example that follows for guidelines on how to complete this evaluation form.

Evaluating All Other Sessions During Instruction:

1. Following the completion of instruction on the targeted leisure skill for a particular session, give the participant another general verbal cue (on line "C") to signal him or her to perform the activity without any assistance.
2. In the column that coincides with the number of that session (session #2: record in column #2), record a plus (+) next to each step that the participant performs independently and a minus (−) next to those steps that are not performed independently during the nonreinforced data probe. A plus or minus should appear in each step of the task analysis at the end of the evaluation.
3. On line "G" write the total number of pluses (+) recorded in that session.
4. On line "H" write your initials.
5. One line "I" write the date that you made your observation.
6. Place a red line across the top of the box or circle the box (in the column that was just recorded) that coincides with the number in the "total # of + 's" box. For example, if the total is 8 correct steps in session #3, place a red line on line #8 in column #3 or circle the box on line #8.
7. These lines will create a graph that will illustrate the participant's level of mastery of the task throughout the program.
8. Locate 2 consecutive minuses in the column in which you just recorded the data. The first, or lower of the 2 recorded minuses is the step of the task analyses at which to begin instruction during the next session.

Evaluation Tool #2—
SOCIAL INTERACTION EVALUATION TOOL

For many individuals with developmental disabilities, an important instructional goal is to initiate and sustain interactions with peers more frequently. A relatively common occurrence may be the presence of several disabled children playing separately from each other during free play (Fredericks, Baldwin, Grove, Moore, Riggs, & Lyons, 1978; Schleien, Rynders, Mustonen, Fox, & Kelterborn, 1986). During these play situations, the potential benefits of social interaction are not accrued.

One way of assessing social interaction is to obtain a simple count of the number of times a child initiates an interaction, receives an interaction, sustains an interaction, or terminates an interaction. Duration assessment may be used to measure the length of the interaction between peers and also between the child and adults in the room. A second means of gathering more information is the coding of specific types of interactions. Carney and her colleagues (1977) have suggested 20 social interaction skills under the 4 interaction categories. In addition to providing sequence, these skills may be task analyzed to determine the individual's proficiency on selected behaviors. These 4 categories of interaction can be employed to code the qualitative nature of the interaction (Hamre-Nietupski & Williams, 1977).

Analyzing the direction of interactions can be helpful in assessing which individuals in the environment are reinforcing to the participant. As Beveridge, Spencer, and Miller (1978) observed, child-teacher interactions occur more frequently than child-child interactions, especially among children with severe disabilities. Structured intervention by an adult is the action usually required to increase child-child interactions (Shores, Hester, & Strain, 1976).

The direction of interactions should be assessed during home visits while observing the child playing with siblings or with neighborhood children. Data on interactions with disabled persons and with nondisabled peers should be recorded. This type of behavioral analysis can be revealing since most children without disabilities do not include disabled children in play unless prompted and reinforced by adults (e.g., Apolloni & Cooke, 1978).

To identify the individuals with whom the participants are interacting during a program, and to determine if participants are increasing or decreasing their interactions toward an individual or a selected group of persons, the *Social Interaction Evaluation Tool* can be used. This evaluation procedure incorporates a data collection method referred to as a "time sampling." The time sampling procedure requires the instructor to momentarily observe (i.e., for 2–3 seconds) a participant at predetermined times, with a minimum of 3 observation times per hour, during the program. These observation times should be evenly distributed within the program time and should vary from session to session. For example, if the program is held from 3 p.m. to 4 p.m. on Mondays and Wednesdays, the instructor may record observations on Monday at 3:05 p.m., 3:35 p.m., and 3:55 p.m. On Wednesday, the observation times may be 3:15 p.m., 3:30 p.m., and 3:45 p.m. At these predetermined times, the instructor should observe the participant for an instant and then record with whom the participant was interacting, and if that interaction was appropriate or inappropriate. Appropriate and inappropriate social interactions, and any other dependent variables that might describe the target behaviors one will be observing must be *operationally defined* in order for the evaluator to have a standard, predetermined criteria in which to make accurate observational judgments. Examples of possible definitions for appropriate and inappropriate social interactions are offered in this chapter. It is important to understand that the more times a participant is observed during instruction, the greater the amount of information that will be obtained from which to evaluate the effectiveness of the program.

Two variations of the Social Interaction Evaluation Tool (Figures 6.3 and 6.4) are included as examples. The first tool could be used to collect information on one participant; the second is used for two or more participants. The directions for using both instruments are identical. This evaluation procedure can be used to gain information on many different social aspects of the community recreation program. For example, if one wishes to evaluate changes in the participants' "sportsmanship" during an integrated softball program, the target behavior, sportsmanship, must be operationally defined (e.g., assisting another participant during the game, not screaming at opponents, taking turns coming to bat). One should then conduct a baseline assessment (refer to the Skill Acquisition Evaluation Tool for this procedure), implement the softball program, observe the participants, record their behaviors, and summarize the results.

Before proceeding, it may be helpful for the reader to become familiar with the completed Social Interaction Evaluation sample forms that follow.

The benefits of implementing the Social Interaction Evaluation Tool could include: 1) identifying the individuals with whom participants are primarily interacting (e.g., staff, nondisabled participant, disabled participant, or no interactions occurring), or 2) documenting changes in the level of interaction between participants.

OPERATIONAL DEFINITIONS

Appropriate Social Interaction (Initiated or Received):

1. *Initiates Positive Interaction:* Participant actively seeks positive contact with peer by touching peer, gesturing to, or vocalizing/verbalizing to peer. Contact must be directed toward a specific peer. Interaction may take the form of facial expression (smiles), vocal tone (pleasant), verbal content (praise, giving directions, or encouragement), nonverbal vocalizations (laughs, giggles), appropriate touch (guidance or assistance, hugs, pats), or gestures or verbal behavior that seeks to recruit peer's attention. *Note: An initiation is any behavior that begins an interaction between two peers.*

2. *Receives Positive Interaction:* Participant is touched, gestured to, commented to, given directions, or questioned by peer in a nonderogatory, nonthreatening manner. Contact must be directed by peer toward participant with a disability. Interaction may take the form of facial expression (smiles), vocal tone (pleasant), verbal content (praise, being given directions, or encouragement), nonverbal vocalizations (laughs, giggles), and/or appropriate touch (guidance or assistance, hugs, pats).

Inappropriate Social Interaction (Initiated or Received):

1. *Initiates Negative Interaction:* Participant touches, gestures to, gives directions, or questions peer in a hostile, derisive, or threatening manner. Interaction may take the form of facial expression (frowns, grimaces), vocal tone (sharp, loud, whiney), verbal content ("No!", punitive, threatening or disapproving remarks, swearing, derogatory, or derisive comments), nonverbal vocalizations (crying, moaning, groaning, or growling), and/or aggressive physical contact (hitting, slapping, flailing at, pushing, pulling, scratching, biting). *Note: An initiation is any behavior that begins an interaction between two peers.*

2. *Receives Negative Interaction:* Participant is touched, gestured to, commented to, given directions, or questioned by peer in a derisive, threatening, or hostile manner. Interactions may take the form of facial expression (frowns, pouts), vocal tone (loud, whiney, sharp, angry), verbal content ("No!", punitive, threatening or disapproving

SOCIAL INTERACTION EVALUATION FOR ONE PARTICIPANT

FIGURE 6.3

A. Program Title: _Talking Art_ C. Name: _Sue Winters_

B. Program Goal: _Increasing social interaction between part._ Evaluator: _E. Fullen_

D. Date: _6-9-87_

E. Level of Interaction

Time (preset)	None	Staff	Dis. Part.	Nondis. Part.	Other	F. Activity	G. Comments
3:05	A					Taking coat off	
3:10				A		Sitting at table	
3:15				I		Throwing clay	Sue was being ignored by staff and peers
3:25		A				Asking for help	
3:40	A					Working on project	
3:45				I		Pushing mess to neighbor's space	Possibly seeking attention from peer in close proximity
3:55				A		Putting coat on	

H. Totals

	None	Staff	Dis. Part.	Nondis. Part.	Other
A	2	1	0	2	0
I	0	0	0	2	0

Key

A = Appropriate Social Interaction
I = Inappropriate Social Interaction

101

SOCIAL INTERACTION EVALUATION FOR TWO OR MORE PARTICIPANTS   FIGURE 6.4

A. Program Title: _Talking Art_

B. Program Goal: _To increase social interactions_   D. Date: _6-11-87_

E. Times to Observe: 1. _3:10 p.m._   2. _3:30 p.m._   3. _3:45 p.m._

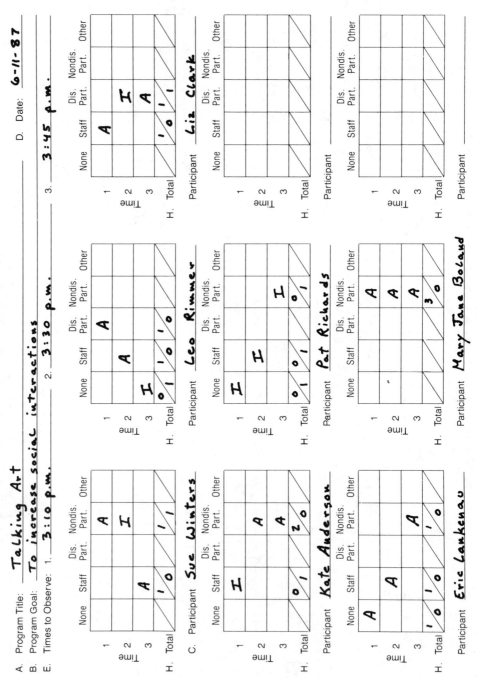

remarks, swearing, or derogatory comments), and/or nonverbal vocalizations (crying, moaning, groaning, growling).

KEY FOR THE SOCIAL INTERACTION EVALUATION TOOL

None = The person with a disability is not interacting with anyone.

Staff = The person with a disability is interacting with a staff person.

Dis. Part. = The person with a disability is interacting with another participant with a disability.

Nondis. Part. = The person with a disability is interacting with a nondisabled participant.

Other = The person with a disability is not present for the observation (e.g., he or she is in the restroom, has gone home early).

DIRECTIONS FOR SOCIAL INTERACTION EVALUATION TOOL (BOTH FORMS)

Before the Program Begins:

1. Write the name of the program on line "A".
2. Write the goal(s) of the program on line "B".
3. Write the participant's name on line(s) "C".
4. Write the date you will conduct the evaluation on line "D".
5. Determine the times you will observe each participant in the session. Write these times in the column labelled "E".
6. Position a clock or wristwatch so that you can accurately observe the participant at the designated times.

Evaluating

1. At predetermined times, observe the participant for a brief moment (approximately 2–3 seconds) and record in the correct column (i.e., **None, Staff, Dis. Part.**) an "A" for appropriate social interaction or an "I" for inappropriate social interaction.
2. If you are observing more than one participant concurrently, list the participants in a predetermined order. At the appropriate observe/record time (e.g., 3:10 p.m.) observe for a brief moment the first participant on the list (e.g., Sue Winters), record her behavior, and then observe the next participant (e.g., Leo Rimmer) on the list. Continue this observe/record procedure until all the participants on the list have been observed. At the next designated observation time repeat this procedure.
3. Write a brief (1–3 word) description of the activity in which the participant was engaged during your observation in column "F". (This description is omitted from the form "for two or more participants" due to space limitations. If possible, write your comment on a separate sheet of paper).
4. Write any comments in column "G" that you believe would clarify the information you recorded. These would be the comments omitted from the form designated for two or more participants' due to space limitations.
5. After the session has ended, determine the total number of appropriate social interactions in each category, and place that number on the left side of the slash in the box (see H) directly beneath that column. On the right side of the slash, place the number of inappropriate social interactions recorded in that column.
6. Finally, transcribe the data from the Social Interaction Evaluation Tool onto the Social Interaction Evaluation Summary Form (see Figure 6.5).

Writing the Social Interaction Evaluation Summary:

1. Write the name of the program on line "A".
2. Write the program instructor's name on line "B".
3. Write the names of other staff persons that assisted in the program on line "C".
4. Write the beginning and ending dates and year of the program on line "D". Include at the end of line "D" the date this Summary Sheet was completed.
5. Write the participant's name on line(s) "E" (bottom of form).
6. In each of the columns (**None, Staff, Dis. Part., Nondis. Part., Other**) add the "A's" (appropriate social interactions) recorded in all the sessions during the first half of the program. Write the totals in the appropriate boxes on line "F". Repeat this procedure with the "I's" (inappropriate social interactions).
7. Color each half of each column up to the number that corresponds to the number in the "total" box.
8. The completed graph illustrates the frequency of interactions by each participant and identifies the persons with whom they were interacting.
9. Repeat steps 6 and 7 after the final session to summarize the interactions of the second half of the program. Write the totals in the appropriate boxes on line "G". A comparison of the graphs from the first to the second half of the program will display an increase, decrease, or stable rate of appropriate and inappropriate social interactions between participants.

Evaluation Tool #3–
SOCIOMETRY EVALUATION TOOL

Several researchers during the last decade have documented gains in social development in persons with disabilities through interaction with peers and adults during leisure education (Schleien, 1984; Schleien & Wehman, 1986; Verhoven & Goldstein, 1976; Wehman & Schleien, 1981). Others have cited a lack of cooperative play skills and of social interaction among peers as the cause for an inordinate amount of isolated play (Pauloutzian, Hasazi, Streifel, & Edgar, 1971). Independent, or isolated, play is a lower stage of social development than cooperative play (Parten & Newhall, 1943; Schleien et al., 1986). In fact, children fail to develop higher level social behaviors, such as cooperative play, when they have little peer interaction during play (Wehman, 1979). Effective feedback cannot be obtained until there are social interactions between children. For these reasons, community recreation professionals need to become familiar with ways to promote the social experiences between participants with and without disabilities. Sociometry is a technique that could help achieve this goal (Ellis, Forsyth, & Voight, 1983; Gronlund, 1959).

The term "sociometry" derives from the Latin term for social or companion measurement. Despite sociometry's widespread acceptance and use in schools, industry, and in recreation camps, schools continue to be the most prevalent setting in which this technique is applied. It has been used by teachers to analyze the social structures of people in group situations and the extent to which individuals are accepted by their peers.

Sociometry is a simple and convenient technique for measuring aspects of a social structure and for generating information about social relations within a group. The ease with which it can be developed and administered makes it a practical and convenient tool for use by community recreation professionals. Furthermore, sociometry can be used to evaluate the attitudes of participants within a group toward each other with respect to a common criterion. The sociometric structure addresses the network of interpersonal relationships between participants. This network is presented in the form of a *sociogram*.

SOCIAL INTERACTION EVALUATION SUMMARY SHEET

FIGURE 6.5

A. Program Title: _Talking Art_

B. Program Instructor: _E. Fullen_

C. Other Staff: _A. Bartlett, R. Thomas_

D. Duration of Program: _6 weeks (6-9-87 to 7-18-87)_   Date: _7-20-87_

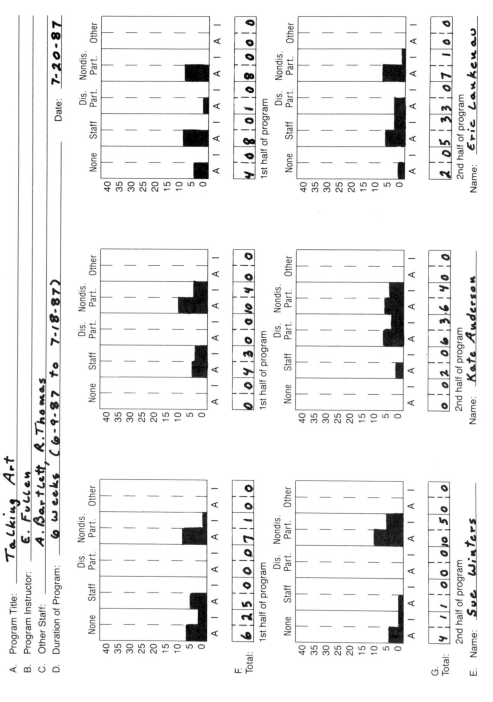

F. Total: | 6 | 25 | 00 | 07 | 1 | 0 | 0 |

1st half of program

G. Total: | 4 | 11 | 00 | 0 | 0 | 5 | 0 | 0 |

2nd half of program
E. Name: _Sue Winters_

F. Total: | 0 | 04 | 30 | 00 | 40 | 0 |

1st half of program

G. Total: | 0 | 02 | 06 | 3.6 | 40 | 0 |

2nd half of program
Name: _Kate Anderson_

F. Total: | 4 | 08 | 01 | 08 | 00 | 0 |

1st half of program

G. Total: | 2 | 05 | 33 | 07 | 1 | 0 | 0 |

2nd half of program
Name: _Eric Lankenau_

Key: A = Appropriate Social Interaction; I = Inappropriate Social Interaction

105

SOCIOMETRY EVALUATION INFORMATION FORM

FIGURE 6.6

A. Program Title: _Exploring Nature_

B. Program Goal: _to learn about nature and people's effect on it_

C. Date of Evaluation: _8-16-87_

D.

Participant	Symbol	G. 1	2	3	4	5	6	7	8	9	10	11	12	13	14	15	16	17	18	19	20
1 _Sue Winters_	△1							x													
2 _Kate Anderson_	◯2				x	x	x														
3 _Eric Laukenau_	◯3					x	x														
4 _Leo Rimmer_	◯4		x			x															
5 _Pat Richards_	◯5		x	x																	
6 _Mary Jane Boland_	◯6			x																	
7 _Liz Clark_	◯7	x		x																	
8																					
9																					
10																					
11																					
12																					
13																					
14																					
15																					
16																					
17																					
18																					
19																					
20																					

TOTAL: | 1 | 2 | 2 | 2 | 2 | 2 | 1 |

E. Question(s) Asked: _Who would you like to go on the hike with?_

Symbol: ◯ = Nondisabled participant; △ = Person with a disability.

F. Evaluator: _E. Fullen_

First, a sociometric question is formulated that will be asked of each participant. For example, each participant is asked "Who would you like to go on the hike with?" Their responses are then documented on the Sociometry Evaluation Information Form. Interpreting and diagramming this information in the form of a sociogram could be completed at other times following the program. The sociometric technique can be implemented on three separate occasions:

1. During the first day of the program to establish the current levels of interaction between participants
2. At the midway point of the program to reveal any changes in levels of interaction, and to identify areas where changes could still be made
3. During the final day of the program to document the total number of changes that have occurred throughout the program

Before proceeding with the directions, the authors suggest that the reader become familiar with the completed Sociometry Evaluation Information sample form that follows.

The benefits of implementing a Sociometry Evaluation Information Tool may include:

1. The internal structure of the group or patterns of interpersonal relationships between participants are determined.
2. Changes in the patterns of social interactions between participants are documented.
3. Any friendships that are being established between participants, especially between individuals with and without disabilities are identified.
4. The emotional climate of the group is determined.
5. The community recreator's personal judgment of the group is supplemented with additional information.

DIRECTIONS FOR SOCIOMETRIC EVALUATION TOOL

Before the Program Begins:

1. Write the name of the program on line "A".
2. Write the program's goal statement(s) on line "B".
3. Write the date of the evaluation on line "C".
4. Write each participant's name in the "participant" column beginning on line "D".
5. Use the number that is to the left of the participant's name for his or her identification number.
6. If the participant has a disability, place a triangle (Δ) in the "symbol" column after their name. If the participant is nondisabled, place a circle ($\bigcirc$) there.
7. Place the participant's identification number inside his or her symbol (e.g., Δ, $\bigcirc$).
8. Generate the sociometric question that will be asked and write it in on line "E". The question must require the participant to name others in the group with whom they would like to play. For example, "If you were the captain of a volleyball team, whom would you choose to play on your team?", or "If I gave you 5 dollars, whom would you like to take to the ice cream shop?" are sociometric questions. The sociometric question(s) must be appropriate for the chronological age of the participants and should reflect realistic situations or concerns for the respondents.
9. More than one question can be asked to check whether the participants respond in a similar manner. This would be a reliability check, and would be an optional procedure. If more than one sociometric question is asked, the response to the second

question should be recorded using a different symbol from that of the first (e.g., use Xs or Os).
10. Write the evaluator's name on line "F".

During the Program: Evaluating

1. During the first, midpoint, and final sessions of the recreation program, ask each participant the sociometric question(s) that is (are) recorded on line "E".
2. Record each participant's response on the Sociometry Evaluation Information Form. For example, if Sue (#1) said she would select Liz (#7), place a mark on line 1 under #7.
3. Repeat this procedure until responses are received and recorded for each participant.

After the Program: Summarizing

1. Tally the number of marks in each column, beginning in column "G", and place the total number of marks in the "Total" box at the bottom of each column.
2. The number at the top of each column coincides with the participant's identification number, and therefore the information in that column pertains to him or her. For example, Column 4 has a total of 2 recorded marks; therefore, 2 participants selected Leo as a companion to take on the hike.

Graphing the Information on a Sociogram:

1. On the Sociogram Evaluation Graphing Form that follows, seven rings can be found; these are numbered 0 to 6. Each ring represents the total number of times a participant was selected by another respondent.
2. Place the participant's symbol, as it appears in the "symbol" column (e.g., Δ), in the ring that matches the number in the "total" box at the bottom of that participant's column. For example, the number in Sue Winter's "total" box is 1. Place her symbol (Δ), with her identification number inside of it (1), in the ring where the Number 1 appears.
3. Place all participants' symbols and identification numbers in the appropriate rings on the Sociogram Evaluation Graphing Form.
4. Using the information recorded on the same line as the participant's name, draw an arrow from that participant's symbol to the individual he or she selected. For example, Sue (#1) selected Liz (#7) in response to the sociometric question. Draw an arrow from symbol #1 to symbol #7. Note: If Liz (#7) also selected Sue (#1), place an arrowhead on both ends of the line that has been drawn between the 2 participants' symbols to illustrate a mutual or reciprocal selection.
5. Graph all the participants' selections.

Interpreting the Sociogram

1. In interpreting these data, one might ask questions that are important to the success of the program such as: Are nondisabled participants interacting with their disabled peers? Are socially withdrawn participants becoming more involved in the recreation program? Who are the most popular participants, and are they being regarded as role models by the other participants?
   Other questions one could ask to interpret the data could include:
   a) Are there any social isolates, that is, individuals who were not selected?
   b) Is there a leader among the group; an individual that many participants did select?

SOCIOGRAM EVALUATION GRAPHING FORM

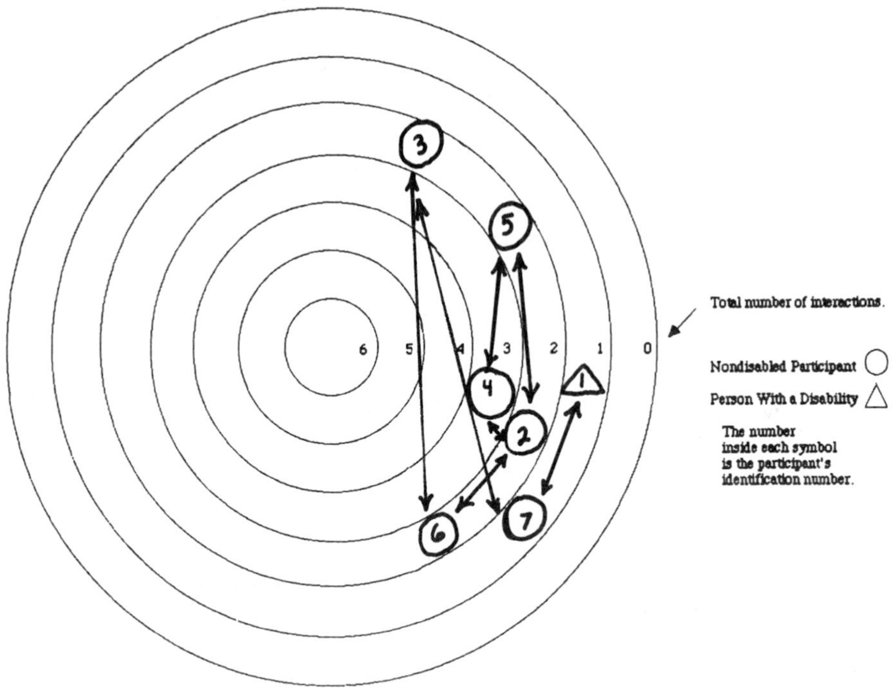

FIGURE 6.7.   Sociogram evaluation graphing form.

c)   Is there a difference in selection rates between nondisabled participants and persons with disabilities?

d)   Are there participants who selected each other in a reciprocal manner?

Evaluation Tool #4—
PEER ACCEPTANCE EVALUATION TOOL

Voeltz (1980; 1982) developed a method to evaluate changes in attitude or in levels of acceptance as demonstrated by persons without disabilities toward their peers with disabilities. The Acceptance Scale survey that is presented on the following pages is a modified version of Voeltz' survey. Within the context of community recreation programs, instructors can improve the level of peer acceptance among the participants with and without disabilities by role modeling, planning cooperative goal-structured activities, and by providing social skills training to the participants.

One method of evaluating peer acceptance is by using a pre- and posttest of acceptance level of others. Prior to the first program session, the Peer Acceptance Survey (see Figure 6.8) can be administered to each participant. The results can be scored (see Figure 6.9, Peer Acceptance Survey Answer Key) and documented outside of class time. During or immediately following the final class session, the same survey can be administered again to the participants; results are recorded on the summary sheet. Similarly, the Peer Acceptance Evaluation Summary Form (Figure 6.10) is easy to implement and provides objective information concerning the attitude changes of nondisabled participants throughout the recreation program.

PEER ACCEPTANCE SURVEY

FIGURE 6.8

Name: _Leo Rimmer_

1. I don't have any friends who are mentally retarded or handicapped.
   Agree ____ Disagree **X** Undecided ____
2. If my sister or brother were retarded, I wouldn't talk about it to anyone.
   Agree ____ Disagree **X** Undecided ____
3. I have talked to people who use wheelchairs.
   Agree ____ Disagree **X** Undecided ____
4. If I found out that someone I hang around with is mentally retarded, I would still be his/her friend.
   Agree ____ Disagree **X** Undecided ____
5. I have talked with some mentally retarded people at the park.
   Agree ____ Disagree ____ Undecided **X**
6. It snows in Minnesota in the winter.
   Agree **X** Disagree ____ Undecided ____
7. There is no reason for me to spend time with anyone who is handicapped.
   Agree **X** Disagree ____ Undecided ____
8. I think that a student who is deaf or blind could be in my recreation program.
   Agree ____ Disagree ____ Undecided **X**
9. I wouldn't want a handicapped person to be my partner in an activity.
   Agree ____ Disagree ____ Undecided **X**
10. I believe that I could become close friends with a person who is handicapped.
    Agree ____ Disagree ____ Undecided **X**
11. I have helped some people who are in wheelchairs.
    Agree ____ Disagree **X** Undecided ____
12. Minneapolis is a large city in Minnesota.
    Agree **X** Disagree ____ Undecided ____
13. Persons who are retarded should not come to the park for activities.
    Agree **X** Disagree ____ Undecided ____
14. I wish I could become friends with a mentally retarded person.
    Agree ____ Disagree **X** Undecided ____
15. I would not like to be around a person who looked or acted different.
    Agree **X** Disagree ____ Undecided ____
16. If someone told me about a new TV program about handicaps, I would probably watch it.
    Agree ____ Disagree ____ Undecided **X**
17. I have never talked with a person who is paralyzed or couldn't walk.
    Agree **X** Disagree ____ Undecided ____
18. I don't say "Hi" to people who are retarded.
    Agree **X** Disagree ____ Undecided ____
19. Minnesota has many lakes.
    Agree **X** Disagree ____ Undecided ____
20. I believe students with handicaps should participate with other people in the recreation department's programs.
    Agree ____ Disagree **X** Undecided ____

Finished! Thank you for completing the survey.

(This questionnaire was adapted from: Voeltz, L. [1980]. Children's attitudes toward handicapped persons. *American Journal of Mental Deficiency, 84,* 455–464.)

1. I don't have any friends who are mentally retarded or handicapped.
   Agree _0_　　Disagree _2_　　Undecided _1_

2. If my sister or brother were retarded, I wouldn't talk about it to anyone.
   Agree _0_　　Disagree _2_　　Undecided _1_

3. I have talked to people who use wheelchairs.
   Agree _2_　　Disagree _0_　　Undecided _1_

4. If I found out that someone I hang around with is mentally retarded, I would still be his/her friend.
   Agree _2_　　Disagree _0_　　Undecided _1_

5. I have talked with some mentally retarded people at the park.
   Agree _2_　　Disagree _0_　　Undecided _1_

6. It snows in Minnesota in the winter.
   Agree _2_　　Disagree _0_　　Undecided _0_

7. There is no reason for me to spend time with anyone who is handicapped.
   Agree _0_　　Disagree _2_　　Undecided _1_

8. I think that a student who is deaf or blind could be in my recreation program.
   Agree _2_　　Disagree _0_　　Undecided _1_

9. I wouldn't want a handicapped person to be my partner in an activity.
   Agree _0_　　Disagree _2_　　Undecided _1_

10. I believe that I could become close friends with a person who is handicapped.
    Agree _2_　　Disagree _0_　　Undecided _1_

11. I have helped some people who are in wheelchairs.
    Agree _2_　　Disagree _0_　　Undecided _1_

12. Minneapolis is a large city in Minnesota.
    Agree _2_　　Disagree _0_　　Undecided _0_

13. Persons who are retarded should not come to the park for activities.
    Agree _0_　　Disagree _2_　　Undecided _1_

14. I wish I could become friends with a mentally retarded person.
    Agree _2_　　Disagree _0_　　Undecided _1_

15. I would not like to be around a person who looked or acted different.
    Agree _0_　　Disagree _2_　　Undecided _1_

16. If someone told me about a new TV program about handicaps, I would probably watch it.
    Agree _2_　　Disagree _0_　　Undecided _1_

17. I have never talked with a person who is paralyzed or couldn't walk.
    Agree _0_　　Disagree _2_　　Undecided _1_

18. I don't say "Hi" to people who are retarded.
    Agree _0_　　Disagree _2_　　Undecided _1_

19. Minnesota has many lakes.
    Agree _2_　　Disagree _0_　　Undecided _0_

20. I believe students with handicaps should participate with other people in the recreation department's programs.
    Agree _2_　　Disagree _0_　　Undecided _1_

(This questionnaire was adapted from: Voeltz, L. [1980]. Children's attitudes toward handicapped persons. *American Journal of Mental Deficiency, 84,* 455–464.)

PEER ACCEPTANCE EVALUATION SUMMARY FORM   FIGURE 6.10

A. Name: _____Leo Rimmer_____

B. Program Title: _____New Games_____

C. Program Goal: _____to participate cooperatively in groups_____

D. Objective: _____Leo Rimmer_____ will increase (his)/her
    (name)
    posttest score __8__ points above (his)/her pretest score after attending __8__ sessions
    (number)   (number)
    of _____New Games_____ .
    (program)

Total number of points possible = 40.

Date	Pretest Score	Date	Posttest Score	Difference between Pretest and Posttest Score
E. 6-17-87	F. 13	I. 7-10-87	J. 34	K. (J. – F.) 21

G. Number of program sessions __8__ .

L. Number of sessions attended by the participant __8__ .

Activities engaged in by the participant:

	Date	Activity	Comment	Initial
H.	6-17	knots	Leo didn't want to hold hands	✓
	6-19	new frisbee	This activity was enjoyed	✓
	6-24	group juggling	Leo found this fun but	✓
	6-26	instant replay	Leo needed much instruction difficult	✓
	7-1	hug tag	Activity was enjoyed by group	✓
	7-3	human pinball	Jim was inapprop. at first	✓
	7-8	taffy pull	Leo played well in his group	✓
	7-10	people pyramids	Leo was very cooperative	✓

Before proceeding with the directions, the reader should become familiar with the completed Peer Acceptance Evaluation Summary Form that is presented following the Acceptance Survey.

The benefits of implementing the Peer Acceptance Evaluation Tool could include:

1. The present attitudes of the nondisabled participants toward their peers with disabilities are determined.
2. Changes in attitudes of the nondisabled participants toward their peers with disabilities are documented.

**DIRECTIONS FOR PEER ACCEPTANCE
SURVEY EVALUATION SUMMARY FORM (FIGURE 6.10)**

1. Write the participants name on line "A".
2. Write the name of the program the participant will be attending on line "B".
3. Write the program goal(s) on line "C".
4. Fill in the blanks to complete the objective, on line "D".

5. During or prior to the first session, administer the Peer Acceptance Survey to each participant. Ask the participants to answer each question individually. Reassure them that there are no right or wrong answers and that their answers are strictly confidential.

6. Score the Peer Acceptance Surveys by referring to the Peer Acceptance Survey Answer Key to determine the point value for the response given to each statement. Add the point values for all 20 statements to arrive at a total pretest score.

7. Write the date that the survey was completed on line "E".

8. Write the participant's pretest score on line "F".

9. Write the total number of program sessions on line "G".

10. On Line "H" write the date of the first session, the activities in which the participant was involved, any comment that may assist with the interpretation of the data (e.g., Leo did not want to hold hands with his partner.), and initial your entry.

11. Repeat step #10 until the program has ended.

12. During the final session, or shortly thereafter, administer the questionnaire, once again, to each participant. Remind the participants that their answers are strictly confidential, that there are no right or wrong answers, and that they must complete the survey individually.

13. Score the Peer Acceptance Surveys (i.e., posttest) in the identical manner as in Step 6 (above).

14. Write the date of the posttest on line "I".

15. Write the posttest score on line "J".

16. Subtract the number on line "F" from the number of line "J" and write the total on line "K" (i.e., J − F = K).

17. Write the total number of sessions that the participant attended on line "L".

Evaluation Tool #5–
SELF-CONCEPT EVALUATION TOOL

One of the most important results of participation by persons with disabilities in recreation programs is the opportunity for participants to develop their self-concept or self-esteem. The Self-Concept Questionnaire (Figure 6.11) is a pre- and posttest measurement tool for determining levels of self-esteem. This 30-item questionnaire is administered to all the participants before the program begins. The scores are then tallied using the Self-Concept Evaluation Answer key (Figure 6.12) and placed on the Self-Concept Evaluation Summary Form (Figure 6.13). There are additional questions on the summary sheet that are to be completed by the instructor. During the final session, or shortly thereafter, the identical questionnaire is once again administered to each participant, and the score placed on the summary form. The Self-Concept Evaluation Tool is simple to implement and to score. It could complement the data collected from the other evaluation procedures described in this chapter. For example, information gained from the Social Interaction Evaluation Tool might illustrate that the participant with a disability only interacts with staff members, and not with his or her peers. The Self-Concept Questionnaire may reveal that this participant has very low self-esteem. Based on these data, the program instructor can encourage the participant to interact with his or her peers and can provide positive social reinforcement such as social praise or back pats and feedback to strengthen the participant's self-esteem.

Before proceeding with the directions, the reader should become familiar with the completed Self-Concept Evaluation Summary Form that follows.

The benefits of implementing the Self-Concept Evaluation Tool can include:

Name: *Sue Winters*

Date: **7-2-87**

1.	I feel like I can improve how I look.	Never	**(Seldom)**	Sometimes	Often	Always
2.	Others think of me as a leader.	**(Never)**	Seldom	Sometimes	Often	Always
3.	I make friends easily.	Never	**(Seldom)**	Sometimes	Often	Always
4.	I learn how to play games fast.	Never	Seldom	**(Sometimes)**	Often	Always
5.	I consider myself smart.	Never	**(Seldom)**	Sometimes	Often	Always
6.	Others tease me.	Never	Seldom	Sometimes	**(Often)**	Always
7.	I want to be like someone else.	Never	Seldom	Sometimes	Often	**(Always)**
8.	I enjoy making decisions.	**(Never)**	Seldom	Sometimes	Often	Always
9.	I get picked last in games.	Never	Seldom	Sometimes	Often	**(Always)**
10.	I feel good when I learn something new.	Never	Seldom	Sometimes	**(Often)**	Always
11.	When I look in the mirror, I like myself.	Never	**(Seldom)**	Sometimes	Often	Always
12.	I am a leader when I am with kids my own age.	**(Never)**	Seldom	Sometimes	Often	Always
13.	I like to play alone.	Never	Seldom	Sometimes	Often	**(Always)**
14.	Others consider me smart.	**(Never)**	Seldom	Sometimes	Often	Always
15.	Others like playing games with me.	Never	**(Seldom)**	Sometimes	Often	Always
16.	Others ask me to be their friend.	Never	**(Seldom)**	Sometimes	Often	Always
17.	I feel bad when my team loses.	Never	Seldom	Sometimes	**(Often)**	Always
18.	Others tell me what to do.	Never	Seldom	Sometimes	**(Often)**	Always
19.	I can make up my own mind.	Never	Seldom	**(Sometimes)**	Often	Always
20.	I enjoy playing by myself.	Never	Seldom	Sometimes	**(Often)**	Always
21.	I only like to play if I win.	Never	Seldom	**(Sometimes)**	Often	Always
22.	I get mad when someone teases me.	Never	Seldom	Sometimes	Often	**(Always)**
23.	I get picked first in games.	**(Never)**	Seldom	Sometimes	Often	Always
24.	I like to play with others.	Never	**(Seldom)**	Sometimes	Often	Always
25.	I feel like I can get things done.	Never	Seldom	**(Sometimes)**	Often	Always
26.	I get what I can from others.	Never	**(Seldom)**	Sometimes	Often	Always
27.	I feel it's my fault when my team loses.	Never	Seldom	Sometimes	Often	**(Always)**
28.	Others enjoy being with me.	Never	**(Seldom)**	Sometimes	Often	Always
29.	I can choose what to do during my free time.	Never	**(Seldom)**	Sometimes	Often	Always
30.	Others like to be around me.	Never	**(Seldom)**	Sometimes	Often	Always

Finished! Thank you for completing the survey.

SELF-CONCEPT QUESTIONNAIRE ANSWER KEY   FIGURE 6.12

#	Item	Never	Seldom	Sometimes	Often	Always
1.	I feel like I can improve how I look.	1	2	3	4	5
2.	Others think of me as a leader.	1	2	3	4	5
3.	I make friends easily.	1	2	3	4	5
4.	I learn how to play games fast.	1	2	3	4	5
5.	I consider myself smart.	1	2	3	4	5
6.	Others tease me.	1	5	4	3	1
7.	I want to be like someone else.	4	5	3	2	1
8.	I enjoy making decisions.	1	2	3	4	5
9.	I get picked last in games.	1	3	4	5	1
10.	I feel good when I learn something new.	1	2	3	4	5
11.	When I look in the mirror, I like myself.	1	2	3	4	5
12.	I am a leader when I am with kids my own age.	1	3	4	5	1
13.	I like to play alone.	1	4	5	3	1
14.	Others consider me smart.	1	2	3	4	5
15.	Others like playing games with me.	1	2	3	4	5
16.	Others ask me to be their friend.	1	3	4	5	1
17.	I feel bad when my team loses.	1	3	4	5	1
18.	Others tell me what to do.	1	3	4	5	1
19.	I can make up my own mind.	1	2	3	4	5
20.	I enjoy playing by myself.	1	4	5	3	1
21.	I only like to play if I win.	5	4	3	2	1
22.	I get mad when someone teases me.	5	4	3	2	1
23.	I get picked first in games.	1	3	4	5	1
24.	I like to play with others.	1	3	4	5	1
25.	I feel like I can get things done.	1	2	3	4	5
26.	I get what I can from others.	1	3	4	5	1
27.	I feel it's my fault when my team loses.	1	5	4	3	1
28.	Others enjoy being with me.	1	2	3	4	5
29.	I can choose what to do during my free time.	1	2	3	4	5
30.	Others like to be around me.	1	2	3	4	5

SELF-CONCEPT EVALUATION SUMMARY FORM   FIGURE 6.13

A. Name: ___*Sue Winters*___

B. Program Title: ___*Just for Me*___

C. Program Goal: ___*To increase personal understanding of 'self'*___

D. Objective: ___*Sue Winters*___ will increase his/(her)
    posttest score _*15*_ points above his/(her) pretest score after attending _*8*_ sessions
    (name)   (number)   (number)
    of _*Just for Me*_ .
    (program)

Total number of points possible = 150.

	Date	Pretest Score	Date	Posttest Score	Difference between Pretest and Posttest Score
E.	7-2-87	F. 66			
I.	7-25-87		J. 104		K. (J. − F.) 38

G. Number of program sessions _*8*_ .

L. Number of sessions attended by the participant _*8*_ .

Activities engaged in by the participant:

	Date	Activity	Comment	Initial
H.	7-2	Interest Survey	Said "I can't do anything right"	
	7-4	Talent Collage	One picture of watching TV	
	7-9	Leadership Skills	Limited but good interaction	
	7-11	New Games	Appeared to enjoy them	
	7-16	Self Portraits	Used bright colors	
	7-18	Being Positive	Made no comments	
	7-23	Growing from Failure	Added to the discussion	
	7-25	Party	Socially involved w/peers	

1. The participant's current view of his or her self-concept is determined.
2. Changes in the participant's view of his or her self-concept are documented.

DIRECTIONS FOR THE SELF-CONCEPT EVALUATION TOOL

1. Write the participant's name on line "A".
2. Write the name of the program on line "B".
3. Write the program goal(s) on line "C".
4. Fill in the blanks to complete the objective on line "D".
5. Administer the questionnaire to each participant. Ask the participants to complete the questionnaire individually. Reassure them that their answers are strictly confidential and that there are no right or wrong answers.
6. Score the questionnaires by referring to the Self-Concept Evaluation Answer Key to determine the point value for the response given to each statement. Add the point values for all 30 statements to arrive at a total pretest score..
7. Write the date the questionnaire was completed on line "E".
8. Write the participant's pretest score on line "F".
9. Write the number of sessions the program is held on line "G".

10.   On line "H", write the date of the first session, the activities in which the participant was involved, and any comment that may assist in interpreting the data. An example of this would be: Sue was not feeling well and did not participate for most of the session and said "I can't do anything right!". Initial your entry.

11.   Repeat Step #10 throughout the sessions.

12.   During the final session, or shortly thereafter, administer the questionnaire to each participant. Remind them that their answers are strictly confidential and that there are no right or wrong answers.

13.   Score the questionnaires in the identical manner as in Step 6 (above).

14.   Write the date of the posttest on line "I".

15.   Write the score of the posttest on line "J".

16.   Subtract the number of line "F" from the number of line "J" and write the total on line "K" (J − F = K).

17.   Write the number of sessions that the participant attended on line "L".

Evaluation Tool #6–NUMERICAL EVALUATION TOOL

Numerical evaluation should be used to complement the other methods of evaluation described throughout this chapter. Numerical evaluation, as the only method of evaluation, usually does not provide sufficient qualitative information to the program leader to allow him or her to make important program decisions and revisions. Numerical evaluation is simply the documentation of the number of persons participating in the program. These data could be compared over time with attendance records of similar programs. In this manner, an understanding of which programs have high registration rates and interest levels could be gained. Numerical evaluation should also take into consideration duration, program costs, and other features that affect successful programs. Numerical evaluations should be used only in conjunction with other evaluation methods.

Before proceeding with the directions, the reader should become familiar with the completed Numerical Evaluation Information Form that follows.

The benefits of implementing a numerical evaluation tool could include:

1.   The number of persons with and without disabilities that are participating in the recreation program can be documented.

2.   An increase or decrease in the number of persons with and without disabilities that are participating in the recreation program over time can be documented.

DIRECTIONS FOR NUMERICAL EVALUATION TOOL

1.   Write the program's title on line "A".

2.   Write the name of the program site on line "B".

3.   Write the goal(s) of the program on line "C".

4.   On line "D" write the requested program information.

5.   On the line in column "E" write the number of nondisabled participants that attended the session.

6.   On the line in column "F" write the number of participants with disabilities that attended the session.

7.   In column "G" write the date that the session was conducted.

8.   If there is any circumstance that causes a dramatic shift in attendance for a given session, write the presumed reason (e.g., snow storm) in Column "H".

NUMERICAL EVALUATION INFORMATION FORM   FIGURE 6.14

A. Program Title: *Me and My Friend*
B. Program Site: *North Commons Recreation Center*
C. Program Goal: *To integrate persons with and without disabilities into a variety of recreation activities at the center.*
D. Program Information (include cost, meeting times, duration, day held, age of participants, etc.):
No charge. Program meets Thursdays from 6:30-7:30 p.m. for 6 weeks. The participants are 8 to 11 years of age.

Session	E. Number of nondisabled participants	F. Number of participants with disabilities	G. Program date	H. Comment
1	17	4	6-5-87	
2	18	4	6-12-87	
3	18	4	6-19-87	
4	18	3	6-26-87	
5	18	4	7-3-87	
6	18	4	7-10-87	
7				
8				
9				
10				

I. Total number of non-disabled participants	J. Total number of participants with disabilities	K. Total number of participants (nondisabled and disabled)
107	23	130

L. Number of sessions conducted	M. Average number of participants per session	N. Number of participants registered
6	21.67	22

9. Repeat steps 5 through 8 following each session until the program's termination.
10. On line "I", calculate the total number of nondisabled participants throughout all sessions.
11. On line "J", calculate the total number of participants with disabilities throughout all sessions.
12. On line "K", calculate the total number of participants (nondisabled and disabled) (I + J = K).
13. On line "L", write the total number of sessions conducted.
14. Write the average number of participants per session that attended throughout the program on line "M". Note: To calculate the average number of participants per session, take the total number of participants (line "K") and divide that sum by the total

number of sessions conducted (line "L"). Place that average on line "M". Thus, Number of disabled participants = 107; Number of participants with disabilities = 23; K (I + J) = 130 participants with and without disabilities ÷ 6 sessions = Average number of participants/session = 21.67).

15.   Write the total number of participants that registered for the program on line "N".

SUMMARY

This chapter discusses the benefits of evaluating community recreation programs and describes six methods for conducting program evaluations. Each method is accompanied by an introduction, step-by-step procedures for implementing the evaluation tool, and directions for summarizing the data. Examples of completed evaluation forms are included in the chapter. Blank forms of all the evaluation tools, suitable for duplication, are found in Appendix H.

Chapter 7

Overcoming Obstacles
to Community Recreation
Integration

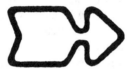

S ince its introduction by Nirje (1969) nearly 2 decades ago, the principle of normalization, as further expanded by Wolfensberger (1972), has become the primary philosophical orientation guiding the development and delivery of community-based services for persons with disabilities. Parents, consumers with disabilities, professionals, and advocacy groups have adopted the normalization tenets, particularly those that enhance opportunities for persons with disabilities to be physically and socially integrated alongside their nondisabled peers. Recent legislation has supported normalization and integration by legally mandating that facilities, programs, and services supported with public monies (e.g., taxes or grants) be open and accessible to everyone, regardless of the extent and level of an individual's disabling condition.

The philosophical orientation of the normalization principle and the intent of the legislation have strong implications for the delivery of community-based leisure services to persons with disabilities. Reynolds (1981) and his colleagues (Reynolds & O'Morrow, 1985) have effectively articulated the relationship between normalization and leisure and the implications for persons delivering leisure services in community and residential settings. Even though many leisure service providers seem to understand, and consequently, to subscribe to the theoretical basis underlying normalization and leisure, significant barriers or obstacles remain that prevent or inhibit persons with disabilities from receiving opportunities for recreation in community-based and integrated leisure environments. Why is this the case? If the philosophical orientation is clear, why can't human services professionals take the necessary steps forward to overcome the obstacles that can be easily identified? Perhaps the answer is that the philosophical orientation is not clear.One has only to look at history to see how poorly persons with disabilities have traditionally been regarded. Before one can critique existing leisure service systems and suggest alternatives that will help to overcome obstacles to leisure participation, one must first examine how society views "differentness," particularly in relation to persons with disabilities.

Hutchison and Lord (1979) provide a useful framework for this discussion. They set forth the problem of negative attitudes as a determinant of major societal handicaps for persons with disabilities. Due to society's negative role perceptions of these individuals, along with a low tolerance for individual differences, persons with disabilities are negatively valued. Therefore, in the authors' opinion, negative attitudes and perceptions directly affect "quality of services, opportunities, and rights" (p. 16). Wolfensberger (1975) provided background on this viewpoint when he described the various ways society perceived the roles of persons with mental retardation. His commentary has clear implications on how persons with any type of disability are viewed by nondisabled persons. Persons with disabilities are often viewed as being "sick" or "ill," and are then assigned as patients or clients to therapy programs where human services professionals "treat" their disabilities in an effort to "cure" them or to remedy the effects of the disabling condition. The print media appear to concur with this view when they describe the person with a mobility impairment as someone "confined to a wheelchair". Additionally, a common way of viewing persons with disabilities is as an object of pity or charity, dependent upon others who will care for, nurture, financially support, and sympathize with their "plight" or "suffering". This over-protective attitude by nondisabled persons, coupled with their low expectations of the capabilities of persons with disabilities, contributes to hierarchical, authoritarian relationships, learned helplessness, and inappropriate dependence on others. Even though the telethons and counter top collection boxes bolster funds to research the cause and prevention of disabilities, these fund-raising drives still present to the general public an image of helplessness that misrepresents the abilities and potentials of persons with disabilities.

If one focuses exclusively on the more visible manifestations of the disabling condition, it is easy to perceive the more overt signs of differentness. Unfortunately, one's first impressions of an individual seem to determine whether or not one will pursue further interactions with that person, or even long-term friendship. One need not move much further than the newspaper, the television, or the magazine rack to perceive what society values most. Physical fitness, blemish-free complexions, active, vital life-styles, affluence, personal independence, professional competence and power, stylishness, competitiveness, sexual attractiveness, and youthfulness are highly valued and are pursued with fervor. Seeking the "ideal" is considered "normal" behavior. Achieving these ideals is difficult for most people. For many people with disabilities, it may nearly be impossible.

To the credit of the many individuals and agencies advocating on behalf of persons with disabilities, a new, alternative view of persons with disabilities is receiving greater attention (Hutchison & Lord, 1979). A person with a disability is being viewed as a developing human being (Wolfensberger, 1975), one who has inherent strengths and abilities, who experiences similar problems, concerns, and weaknesses as nondisabled persons, and who has the potential to try and to succeed, or to fail, as anyone else. Even labels currently deemed appropriate such as: "integrated groups of persons with and without disabilities" are being changed to reflect more positive perceptions such as: "mixed-ability groups". Even further, persons with disabilities have begun to label otherwise able-bodied persons as "TABs", or temporarily able-bodied, to underline the potential of anyone to be severely and traumatically injured in a moment's occurrence or to experience the potentially debilitating effects old age may have on one's body and mind. It is also encouraging to note that there are many national and grassroot efforts to alert communities to the presence of barriers that prevent integration of citizens with disabilities. In addition, significant attempts are being made to alert media professionals to more appropriate ways of portraying persons with disabilities in articles, photographs, and in advertising. When internationally known corporations such as fast-food chains or clothing manufacturers use actors with disabilities to market familiar goods and services, without focusing on the person and/or their disabling condition, this presents to the viewing public a positive portrayal of these persons. This may ultimately change opinions and stereotypes, clearing the way for more open and accessible service systems for persons with disabilities.

OBSTACLES TO COMMUNITY RECREATION INTEGRATION

It is not difficult to understand how societal attitudes and perceptions are reflected in the types of leisure service delivery systems that are established in communities. Sessoms (1984) pointed out that in complex societies, delivery systems are developed in order to meet specific societal needs. For example, leisure service systems were created to answer society's need to engage in recreational activities that permit one to escape the demands of work or of everyday life. But society is made up of diverse individuals with varying recreational interests and needs. It is the task of the community recreation planner to endeavor to meet these diverse needs.

In training, community recreation professionals are cautioned that a primary issue in the provision of community recreation services deals with priorities (Sessoms, 1984). Specifically, community recreation personnel need to make it a priority to regard themselves as "generalists" endeavoring to meet the leisure and recreation requirements of a demographically and culturally diverse constituency. Even with such efforts, the community recreation professional knows that not everyone will get all of his or her needs met. He or she seeks an appropriate compromise, trusting that the community will recognize his or her efforts to provide services that meet the community's needs.

Priorities become an even greater issue when considering programs that will include persons with disabilities. Often, the community recreation professional is unaware that persons with disabilities live in the community and desire recreation and leisure services. Or the recreation professional may assume that parents and careproviders are meeting the leisure needs of individuals with disabilities in the residential setting. These professionals have not made it their top priority to know the demography and the needs of their communities. Another situation where recreation professionals can manifest misplaced priorities is in the "special recreation" program that attempts to "take care of" all persons with a similar disabling condition. Notable examples of activities from such programs include the Saturday morning program for the "autistic," the Friday night dances for "the retarded," and "the deaf" volleyball league. These are cases of putting the burden of responsibility for service delivery on other persons or agencies. When questioned about service delivery to persons with disabilities, community recreation personnel in the above situations may respond with: "I didn't know they lived in my community"; "Sunshine Park does all the programming for the retarded"; "I didn't know they wanted to come to my park"; "Their careproviders play with them at home"; and so forth.

Hayes (1978) provided some insight into the way leisure services for persons with disabilities may be approached. In his provocative report on the problems of mainstreaming recreational services, Hayes remarked that individuals with disabilities are further handicapped by negative attitudes. The negative attitudes represent a lack of acceptance by a society that is unable to fully accept individuals it regards as "deviant." The result is that community stigma, that is, negative attitudes toward participation by persons with disabilities in community recreation and leisure activities and settings, begins to attach itself to persons with disabilities. These discriminatory attitudes and beliefs are further reinforced as persons with disabilities, their parents, careproviders, and advocacy groups, receive the message that they clearly "do not belong." It is much easier to maintain the status quo by not thinking about the recreational needs of persons with disabilities or by assuming that other persons or agencies are meeting these needs, somewhere and somehow.

Additionally, recent interviews with community recreation personnel revealed that resistance to provision of leisure services to persons with disabilities may be a result of "organizational stigma" (West, 1982). "Organizational stigma" refers to the situation wherein recreation professionals attach their own preconceived values about a person's leisure needs and abilities to the type and extent of services offered, thus limiting service diversity and flexibility. Interestingly, West (1984) also found that persons with disabilities are able to perceive this stigma and thus tend to maintain a "self-imposed exile from active participation in community recreation" (p. 41). One can readily see how each view reinforces the other and prevents successful integration from taking place. For example, the recreational professional offers primarily athletic programs. Persons with physical disabilities are unable to participate in such programs. The professional assumes "handicapped people" are not interested in these programs because they are never heard from, nor are they seen at the park. Furthering this process, the same programs are offered each year. Persons with disabilities continue to stay away from the park because they cannot participate. Community and organizational stigma are thus reinforced. Persons with disabilities disappear into the home or are shunted into segregated, special recreation programs for an indefinite period of time.

Few exemplary recreation and leisure service strategies exist that set forth a systematic and comprehensive approach to making community recreation settings and programs integrated and accessible. This text is a direct response to this need. Other recent books (Kennedy et al., 1987, for example) justify and describe guidelines for developing special recreation service models within communities. Even if human services personnel highly value the normalization principle and its chief corollary, integration, these professionals may still lack the competencies to translate these values into practice. As Horner, Meyer, & Fredericks put it (1986): "It sounds good, but how does it work?" (p. xv). Professional human services preparation programs, which traditionally have not addressed the issue of leisure service provision to persons with disabilities, are beginning to introduce students to the various concepts, philosophies, and strategies for making programs and services accessible. An example of such a program can be found at the University of Minnesota Twin Cities Campus. The University's Division of Recreation, Park, and Leisure Studies requires students who are enrolled in the Leisure Services Management program to register for a course entitled "Community Leisure Services and Special Populations." This blending of emphasis areas (i.e., Leisure Services Management and Therapeutic Recreation) has the potential for substantially improving leisure service delivery for persons with disabilities in a variety of generic, community-based recreation settings.

Even though clear strategies for program integration have not been forthcoming, there have been attempts by professionals and academics to identify the specific obstacles that prevent or inhibit community recreation participation by persons with disabilities. A comprehensive literature review presented in Chapter 1, for example, reveals results of surveys given to leisure service providers and consumers with disabilities. While some studies seek to broaden awareness of issues surrounding specific barriers (Smith, 1985), others examine specific approaches to alleviate barriers commonly experienced by community recreation agencies (Vaughan & Winslow, 1979). Research on obstacles to community leisure participation has also focused on a number of areas, including: the needs of groups represented by specific disabilities such as mental retardation (Putnam, Werder, & Schleien, 1985; West, 1984), the attitudes held by park and recreation organizations toward disabled persons (Austin et al., 1977; West, 1982), and the relationships between organizations (e.g., municipal park and recreation departments, community education agencies, schools) that provide community leisure services to persons with disabilities (Schleien & Werder, 1985; Wheeler, Lynch, & Thom, 1984). The barriers most commonly cited by these authors include: architectural inaccessibility; lack of transportation; lack of personal and/or public funding support; social and leisure skill deficits of participants with disabilities; negative community attitudes; lack of organizational and instructional skills by recreation staff; lack of volunteers; lack of knowledge about needs and preferences of persons with disabilities; lack of communication and collaboration among individuals and agencies.

SURVEY OF LEISURE SERVICE DELIVERY SYSTEMS

Prior to developing, implementing, and validating key integration strategies that were presented in the preceding chapters, and as part of a personnel preparation grant to PIRC (Project for Integrated Recreation in the Community) funded by the Office of Special Education and Rehabilitative Services, U.S. Department of Education, the authors conducted a survey of 46 community recreation professionals within a large Midwestern metropolitan area to assess the current extent and level of leisure service delivery to community residents with disabilities (Ray, Schleien, Larson, Rutten, & Slick, 1986; Schleien & Ray, 1986). The surveys were audiotaped so that investigators could record and study responses in order to obtain a clear and comprehensive understanding of the exact nature of service delivery as perceived by the respondents. It is quite apparent that, even within one service delivery system or agency, a wide variety of opinion exists regarding the factors that inhibit integration. In addition, responses reveal a lack of clear understanding on the part of respondents as to why programming for persons with disabilities is even an issue.

Of the 46 respondents, approximately 70% stated that they had, at some time in the past, conducted programs designed specifically for members of special populations. Programs were typically segregated in nature and conducted on a limited basis. Only 50% of the respondents stated they currently administer programs like this. A large percentage of respondents (85%) were aware that persons with disabilities were using their buildings and outdoor areas. A number of special population groups (Table 7.1) were identified as frequent participants in municipal park and recreation services. The reader should note that interpretations by community center directors of what constitutes "special populations" vary in definition, and are not limited to traditional disability groups. This changing perception of who these persons with "special needs" are, may have implications for future community recreation programming (Kunstler, 1985).

An important component of this survey concerned the identification of barriers encountered when developing or implementing recreation programs. Respondents were asked to identify barriers as either being administrative or programmatic in nature. The responses revealed that the community center directors had a difficult time differentiating between the two barrier types, with several barriers identified as being both administrative and programmatic. Barriers are listed below within specific "community integration markers" (Table 7.2). Meyer and Kishi (1985) provide support for the identification of integration markers which, when utilized, allow program personnel to examine areas where barriers may be found and to develop strategies to overcome identified barriers. The reader should note that each integration marker and cited barrier represents the perspective of the center director who is responding in the survey, and should not be compared to, or combined with,

TABLE 7.1. *Special populations[a]* as identified by community recreation center directors

1. Mentally Retarded (30)	17. Learning Disorders (2)
2. Physically Disabled (23)	18. Diabetic (1)
3. Hearing Impaired/Deaf (14)	19. Multiple Sclerosis (1)
4. Elderly (14)	20. Multiply Handicapped (1)
5. Visually Impaired/Blind (8)	21. Developmentally Disabled (1)
6. Chemically Dependent (7)	22. Brain-injured (1)
7. Chronic Mentally Ill (5)	23. Autistic (1)
8. Epilepsy (4)	24. Single parent families (1)
9. Cerebral Palsy (3)	25. Battered women (1)
10. Severely Handicapped (3)	26. Juvenile Delinquents (1)
11. Emotionally Disturbed (3)	27. Adults who can't read (1)
12. Wheelchair users (unknown etiology) (3)	28. "The poor" (1)
13. Don't know/Not aware (3)	29. Street people (1)
14. Alcoholics (2)	30. Hospital patients (1)
15. Muscular Dystrophy (2)	31. Not appropriate to ask (1)
16. Behavioral problems (2)	

[a]The terms used here are how they were reported by the respondents and may not be the preferred nomenclature. The number in parentheses denotes the total number of Center Directors who identified this special population group ($N = 46$).

barriers identified in previous studies. Each integration marker is accompanied by a relevant question and paraphrased examples of barriers cited by the center directors.

One additional survey was conducted during the PIRC grant project period. For this survey, the authors were particularly interested in determining whether there were regional similarities in barriers (e.g., transportation, lack of funds, unskilled staff) encountered when developing and implementing community recreation services for persons with disabilities. These data were then compared to data obtained in other studies, including the PIRC survey. The purpose of this survey was to determine the status of community recreation services for persons with disabilities within cities and towns of varying population sizes. The specific municipalities under investigation were those with populations of 10,000 and under; 10,001–25,000; 25,001–50,000; 50,001–100,000; and those over 100,000 in a 7-state area within the Great Lakes region. The states included in the survey were: Illinois, Indiana, Iowa, Michigan, Minnesota, Ohio, and Wisconsin.

A total of 70 survey forms were mailed to a randomly selected group of cities and towns in each state within the study region. For example, Ohio received 10 surveys: 2 for each population size category. Of the surveys distributed, 69% were completed and returned. The respondents represented various positions within their organization, such as agency director, assistant director, program director, community center director, or therapeutic recreation specialist. Respondents also included a mayor, city clerk, director of public service, and a park superintendent or supervisor; the greatest response was received from agency directors (56%).

Findings revealed that 83% of the respondents "somewhat agreed" or "strongly agreed" that municipal park and recreation agencies should provide leisure services for persons with disabilities. When asked to identify agencies or individuals having primary responsibility for leisure service provision, 29% identified municipal park and recreation agencies, nearly twice the number identifying the nearest service delivery competitor (schools, 15%; advocacy groups, 12%; others, 12%). It is encouraging to note that 73% of

TABLE 7.2.   Community integration markers as perceived by community recreation center directors

1. **Consumer/Community Awareness** (Who are potential users? Where do they live?)
   - Unclear definition of "handicapped," "special populations"
   - Where do members of special populations live?
   - Participants of segregated (e.g., handicapped-only) after-school programs at parks who are not members of that community

2. **Consumer/Community Needs** (What programs and services are needed? Preferred?)
   - Center Director, as a "generalist" is expected to meet everyone's needs
   - Lack of needs assessment conducted with special population groups in community
   - Little or no outreach, networking, or linkages
   - Personal/professional exposure to special population groups limited; therefore, not aware of needs

3. **Staffing** (What qualifications do staff need? How many staff should there be per program?)
   - Lack of qualified instructors who can adapt programs
   - Job responsibilities of Center Director limit ability to develop new, specialized programs
   - Need staff with specialized backgrounds (e.g., Therapeutic Recreation Specialists)
   - Lack of volunteers or of time commitment by volunteers

4. **Attitudes**

   How do "regular" consumers view participation by members of special populations?
   - Center Director reactions: "Fear of the unknown"; "intimidation"; "scared at first"; programming for special populations is "spooky"
   - Nonhandicapped participant reactions: "resentment"; "discomfort"
   - Neighborhood complaints regarding noise from a segregated program (e.g., Friday night dances)
   - Instructional time per participant is diminished if staff needs to "work" with handicapped person

   How do members of special populations and their parents/careproviders view community recreation activity participation within "regular" program offerings?
   - Once solicited, handicapped refuse to come to the park
   - Parents not used to having their handicapped children in park programs
   - Handicapped persons prefer segregated programs
   - Special population groups "have a lot going on" and can't join into park programs

5. **Current Program Practices** (What is the nature of currently offered programs and services at the park [e.g., sports, crafts, dance, outdoor recreation, cooking]?)
   - "Other parks nearby are providing programs for members of special populations, why should I?"
   - Trouble getting the "regular" community to use the park
   - Most programs geared to children, not adults
   - Programs too "physical" in nature; level of competitiveness high; activities require high ability levels
   - Image of the parks and their programs and services to members of special populations not projected well

6. **Physical and Fiscal Resources** (How is park accessibility affected by facility design, transportation, and allocation of money?)
   - Inaccessibility of park building/grounds
   - Lack of transportation alternatives
   - Specialized equipment needed
   - Specialized staff (e.g., TRS, sign language interpreters) cost large sums of money

the respondents stated that their agency currently had programs designed for persons with disabilities. The programs offered were either segregated (15%), integrated (14%), or both segregated and integrated (44%). No response was indicated for this question in 27% of the surveys returned.

The administrative and programmatic barriers cited by the respondents were listed and tallied for each population (Table 7.3). The five most frequently cited barriers were:

1. financial or budget constraints (19%)
2. lack of qualified staff (14%)
3. lack of transportation (10%)
4. lack of facilities to conduct programs (7%)
5. lack of communication (5%)

The findings from these surveys of municipal park and recreation agencies in the 7-state Great Lakes Region, along with interviews with community recreation professionals, confirm the presence of a diversity of barriers found within community recreation settings. The findings also affirm the findings of previous studies. The fact that there is no clear, fixed definition by recreation personnel of what constitutes a programmatic or administrative barrier in community recreation programs underscores the widespread need to develop effective ways of preventing and/or overcoming obstacles to participation by persons with disabilities.

OVERCOMING OBSTACLES

Those recreation professionals with experience in providing recreation services to persons with disabilities realize that barriers may be encountered at any stage of the recreation service delivery process. Problems encountered could be a result of any number of circumstances related to the organization of recreation services, to personal or professional attitudes, to individual skills, and to the disability characteristics of the potential user. The strategy selected by the recreation professional to resolve these barriers determines the success of that program.

One must not be discouraged by the presence of barriers, since it is unusual for an agency not to encounter them. In fact, persons without disabilities may also experience conflicts or difficulties when attempting to participate in recreation activities, even though they are not handicapped by a disability or do not typically experience negative stigma from the community. Examples could include: lack of skills to enroll in an art class, lack of sufficient physical fitness to join a jogging program, lack of funds needed to pay class fees, or lack of convenient transportation to and from the program.

Empathizing with persons with disabilities may be an effective means of understanding barriers that everyone might experience at one time or another as he or she attempts to enter into community recreation settings. A professional approach to understanding barriers should be tempered with this personal awareness of the potential for encountering barriers. This will permit the recreation professional to assess each situation as unique. However, a word of caution about this approach is in order. One must be careful not to empathize with persons with disabilities to the point of becoming patronizing or paternalistic. These behaviors, which can be manifested as talking "down" to a disabled person in a parent-to-child manner, can further "devalue" the person with a disability by making him or her feel helpless, dependent, and possibly, humiliated. Recreation professionals must be just that—professionals: persons who bring skills, training, motivation, enthusiasm, and commitment to their jobs, in this case, the systematic approach to providing barrier-free community recreation services.

TABLE 7.3. Great Lakes regional survey of barriers to community recreation participation by persons with disabilities according to population size

Barrier cited	Total responses by population size					
	10,000– under	10,001– 25,000	25,001– 50,000	50,001– 100,000	Over	TOTAL
1. budget/financial contraints	1	3	4	4	11	23
2. lack of qualified staff	1	5	5	1	5	17
3. transportation			2	2	8	12
4. lack of facilities		2	3	1	3	9
5. lack of communication				2	4	6
6. lack of support from referral agencies and families	1		1	1	2	5
7. inaccessible facilities	1		2	1	1	5
8. no support for integration			1	2	1	4
9. lack of adapted equipment		1		1	2	4
10. unclear role definitions			2	2		4
11. negative attitudes by community					3	3
12. lack of community awareness		1			2	3
13. unable to identify potential users and their needs			1		2	3
14. unable to "secure" enough participants for segregated programs			1	1		2
15. lack of volunteers	1					1
16. staff lack recreation skills in general	1					1
17. parents prefer integrated programs (note: respondent referred to this as a "parental problem")			1			1
18. parents lack awareness of child's leisure needs			1			1
19. lack of interagency coordination			1			1
20. programs discontinued because of duplication				1		1
21. lack of staff inservice training			1			1
22. unclear program philosophy and agency mission				1		1
23. persons with disabilities prefer segregated programs				1		1
24. needs of participants too diverse				1		1
25. inability to reach people with program information				1		1
26. lack of programs for severely handicapped persons					1	1
27. disability groups are mixed in programs					1	1
28. "no-shows" in special population programs					1	1
29. participants lack skills					1	1
30. no barriers encountered				1	1	2
31. no response to this question	4		1		1	6
Grand Totals	10	12	27	24	50	123

There are many ways to categorize sources of barriers to accessible community leisure services (Goffman, 1963; Kennedy et al., 1987; Smith, 1985; Vaughan & Winslow, 1979). For example, barriers may stem from the nature (i.e., the level and extent) of the person's particular disability. *Individual* barriers pertain to such issues as deficits in social or recreational skills, extent of dependency on others for assistance to participate, health or fitness levels, knowledge of recreational opportunities, and motivation to participate. A second, and more powerful category of barrier arises from *external* forces that further handicap persons with disabilities and that inhibit their full participation in community recreation experiences. External barriers are the most common barrier type cited by recreation professionals and others. Examples include: financial constraints, lack of qualified recreation staff, lack of accessible and available transportation, lack of accessible facilities, poor communication, negative attitudes, and ineffective service systems. Granted, the person's disability may inhibit his or her access to the full range of community recreation services and settings. However, external forces place additional pressure on the individual, making the disability, and consequently the individual, the problem. This creates further barriers. People, agencies, and social systems can thus further handicap and stigmatize persons with disabilities. Because the municipal park and recreation agency has the ultimate responsibility for providing recreation services to all members of the community (Schleien & Werder, 1985), and because external or environmental barriers are the leading factors that inhibit accessible and integrated recreation services for persons with disabilities, external barriers will be addressed first with proposed solutions. A discussion of individual barriers will follow in a similar form. The recreation professional is challenged to identify and eliminate external barriers in his or her own community, and to avoid the assumption that the individual with disabilities is the primary cause of obstacles to integrated and accessible services. Working collaboratively with key players is the most successful strategy for arriving at solutions to common barriers encountered in recreation service delivery.

EXTERNAL BARRIERS

Financial Constraints

Financial constraints can relate to one or more of the following: 1) potential participants, 2) staff, and 3) facilities and materials. Persons with disabilities might have less discretionary funds to spend on recreation and leisure activity participation. The cause may be lack of employment, low pay, limited assistance from social service agencies such as Medicare or Welfare, and greater expenses due to the need to purchase specialized or adapted equipment such as vans with wheelchair lifts and/or custom-made clothing. Municipal park and recreation departments are further constrained when public funds are restricted, thereby limiting development or acquisition of new services, equipment, facilities, accessible buildings, and qualified staff. Several solutions to this barrier may be proposed.

If the financial constraints are participant-centered, a sliding fee schedule for all participants, based upon ability to afford the cost of the activity, could be implemented. If volunteer advocates are needed for the person to participate, let them attend for free or at substantially reduced rates. Participants with disabilities could also donate services (e.g., reception or secretarial duties or horticultural work) to park and recreation departments in exchange for program fees. Perhaps a scholarship fund could be created for persons with financial needs. Various civic or corporate organizations can sponsor potential participants by assisting with fees or transportation. Donated in-kind services (e.g., photocopying, printing, mailings) by these same agencies could release monies to be applied to scholarships and fee reductions.

If an agency believes that additional staff are necessary to implement programs but lacks funds to hire them, a consortium between agencies could be created to hire a "travelling" or itinerant Therapeutic Recreation Specialist, that is, a TRS consultant, to work with various park and recreation agencies and to provide assistance in such areas as activity modifications, or evaluation when needed. Rather than relying on several expensive specialized staff, it might be more cost-effective for the agency to create and fund a Volunteer Services Coordinator staff position. The return on investment will occur when an extensive network of volunteers is developed and available for resource staff to train and use as volunteer advocates. Additionally, provision of ongoing inservice training for existing staff should eliminate the need for specialized staff.

Sometimes facilities must be made more accessible to mobility-impaired persons. Also, adaptive materials and equipment may enhance program accessibility and partial participation. Agencies should pursue donations or corporate funding to purchase necessary equipment and materials such as accessible vans or bowling ramps. Private donations or corporate funding can also be utilized to produce media presentations such as slide shows or videotapes for use as promotional or staff training aids. Additionally, communities could earmark funds from the municipal park and recreation department budget to improve the accessibility of recreation services. Since approximately 10% of the nation's population are classified as disabled, a comparable amount of funds should be allocated to serve these persons. Currently, state and federal grants are available to upgrade personnel development from the U.S. Department of Education, Office of Special Education and Rehabilitative Services. Furthermore, the U.S. Department of Transportation provides funds for upgrading facilities, and the State Developmental Disabilities Council provides grants for program development. Select agency personnel could develop grant writing skills to pursue new funding sources.

Collaboration between public and private sector leisure service agencies is a viable method of coping with scarce resources. Cosponsoring programs with other agencies can provide access to additional resources such as materials, equipment, and funds. Finally, agencies should be challenged to develop simplified, homemade equipment and material adaptations to replace commercially marketed adapted equipment that can cost significantly more money to purchase and maintain.

Lack of Qualified Staff

Even though community recreation professionals claim to be generalists and are empowered to plan and provide programs and services to constituents within a particular geographic area, they often do not possess the skills, knowledge, or motivation to adequately or appropriately include persons with disabilities in these programs. Due to these factors and for reasons related to attitudes and past practices, municipal park and recreation agencies may think that special population groups require special services. Therefore, special staff must be hired to provide these services. However, agencies must be willing to provide more training to generic leisure service personnel in order to eliminate unnecessary reliance on specialized staff.

Inservice training programs for current staff and volunteers must be ongoing, comprehensive, and relevant. Agencies may wish to hire a TRS consultant to conduct this training and to facilitate the process of developing and implementing accessible leisure services. Trained volunteers and student interns could be incorporated into programs and services to expand staff and, consequently, opportunities for participants with disabilities. More practicum and internship sites must be developed within the municipal park and recreation agency to enhance this potential. Job descriptions must be developed or revised to affirm the role of the community recreation professional as a facilitator of accessible leisure services. Special education teachers and part-time assistants from local schools may wish to serve as staff or consultants during the summer months. Equally important, there must be additional training provided at the preservice level to university undergraduate and graduate students on those competencies needed to be an effective community recreation professional. This instruction should include training methods for integrating persons with disabilities into recreation programs and settings.

Lack of Transportation

Some of the most prevalent concerns that persons with disabilities have are the availability and quality of transportation services to community recreation settings. Also, transportation systems such as public buses or taxis may not be physically accessible. Additionally, taxis may be too expensive. If adapted vehicles are used, they may only be available on a limited, reservation-only basis. Due to the large amounts of segregated programs being offered in centralized locations, and the apparent lack of accessible neighborhood recreation programs and facilities, persons with disabilities must rely totally on alternative transportation systems. However, alternative transportation options are not always available.

Several solutions may be offered. The disabled person or advocate could contact public (e.g., city transit authority) and private (e.g., ambulance service) transportation agencies to determine the availability of handicapped-accessible vehicles, costs, and scheduling information. Corporations that use employee van pooling and that have corporate-owned vehicles may be willing to donate transportation services during times when the vehicles are not in use. Privately owned taxi cab companies could offer rate reductions and convenient services for users of community recreation services. Additionally, organizing car pools utilizing volunteers, parents, and careproviders is a proven method of overcoming transportation barriers for persons with disabilities. Churches often own buses and vans and may be contacted to determine if these vehicles are available during slow times. Finally, potential participants must be taught how to independently take advantage of available transportation systems. This is an extremely important leisure skill which parents, careproviders, teachers, and therapeutic recreation specialists should teach to persons with disabilities.

Lack of Accessible Facilities

Federal laws mandate that public facilities and services, including those providing recreation in the community, must be architecturally accessible for persons who have disabilities such as mobility and visual impairments. Individuals with disabilities cannot successfully participate in park and recreation programs if they are unable to enter or to make their way around facilities and park areas. Physical obstacles in the outdoors (e.g., obstructed trails, or walkways, fallen trees) cannot be completely regulated by the government. However, architectural barriers in the environment can be minimized in the following ways.

Architectural accessibility surveys of indoor and outdoor environments should be conducted under the direction of the leisure service agency and the recreation staff. State (e.g., Council for the Handicapped) and national (e.g., Architectural and Transportation Barriers Compliance Board) boards and commissions may be contacted for standards and recommendations regarding physical accessibility of facilities (also see Appendix F). Federal and state money may be available for use in removing existing physical barriers. In several instances, low-interest (e.g., 3%) loans are offered by communities to businesses that seek to comply with accessibility standards.

In the event that facilities and areas cannot be made totally accessible, program modifications such as conducting nature hikes on blacktop trails or switching classrooms must be considered. If outdoor environments are being used, small teams of individuals can be created to assist each other to move through the natural environment. For example, two people can walk with one person in a wheelchair, or a sighted guide can accompany a blind skier. If necessary, arrange with other leisure service organizations such as YM/YWCAs, churches, or sports and health clubs to use their facilities, if these are more accessible.

Poor Communication

For those individuals whose speech and language abilities are affected by certain developmental disabilities, by cerebral palsy, or by hearing impairments, communication may be limited. Unfortunately, recreation planners can compound this problem if they lack necessary skills (e.g., sign-language, interpreting communication boards) to "talk" with them.

Speech impediments are only one manifestation of poor communication. Unclear communication may also be found in those situations where recreation professionals are "hearing" but not "listening" to potential participants. Because persons with disabilities represent only a small minority group within a community, recreation professionals usually design most of their programs for the majority, nondisabled population. Potential users with disabilities may express their needs, preferences, and suggestions, but, if community recreation professionals are not "listening," accessible programs will not result. Thus, unclear lines of communication can be a significant obstacle.

In addition to unclear interpersonal communication, lack of communication across agencies can also be a problem. For example, ineffective networks can "muddy" lines of communication. This can result from a lack of a unified process that involves active collaboration and communication or networking between individuals and agencies with similar interests and missions. Several solutions are suggested to alleviate these communcation barriers.

One solution to poor "networking" would be for community recreation professionals to invite an allied health professional such as a Speech Pathologist or a Communication Disorders Specialist to make an inservice presentation on communication disorders and alternative communication systems (e.g., sign language, bliss symbols, word boards, electronic devices). Additionally, recreation staff may wish to enroll in sign language classes at the local technical-vocational institute or at the university. A meeting between potential participants and recreation staff may also be useful. The person with disabilities and/or their careprovider should explain to recreation staff the participant's communication needs for the recreation activity in which he or she is planning to participate. Volunteer advocates, who understand the participant's communication system, may serve as liaisons or intermediaries between recreation staff and the participant with the speech impairment. Community recreation professionals should also avoid the use of jargon and professional terminology when meeting with parents and careproviders. As a final approach to solving interpersonal communication barriers, the community recreation professional should heed the following guidelines: Be an active listener, maintain direct eye contact, talk to the individual (not the volunteer advocate or careprovider), ask for clarification if what is being said is unclear (if necessary, have the person repeat him or herself), speak in 2–3 word phrases, invite the volunteer advocate to assist when appropriate.

To further enhance communication across individuals and agencies, the following solutions are proposed. The community recreation professional should communicate regularly with parents and careproviders to provide feedback on participation by persons with disabilities in the recreation program and to determine if skills learned at the recreation site are being generalized to the home. Community recreation personnel could also help to create a community advisory board made up of key players in the integration process. Recreation personnel can be advocates of accessible community leisure services, as well as personal advocates for specific individuals with disabilities, at local government meetings and state legislation sessions when decisions concerning community recreation funding or service delivery are being made. Additionally, personnel may plan to participate in advocacy group meetings or to serve on associated task forces such as ARC Leisure Advisory Committees. Clearer communication through networking will occur if participants express care, concern, and understanding of others.

Negative Attitudes

Persons with highly visible disabilities such as mobility impairments, cerebral palsy, or profound mental retardation may be less valued than nondisabled persons because of their disabilities. Nondisabled individuals may accentuate these differences in the manner in which they interact, or choose not to interact, with persons with disabilities. Included among the variety of unpleasant behaviors that may be manifested by a nondisabled person toward a disabled person are: paternalistic behaviors (e.g., head patting, age-inappropriate talk, excessive praise), avoidance (not acknowledging their presence), or negative behaviors such as mocking or name calling. Since negative attitudes are, perhaps, the most pervasive of obstacles, it is extremely important that significant efforts be made to arrive at solutions that minimize these barriers. One general suggestion is to have local advocacy groups such as the Association for Retarded Citizens, the Multiple Sclerosis Society, or parent groups present workshops on disability awareness. Professional/educational associations such as the Division of Recreation, Park, and Leisure Studies at local universities could present workshops, conferences, and courses on leisure and disability issues. Also, it might be helpful for recreation personnel to visit neighborhood group homes, nursing homes, and "natural" homes of disabled persons in order to understand how persons with disabilities experience their lives (i.e., through observation, naturalistic inquiry, interviews, surveys). Agency supervisors should make every effort to educate and to train staff on the importance of demonstrating accepting and caring behaviors to all people. Hiring qualified individuals who have disabilities as staff is another useful way to help dispell negative attitudes, because these individuals can serve as appropriate role models to other individuals with disabilities. An additional suggestion would be to have disabled volunteers lead awareness programs or training workshops. These activities have proven to be effective in heightening staff awareness of the needs of special population groups.

Ineffective Service Systems

While community recreation professionals may support the tenets of normalization and integration, often the park and recreation systems within which they operate can confound their efforts by being slow to change traditional service delivery processes. Ineffective service systems may result from a combination of obstacles in the environment, including barriers of omission, and rules and regulation barriers. Often it is what is not provided by a service system that limits participation by persons with disabilities. Because persons with disabilities are a minority and generally not as visible in the community, they may not be remembered or included when new programs and services are being developed by recreation departments. The result: barriers of omission.

Rules and regulations are typically developed by persons who are nondisabled, and who seldom take into account the needs of persons with disabilities. The result is that participation by persons with disabilities in recreation is often limited. Examples include:

1. People in wheelchairs must often sit in aisles and walkways when attending events at inaccessible theatres and sports complexes. This action is against fire regulations.
2. Most games, whether board games or athletics, have prescribed rules for participants or else penalties are imposed. Rather than deviating from the rules, persons with disabilities frequently choose to become spectators rather than participants.
3. The separate restrooms and locker rooms provided for men or women can present problems for the disabled person whose attendant is not of the same sex.

There are many solutions to barriers imposed by ineffective service systems. Administrators and recreation programmers should make a careful assessment of their roles and responsibilities to determine the optimal approach to overcome these significant barriers. For example, professionals can work to become aware of the unique needs of persons with disabilities by examining the present system of leisure service delivery to identify obstacles created by service gaps. Also, professionals can take "preventive measures" by actively implementing a systematic process for service delivery to all persons with and without disabilities. This will prevent obstacles from occurring in the first place. Additionally, they can develop and assume an active role on a Community Advisory Board to enhance awareness and interpersonal and interagency communication through networking with schools, municipal park and recreation departments, and community education agencies. Board members could use brainstorming meetings as a forum to exchange ideas on program delivery and activities. This process will be beneficial for a number of reasons: participation and advocacy may be increased; professional staff, educators, students, and advocacy groups such as the Association for Retarded Citizens may be encouraged to do research to examine the effectiveness of implementing the integration strategies within the Accessible Community Leisure Service Process; and service providers could receive current information on consumer needs with regard to programmatic and architectural accessibility.

There are a variety of ways to advertise recreation and leisure services in order to ensure that people are aware that services are open and accessible. These methods include: advertising on gas, water, or electric bills or in bank statement envelopes; inserting program brochures into newspapers and advocacy group newsletters; creating public service announcements to be broadcast on the radio and TV; inviting media coverage of integrated programs; or leaving brochures with neighborhood businesses such as laundromats, grocery stores, or banks for distribution.

Finally, a concern expressed by parent groups to PIRC staff during their study is worth noting: that the "legalese" nondiscrimination statements on program brochures are impersonal and tend to discourage participation. Therefore, agencies must develop a more personal nondiscrimination statement to be included in all program brochures and advertisements. Examples may be found in Appendix C. Recreation professionals may also need to take the initiative to contact local and statewide social service agencies, especially those that provide services to persons with disabilities, for assistance in locating potential consumers of leisure services. Also, a recent concern of recreation and parks professionals has been in the area of liability and risk management. The recreation professional may wish to investigate current insurance and liability coverage to determine if policies can be obtained to cover programs that employ volunteers, and that use specialized equipment and vehicles.

INDIVIDUAL BARRIERS

Skill Deficits

Because persons with disabilities have traditionally been excluded from opportunities to socially interact with nondisabled peers, they often lack the interpersonal skills that promote positive and appropriate interactions within community recreation settings. The community recreation setting is an ideal place for an individual with disabilities to gain social skills and, perhaps, to develop genuine friendships within the context of an enjoyable recreation activity.

Additionally, persons with disabilities lack sufficient opportunities to develop expertise in recreation activities. Even if they possess the fundamental social, motor, and cognitive skills to participate in an activity, persons with disabilities may not have sufficient opportunities to engage in these activities. If persons with disabilities do not possess sufficient leisure-related skills and are not being taught those skills by recreation staff, they may be relegated exclusively to activities that require passive, low-level skills or that are age-inappropriate (e.g., adults participating in cut and paste activity rather than in an art appreciation class). Because a person may be perceived as being "not-ready-for" integrated programs due to his or her skill deficits, he or she may participate very little or not at all in community recreation settings.

Because leisure skill instruction is vitally important, the authors suggest several solutions for overcoming obstacles related to skill deficits. Teachers and parents or careproviders should be encouraged to provide social and leisure skills training in age-appropriate, leisure activities at school, at home, and in community settings. Also, programs should be designed to encourage socialization among participants, for example, through cooperative grouping arrangement strategy, table games, and noncompetitive team games. Appropriate social skills (e.g., greetings, shaking hands, social praise) and leisure skills should be modeled during the program in the recreation setting and should be consistently practiced with participants at home and throughout the length of the program. Through participation in integrated programs, persons with disabilities could learn skills by imitating their non-disabled peers. Nondisabled children and adults can be taught to be "Special Friends" using narrated slide presentations, puppets, and question/discussion sessions. These volunteer advocates may be needed as facilitators of socialization and leisure skill development in programs to enhance integration. Structured programs over 1 hour in length may need to have breaks part of the way through the activity to enable participants to have opportunities to informally socialize with peers.

Finally, prerequisite core skills, those that are basic and vital to participation, should not be exclusionary in nature. Therefore, participants could develop core skills within the context of age-appropriate activity. Thus, activities could be task analyzed to determine the participant's strengths, general abilities, and skill deficits. Programs could be designed to be sufficiently flexible to permit participants to enter them at different skill levels, yet offer opportunities to improve over time (e.g., bowling, video games, art, music, aerobics).

Dependency on Others

Whether limited by disability, by restrictive social service systems, or by overprotective families and acquaintances, persons with disabilities either lose, or never gain the ability to function independently in the community. Personal growth and development are not achievable if persons with disabilities become "handicapped" by a lack of control over their environments. Therefore, they become deficient in their abilities to make decisions and choices and must depend on significant others to have their recreation needs met. The following provide some guidelines for decreasing or eliminating barriers caused by dependency.

First, persons with disabilities should be accorded the same respect and understanding as anyone else. One should relate to the person with disabilities in an age-appropriate manner; one should never "talk down" to the person. Give the participant opportunities to make decisions. If necessary, provide decision-making training to individuals with disabilities (Dattilo & Rusch, 1985). Second, one should encourage family members and care-providers to allow the individual with disabilities to independently use a community recreation setting with only minimal assistance. Other persons should assist only if necessary. Third, the recreation professional can determine, through use of the Environmental Analysis Inventory, those times when personal assistance for the disabled individual is absolutely necessary for such tasks as toileting, dressing, self-care, and eating. Program modifications can then be made that permit appropriate levels of interdependence while allowing opportunities for maximum independence.

Health and Fitness

The health and fitness needs of a person with disabilities are generally determined by the nature of his or her disability. For example, persons with multiple sclerosis may fatigue easily, and persons with quadriplegia are susceptible to hypothermia due to poor blood circulation. Endurance, stamina, and strength to participate in a variety of activites may be severely limited due to health and fitness barriers.

There are several strategies a recreation professional can use to assess the health and fitness needs of potential participants to maximize their safety, welfare, and enjoyment during the recreation experience. Initially, and if it is an obvious concern, the recreation professional should discuss with participants, physicians, advocacy groups, parents or care-providers, and other pertinent allied health professionals, the general health concerns of persons with disabilities. If the professional requires information on a specific participant's health status during registration, the following should be considered: extent and level of disability; current medications; fitness level (e.g., flexibility, coordination, strength, balance); emergency notification procedures; and allergies. Throughout the duration of the recreation program, instructional and program staff should monitor physical status (e.g., skin color, fatigue, breathing) of persons with disabilities (e.g., multiple sclerosis, diabetes, or epilepsy) who have been determined, through the initial assessments, to be at some health or fitness risk. Prior to enrollment in any active sports program, participants should undergo a physical examination by their physician. Also, recreation professionals could contact the American Red Cross and/or specific advocacy groups to determine what, if any, appropriate measures should be taken with persons with disabilities concerning administration of cardio-pulmonary resuscitation (CPR) or first aid. When in doubt, always ask the participant with the disability first.

Lack of Knowledge

If persons lack information about community recreation programs and services, or knowledge of the support systems available to help make recreation opportunities accessible, their participation will be inhibited or nonexistent. A leisure education program, sponsored by the recreation agency or initiated in collaboration with a school system or community education organization, could be instituted to develop awareness of accessible and integrated recreation programming. Facilitating a leisure education program could be a primary responsibility of the TRS consultant. Another suggestion would be to develop a resource booklet that describes integrated and specialized community recreation programs. This could be a specific task of the Community Advisory Board, who could then disseminate it to persons with disabilities. Other suggestions include the development of a seasonal program brochure outlining all programs offered, including descriptions, dates, times, fees, and skill and clothing requirements. Other suggested activities include advertising programs in the local media (e.g., community newspapers), and posting program brochures or flyers in public places (e.g., grocery stores) that are frequented by many people, including persons with disabilities. Finally, volunteers could be trained to serve as communication links between community recreation centers and other agencies serving persons with disabilities such as residential facilities, day activity programs, or counseling services to make sure that program and resource information is being shared.

SUMMARY

It has become increasingly apparent that the philosophical, theoretical, and legislative support for the principle of normalization and its chief corollary, integration, provide strong support for community recreation services to be accessible to persons with disabilities. While the mandate for accessible services seems clear, there continue to be any number of barriers that may impede progress towards achieving the goal of integrated, accessible leisure services in the community. Society's negative role perceptions of persons with disabilities, as well as its low tolerance for individual differences, increase the likelihood that obstacles such as community and organizational stigma and negative attitudes will continue to decrease leisure service delivery and to diminish rates of participation by persons with disabilities. However, a new and more positive view that the disabled individual is also a developing human being may help change societal perceptions. A change toward more open and accessible service systems could be a reflection of these perceptual changes.

The primary thrust of this chapter is to underscore the work of various field investigators who, through a variety of survey methods, have identified persistent obstacles to the community recreation integration of persons with disabilities. Several obstacles are discussed in the chapter and are then categorized. Barriers are attributed either to the individuals, themselves, or to any number of external, environmental factors. Environmental factors are cited as the leading cause of inaccessible and nonintegrated recreation services. Each obstacle or barrier is addressed individually with a number of solutions proposed.

It is the authors' firm belief that many of these obstacles could be avoided or eliminated if community recreation agencies incorporate the strategies presented in this text to change and improve existing leisure service delivery systems. Ongoing communication and collaboration with key others will ensure that the recreation needs of persons with disabilities are being met in the community, where physical and social integration with nondisabled peers is stressed and the intent of the normalization principle is realized. Community recreation professionals are also reminded to take a "proactive" rather than a reactive approach to systems and personnel change, and to avoid making the erroneous assumption that barriers to integration and accessibility are created or caused by the individual characteristics of persons with disabilities.

Chapter 8

Integrating Community Recreation
Exemplary Programs

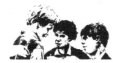

T he responsibility for ensuring appropriate recreation activity participation by persons with disabilities does not rest solely with community residential care-providers, teachers, and families. Due to deinstitutionalization and the normalization movement, there are increasing numbers of individuals with disabilities living in community environments. Because of this trend, the responsibility for the provision of leisure services has increasingly shifted to community organizations such as municipal park and recreation agencies. Thus, in order to optimally meet the needs of persons with disabilities, the responsibility for improving and expanding recreation services in park and recreation, community education, and school environments should rest not only with educators, and families, but with professionals as well. However, if responsibilities are spread too widely among agencies, there is the possibility that no one organization will guarantee that services are carried out. Additionally, lack of communication could result, leading to redundancy or gaps in services. Thus, it is advisable to designate a lead agency to assume overall programming responsibility, to ensure that comprehensive recreation services are provided in an efficient and effective manner. Services can be provided on the basis of the age groups of community residents with disabilities, or on the basis of available community resources. For example, the responsibility for educating young people (up to age 21) in recreation and leisure skills can be assumed by public schools and by specific community recreation agencies such as public recreation and park departments and community education agencies. Or, responsibility could fall with the agency best equipped in terms of facilities, staff, and funds to provide special recreation services. However, the success of dividing responsibilities depends upon the quality of communication among the agencies (Putnam, Werder, & Schleien, 1985; Schleien & Werder, 1985).

If, for any of a variety of reasons, local agencies fail to take responsibility for providing quality recreation services for persons with disabilities, one agency should assume leadership. Robb (1979), in discussing the movement of persons with disabilities from institutions to community settings, suggested that park and recreation agencies should assume responsibility for delivering recreation services. Since it is the public recreation and park department's responsibility to meet the needs of all citizens within the political jurisdiction, it would follow that this agency should assume a primary leadership role in the trans-agency model of special recreation service delivery. As a leading agency, park and recreation departments can bridge the gap between public schools—which provide prerequisite recreation skill instruction—and community settings where participants with disabilities can generalize leisure skills in actual recreation situations. In this vital role, park and recreation departments can provide practice and experience opportunities needed by persons with disabilities if they are to develop leisure preferences and refine recreational skills.

Normalization calls for the delivery of services in environments under circumstances that are as culturally normal as possible. That is to say, leisure services programs for persons with disabililties should include a broad array of activities and programs similar to those available to the nondisabled residents of the community. Integration with nondisabled peers can lessen the social isolation experienced by many disabled persons and can provide more positive role models than those present in handicapped-only programs. This book has so far been devoted to instructional techniques to prevent and overcome barriers to community recreation participation by persons with disabilities. However, the true test of community integration, as shall be argued below, is the success with which the participant with disabilities uses recreation and social skills alongside nondisabled participants in community settings.

Research documenting the benefits of recreation activity participation for individuals with disabilities is reviewed in this chapter. It must be emphasized, however, that meaningful participation in recreation activities is also recognized as a basic human right. The research findings appear promising on the contribution of active recreation programs to the enhancement of community integration and to the improvement in behavior functioning of persons with disabilities. Despite limited work in this area, it seems obvious—indeed, essential—that the scope of research and program development needs to be upgraded, and that opportunities for constructive recreation participation for children and adults with disabilities need to be increased. In a society that places so much focus upon education and vocational training, it is important that persons with disabilities have sufficient opportunities to express and develop their skills through participation rather than in isolation. This chapter reports the procedures and results of programs that unequivocally answer the question: "Could persons with disabilities successfully participate in integrated community leisure services?" The authors respond to this question with a strong "Yes".

EXEMPLARY PROGRAM I

Adult Leisure Education for the Independent Use of a Commmunity Recreation Center

Stuart J. Schleien and Angela Larson

As previously institutionalized individuals return to community environments, therapeutic recreation specialists, community recreation professionals, community educators, and special education classroom teachers (via therapeutic recreation consultation) will increasingly be asked to provide recreation and leisure skills training to persons with special needs. This demand for recreation skill training will require recreation services agencies to develop functional, age-appropriate recreation and leisure education for the generalization of skills to natural environments (Schleien, Certo, & Muccino, 1984).

The purpose of this study was to implement and evaluate a leisure education training program designed to teach adults with severe mental retardation the complete and functional use of a community recreation center. Since these individuals resided in a group home just six blocks from the park, thus eliminating the need to arrange transportation, this program was deemed viable by group home and park board staff. Community recreation center use by the nondisabled citizens of the neighborhood was utilized in this program as the training standard.

METHODS

Setting and Participants

Two adults with severe mental retardation served as participants. The community recreation center in Minneapolis, MN, which was the intervention site, offered leisure skills training, recreational equipment, and a social environment that afforded opportunities for peer interactions.

The participants, Charles and Lawrence, were selected for the program based on their preference for participation, their need for appropriate leisure skills, and their availability for participation. Charles, age 29, had Down syndrome and had received an IQ score of 23 on the Stanford-Binet Intelligence Scale. His speech was incomprehensible, due to a cleft palate, and he used sign language only when prompted. His leisure skill repertoire consisted of placing dashes in notebooks and paging through pamphlets of information. Lawrence, age 27, also had Down syndrome. His IQ, according to the Stanford-Binet Intelligence Scale, was 33. He spoke in short phrases, seldom using sentences. His leisure repertoire consisted of listening to music and singing in front of a mirror. Both participants demonstrated adequate dynamic balance and coordination during activities but found it difficult to comprehend and apply rules to the games and activities. Prior to this study, recreation opportunities for the two participants typically consisted of attending segregated dances and segregated social clubs as part of a group that included all six residents of the group home where they lived.

During an initial visit to the community recreation center, a general verbal cue (e.g., "Use the recreation center.") was given to the participants by the instructor as a pre-baseline measure. Charles and Lawrence immediately walked to the "tot lot" area and played on the animal springs and animal swings. Even though the recreation center was only six blocks away, none of the residents from the group home had ever used the center during the 8 years they had resided in the neighborhood. The participants were believed to be familiar with simple playground equipment (e.g., animal springs, seesaw) through exposure to similar equipment at the institution where they had lived prior to the group home.

Program Goals

The goals of the program included: 1) to walk appropriately with a peer to and from the recreation center, 2) to select a chronologically age-appropriate activity and to participate in the activity appropriately at the recreation center, and 3) to generalize acquired skills in choice making and appropriate recreation behavior to another community recreation center in the city.

Procedure

The program was implemented during 3-hour sessions once a week for 20 weeks. A multiple baseline design (Hersen & Barlow, 1976) was used to teach three recreation skills in succession throughout the duration of the program. Methods incorporated into leisure education instruction to facilitate generalization and independent participation included conducting sessions on varying days and at different times of the day. In addition, sessions were conducted over two seasons in order to expose participants to different recreational equipment. For example, in the fall, participants can use basketballs; in the winter, they can walk in the snow using snowshoes.

An environmental analysis inventory was conducted to determine the skills and procedures necessary for Charles and Lawrence to participate in the community recreation center independently and in a fashion similar to their nonhandicapped peers. From this information the task analyses for three center activities were derived: playing fooseball, selecting a game from the check-out desk and playing the game, and walking to and from the recreation center.

Instruction

Each instructional session consisted of two training periods following by a nonreinforced data probe. During the nonreinforced probe, a general verbal cue such as "Play fooseball" was given to the participant; the number of steps of the task analysis performed independently was recorded. Each instructional session began at the step of the task analysis that had not been performed correctly or independently for two previous consecutive sessions.

An instructional cue hierarchy/error correction procedure was employed to facilitate learning of the three leisure skills. This consisted of giving the verbal cue for the step being taught (e.g., "Charles, release the ball onto the table.") and socially reinforcing the correct response by, for example, verbal praise or a pat on the back. If the verbal prompt did not result in an independent response, the verbal cue was repeated. This cue would be accompanied by a demonstration of the appropriate behavior and followed by a verbal prompt to "Try again." If the desired behavior was exhibited, the participant was socially reinforced. If not, the instructor again repeated the verbal cue and physically prompted the participant with the correct response followed by social reinforcement for the prompted response.

To facilitate participant selection of recreation equipment, an illustrated booklet of available recreation equipment was compiled and left at the check-out desk of the recreation center. By pointing to the desired item in this book, the participants could select equipment without gesturing the motions of a particular activity as they were accustomed to doing. No other special modifications were made during the program.

Instruction continued until the participant was able to perform each step of the activity task analysis for three consecutive sessions with only the general verbal cue. Generalization probes were conducted in three other community recreation centers in Minneapolis during a 3-month period after instruction ended. No social reinforcement was delivered during generalization probes.

All three recreational skills were mastered within the 20-week period. More specifically, Skill 1 was mastered after 13 weeks of instruction (Session 17) by both participants; Skill 2 was mastered by Charles after 8 weeks of instruction, and by Lawrence after 9 weeks (Sessions 17 and 18, respectively); Skill 3 was mastered by both participants after only 6 weeks of instruction (Session 20).

Nonreinforced generalization probes were conducted in three different community parks throughout the city. In all but one generalization probe, 100% criterion was met by both participants. During the session in which 100% criterion was not met, Lawrence did not play fooseball until 10 goals were scored and the game completed. The three generalization probes were not conducted on the third skill (that of walking to the recreation center independently) because the community parks used as generalization sites were not within walking distance from the group home.

Finally, a 7-month follow-up maintenance probe, with only a verbal cue provided by the careprovider to prompt the participant's use of the recreation center, was conducted at the original training site. During the maintenance probe, 100% and 95% of the steps for the first skill, fooseball, were completed independently by Charles and Lawrence, respectively. Upon entering the recreation center, Lawrence approached the counter at the same time that a nondisabled peer was returning a fooseball. Lawrence picked up the fooseball from the counter and, therefore, did not request to check it out as depicted in the task analysis. In the second skill, (game selection), Charles independently achieved 95% of the steps of the task analysis. At this time, Charles and Lawrence were the only visitors in the park. Lawrence only engaged in his selected activity for 8 of the required minimum 10 minutes and thus achieved 90% of the steps of the task analysis. In the third skill, walking to center, both participants successfully performed 100% of the task analysis during the 7-month follow-up maintenance probe.

CONCLUDING REMARKS

During baseline probes, the nontrained, unskilled participants immediately demonstrated a preference for the chronologically age-inappropriate playground equipment (i.e., animal swings). At that time, interactions with nondisabled peers were nonexistent. Only following leisure skill education did the participants select activities similar to those that other young adults engage in. During participation in these activities, such as fooseball and table tennis, nondisabled persons concurrently using the recreation center initiated interactions and joined them in the activity. The findings suggest that personal preferences were governed by an existing repertoire of skills and past exposure to the activities. These data are consistent with findings by Birenbaum and Re (1979) and Matthews (1982) in which differences in recreational preferences and participation between persons with and without mental retardation have been found and interpreted differently. When persons with mental retardation do not take part in particular recreational activities, it is usually for the same reasons that nonhandicapped individuals would have for not participating.

Results demonstrated that individuals with severe mental retardation could: 1) acquire age-appropriate leisure skills to independently use a recreation center, 2) utilize a neighborhood center in the absence of the residential careprovider, and 3) effectively interact with community recreation center staff concerning personal preferences of recreational activities.

Local community recreation and leisure programs and services are either limited or are nonexistent for many individuals with severe disabilities. As a majority of persons with disabilities reside in the community, and not in segregated public facilities, they become part of the community citizenry and can be expected to engage in recreation and to use other community services alongside their neighbors and peers. Even though individuals with disabilities reside in proximity to a variety of recreational facilities and resources, their participation in programs with nondisabled peers has not always occurred. This lack of participation could be due to the dearth of recreational support skills to independently participate in an integrated program, the lack of careprovider support to enable residents to use community facilities, the scarcity of adequately trained staff in generic recreational facilities, and to attitudinal barriers to community recreation participation. Transportation to the community program is often an additional barrier. Teaching individuals to independently utilize local, neighborhood recreation facilities (i.e., community recreation centers and parks, bowling alleys, movie theaters, roller skating rinks, sports stadiums, community education, or youth service agencies) can help to eliminate this attitudinal barrier. With newly acquired recreation (e.g., fooseball) and related support skills (e.g., walking to the center), an individual who was previously dependent upon special transportation arrangements could participate locally in an independent or partial fashion (Ford et al., 1984).

EXEMPLARY PROGRAM II

The Effects of Integrating Children With Autism Into a Physical Activity and Recreation Setting

Stuart J. Schleien, March L. Krotee, Theresa Mustonen,
Bonnie Kelterborn, and Anita D. Schermer

The deprivation of systematic physical education and leisure experiences, combined with the lack of opportunity for integrated physical learning experiences, can restrict the disabled child from developing basic motoric patterns, psychomotor competency, psychosocial awareness, and physical strength and fitness (Barrow, 1971; Krotee, 1980; Krotee & Bart, 1986). Similarly, this lack of opportunity denies the nondisabled child the opportunity to gain knowledge, understanding, and appreciation of the disabled individual through personal contact in a nonrestrictive, integrated environment. Direct contact and frequent interaction between disabled individuals and their nondisabled peers have been shown to stimulate the formation of more positive attitudes (Hamilton & Anderson, 1983; Handlers & Austin, 1980; Voeltz, 1982).

One way to bring about these face-to-face learning experiences is through participation in integrated physical activity and recreation programs. Clearly, it should be a goal of the recreation and physical education professions to provide such planned, positive learning environments in integrated and cooperative settings. Such settings may potentially enable each individual to develop to his or her fullest potential. It is with this objective in mind that the following exploratory study was formulated. The focus of the study was to examine the effects of participation in a planned physical activity program on the social, leisure, and adaptive behavior skills of children with autism. A secondary goal of the study was to assess the attitudes of nondisabled peers toward the children with autism involved in the program.

METHODS

Setting and Participants

The subjects involved in the study consisted of two severely disabled autistic children age 8 years, 5 months (female S[1]) and 11 years, 2 months (male, S[2]) as well as 67 nondisabled children ages 7–12 who were enrolled in the University of Minnesota Children's Sport Fitness School (CSFS). S[1]'s overall mental age, 27–31 months, was classified by the Psychoeducational Profile (PEP), a developmental assessment tool for evaluating children with autism and other disabilities (Schopler & Reichler, 1979). S^2 received a PEP score of 35–38 months.

The two autistic subject's total scores on the Topeka Association for Retarded Citizens assessment system (TARC), a behavioral assessment inventory for children with severe disabilities concerning education-related skills (Sailor & Mix, 1975), were $S^1 = 124$ and $S^2 = 151$ respectively, out of a possible 194. S^1's TARC skills assessment included scores of 41 in self-help skills, 46 in motor skills, 14 in communication skills, and 23 in social ability, while S^2's TARC rating included a 46 in self-help skills, 48 in motor skills, 27 in communication skills, and 30 in social ability.

S^1's target excess behaviors, as measured by the Social Interaction Observation System: SIOS (Voeltz, Kishi, & Brennan, 1981), a multi-variable observation system, included crying, moaning, and tantrums characterized by thrashing of arms and throwing the body to the floor. S^2's target excess behaviors included grabbing objects from peers without provocation, screaming in high-pitched tones, and self-injurious behavior, including repetitive striking of the chin. Each subject attended a special wing for autistic children in a Minneapolis, Minnesota public elementary school during the regular school year. Additionally, each student was enrolled for the summer in the University of Minnesota's Children's Sport Fitness School (CSFS) together with 67 nondisabled students from the metropolitan area.

The setting for the study, a 3-week summer program sponsored by the School of Physical Education and Recreation at the University of Minnesota, was the CSFS. The program was conducted at four proximate locations on the University campus: 1) a large gymnasium with various standardized and modified courts (e.g., badminton, basketball, volleyball) marked on the floor; 2) a smaller gymnastics room equipped with mats, mirrors, balance beam, side horse, parallel and horizontal bars; 3) an adjacent outdoor sports field, and 4) a swimming pool.

Supplemental equipment appropriate to the planned activity, including balls, bats, rackets, scooters, and nets were provided by the CSFS. Classrooms, human performance laboratories, tennis, squash, and racketball courts, as well as an indoor field house, were also made available for utilization.

Procedures

The two autistic children who were chosen for the study were selected in part because their parents expressed the desire to enroll their children and have them participate in the program. Parents were briefed regarding the nature of the integrated program and research study. Each subject's physical activity and recreational preferences were identified by their parents, the adapted physical education teacher, and the special education classroom teacher. All of the children with and without disabilities were registered, and standard uniforms were distributed to the participants.

During the first week, an environmental analysis inventory was conducted to determine the physical activity skill and behavioral requirements for the subjects with autism. As part of the ecological analysis conducted over a period of 2 days, the nondisabled children were observed in the four settings: large gymnasium, small gymnastics room, outdoor sports field, and swimming pool. Using this inventory and a preprogram and postprogram attitude acceptance scale, functionally age-appropriate skills and social performance levels and attitudes were assessed to obtain reference points for the expected integrative performance level of the autistic children.

Prior to the start of the program, a "Special Friends" audiovisual presentation was made to the nondisabled children and the CSFS staff. The presentation, which depicted children with severe disabilities interacting with their "special friend" peers in regular classroom settings, was shown separately to each of the school's three age groups. A brief question/answer and discussion period followed the presentation. At that time, the children were informed that two severely disabled autistic children would be enrolled in the 3-week CSFS program. "Special Friends" were solicited to assist the autistic children, and those children who first volunteered to assist, and who matched the disabled children in age and gender, were selected as "buddies." Three buddies were selected for each disabled child—one friend for each week.

Analysis of Data

In order to determine the effects of participation in an integrated physical activity and recreation program on the behavior patterns of severely disabled autistic children, a number of evaluations were made. An attitude acceptance scale was administered before and after the program intervention in order to assess changes in acceptance by nondisabled participants toward their autistic peers. Observations of the participants' behavior, including appropriate and inappropriate play behavior and orientation to play objects and peers, were assessed using the SIOS system and were statistically treated to determine if significant differences in behavior from Week 1 to Week 3 occurred. In addition, t-tests were applied to the data to determine if significant differences in attitudes and behavior were exhibited before and after program intervention.

Attitude Acceptance Scale

An attitude acceptance scale for grades 3–6 (Voeltz, 1980; Voeltz, 1982), measuring social contact willingness, deviance consequation, and actual contact was administered to the nondisabled children before and after implementation of the integrated physical activity and recreation program. Thirty-four randomly varied positive and negative statements concerning individual differences and disabling conditions were presented in paper form and were also read aloud to the children. In response, the children marked "yes," "no," or "maybe", depending on whether they agreed, disagreed, or were not sure about each statement. The investigators addressed any questions raised by the students.

Behavioral Observations

Observations of participants' behavior were recorded of interactions between the disabled children, "Special Friends," and the environment through employment of the Social Interaction Observation System. The SIOS system was used to record four major categories of behavior and was adapted from the original instrument that recorded seven behavioral categories, including information on over 44 individual behaviors for disabled and nondisabled children (Voeltz, et al., 1981). Participants' behaviors in the areas of appropriate and inappropriate play, and orientation to play objects and peers were observed and recorded for both autistic and nondisabled children.

A fourth category, individual target behaviors (i.e., crying and throwing tantrums for S^1; hitting of the chin, screaming, and grabbing objects for S^2) was noted and recorded. These behaviors were identified by the subject's respective special education classroom teachers. A target behavior was recorded if it occurred at any time during the 10-second observation period.

Program Implementation

The 3-week physical activity and recreation program, scheduled between 1:00 and 4:00 p.m., consisted of three 40-minute activity periods that included cooperative sports and games, swimming, gymnastics, and an open recreation session. The CSFS participants were divided into three age groups (7–8, 9–10, 11–12) and received instruction in physical activity and recreational skills, as well as health and fitness concepts. The first activity period was followed by a 10-minute break; the second activity session was followed by a 15-minute break; and the third activity was followed by 30 minutes of supervised open play and/or individualized instruction. Each age group rotated from activity to activity throughout the afternoon, but merged during the open recreation period.

Recreational activities for each group were generally located in the outdoor sports field, the large gymnasium, the small gymnastics room, or in the swimming pool, depending on the weather and the particular activity planned for that day. These physical and recreational activities included cooperative, competitive, and individualized play and games, including modifications of traditional sports such as volleyball, badminton, soccer, and floor hockey, as well as fundamental movement, gymnastic, and aquatic skills. Acquisition and improvement of leisure and motor skills and cooperative play were emphasized. The planned activity program also included exercises promoting awareness of such factors as heart rate, blood pressure, body composition, relaxation, stress management, posture, and nutrition.

Results

Each subject was observed in three physical education and recreation-specific activities for ten 15-second intervals per day throughout the duration of the investigation. Paired t-tests were employed to determine if significant differences existed between Week 1 and Week 3 observations on the following four variables: appropriate play, inappropriate play, orientation to play objects and peers, and target behaviors.

Subject 1 The mean number of intervals during which S^1 played appropriately increased in all three activities from Week 1 to Week 3. During Week 1, her behavior varied daily, but over time, her appropriate behavior stabilized. S^1's inappropriate play decreased from Week 1 to Week 3. In orientation to play objects and peers, the mean number of intervals increased over the weeks for all three activities. S^1's target behaviors for two of three physical activity and recreational settings were found to decrease, but in a nonsignificant manner (i.e., gymnastics and swimming), with no recorded change in the sports setting.

Subject 2 The mean number of intervals during which S^2 played appropriately increased significantly ($p < .05$) in all three activities from Week 1 to Week 3. At the same time, his inappropriate play decreased significantly in all three activities. His orientation to play objects and peers increased dramatically from Week 1 to Week 3 in all 3 activities. Target behaviors were also observed to decrease significantly in gymnastics. Target behaviors were found to increase, but at a nonsignificant level, in the sports setting. In swimming, target behaviors decreased slightly from Week 1 to Week 3.

The attitude acceptance scale administered to the nonhandicapped peers revealed a nonsignificant ($p < .05$) but positive change ($\overline{X}_{pre} = 35.4$, $\overline{X}_{post} = 37.8$). This result may have been influenced by the unusually positive pretest measures regarding acceptance of children with disabilities by the nondisabled participants of the CSFS as compared to the national pretest norm ($\overline{X}$ pre = 26.6) and posttest norm ($\overline{X}$ post = 27.7).

CONCLUDING REMARKS

The results of the study indicated that appropriate play behavior and orientation to play objects and peers positively increased in all of the CSFS children's physical activity and recreational settings. Appropriate play behavior was found to increase significantly in two of three physical activity and recreational settings for S^1 and also increased in each of the three settings for S^2. Significant increases occurred for the most part in the subject's preferred physical activity (S^1's preferred activity was swimming; S^2's preferred activity was gymnastics).

Concomitant with the positive increases in appropriate play behavior and orientation to play objects and peers, the study revealed substantial decreases in inappropriate play behavior for each subject. Significant decreases in inappropriate play behavior were found in swimming, the most preferred activity of Subject 1, and in all of Subject 2's physical activity and recreational settings.

The positive behavioral and attitudinal changes revealed in this study suggest that the integration of children with and without severe disabilities into physical activity and recreational settings is a viable goal. However, it would be remiss to attempt to integrate the severely disabled individual without implementing certain program strategies to ensure that there will be positive physical and psychosocial integrative results. The crucial program strategies employed in this investigation included the concern for personal activity preferences by the severely disabled participants, and the employment of cooperative group structures and the "Special Friends" training techniques.

The results of the study suggest that integration of students with severe disabilities into physical activity and recreational settings is both feasible and beneficial for all participants. Not only did positive and significant behavior changes occur in regard to appropriate and inappropriate play behavior, in orientation to play objects and peers, and in target behaviors, but acceptance by nondisabled participants toward their severely disabled peers changed in a positive direction as measured by the attitude acceptance scale. These positive integrative experiences support the argument that more recreation and physical activity settings as well as other dynamic social environs should open their doors to individuals with severe disabilities and other persons with special needs.

EXEMPLARY PROGRAM III

Using Applied Behavior Analysis Approaches to Integrate Children With Severe Handicaps Into an Outdoor Education Environment

Stuart J. Schleien, John E. Rynders, and Theresa Mustonen

An integrated outdoor education experience offers important learning opportunities to campers with and without disabilities alike. In an integrated environment, campers with disabilities can improve their recreational skills and their functional learning and socialization abilities as well (Mitchell, Robberson, & Obley, 1977; Schleien & Ray, 1986; Wehman & Schleien, 1981). Nondisabled campers, in interacting positively with individuals who have severe disabilities, can develop an appreciation of companions with disabilities (Brown, Branston, Hamre-Nietupski, Wilcox, & Gruenwald, 1979; Voeltz & Brennan, 1984), and disabled persons can develop the ability to estimate their own self-worth more realistically (Donder & Nietupski, 1981). In spite of these potential benefits, only a handful of reports describe the virtues of integrated camping and outdoor education experiences (Byers, 1979; Carter, 1954; Carter & Farley, 1978; Feldman, Wodarski, & Flax, 1975; Flax & Peters, 1969; Hayes, 1969; Lupton, 1972; Rosen, 1959; Rosen, 1974; Shea, 1977).

In the study reported, the impact of an integrated camping experience on the social, leisure, and attitudinal development of children with and without severe disabilities was evaluated.

METHODS

Setting and Participants

Three children described as having severe disabling conditions participated in the outdoor education program. All three lived at home with their parents and attended self-contained special education classes in regular elementary schools. All were selected on the basis of their scores on the TARC, a brief adaptive behavior rating with a possible maximum score of 196, and their parents' willingness to allow participation in an integrated camping experience. The norm reference was a group of moderately and severely disabled children, ages 3–16 (Sailor & Mix, 1975).

One of the children, Molly, was a 9-year-old girl diagnosed as autistic. She did not actively seek interactions with adults, except to sign for assistance. She also tended to ignore her peers. Molly needed assistance with personal hygiene and dressing and exhibited tantruming behavior from time to time. She was nonverbal, although she had a limited sign language repertoire. Her score on the TARC was 130.

Mary, an 11-year-old girl, had severe mental retardation and a profound bilateral hearing loss that was partially corrected with a binaural hearing aid. She was able to follow one-step directions and seemed to understand simple phrases. Mary did not actively seek interactions with peers or adults. Her interactions with others were described as appropriate, although she responded to adults more than to her peers. She needed reminders to toilet herself and required assistance with personal hygiene and dressing. She achieved a TARC score of 123.

John, a 9-year-old boy, had severe mental retardation and arrested hydrocephaly. Although John was nonverbal, he tried to imitate spoken words and sounds, and had an extensive sign language repertoire. He also cried easily. John interacted with adults and peers, although he tended to seek out adults for interactions more than peers. He required little assistance with dressing, grooming or personal hygiene, though he did require prompting to initiate and maintain these skills. His score on the TARC was 142.

Participants in the study who were without disabilities consisted of three boys and five girls ranging in age from 10 to 13 years. These nonhandicapped participants attended public or parochial schools throughout the Twin Cities, Minnesota metropolitan area.

Wilder Forest, operated through the Amherst H. Wilder Foundation, was the site for this study. Wilder Forest is a 980-acre outdoor education environment near St. Paul, Minnesota serving a variety of human services agencies from the Twin Cities area and the upper Midwest. Facilities include campgrounds, handicapped-accessible earth shelter lodges, a dining hall, a 70-acre farm, a greenhouse, an orchard, gardens, and a swimming beach and boating area. During the study, participants resided in an earth shelter lodge that contained two large sleeping rooms—one for boys and one for girls—kitchen, dining, and living areas, and two bathrooms. All participants lived together as a group, on a 24-hour basis, for 2 weeks.

Training of Nondisabled Peers

Although an introductory meeting was held during the first day, a more extensive informational session took place during the second day of camp. Participants with disabilities were not present during this second session. The nondisabled campers viewed a slide show that depicted children with and without severe disabilities engaged in a variety of leisure activities. The accompanying audiotape described the positive attributes and challenges of friendship with a child who is disabled. The researchers emphasized that the campers with disabilities had come to camp for the same reasons the nondisabled campers had, namely: to make new friends, to learn outdoor skills, and to have fun. Similarities between the two groups of campers in terms of their leisure time interests and comparable school curricula were discussed. Campers practiced signs (i.e., sign language) used at home by the disabled childrens' parents and signs that were also appropriate for use during camp activities. Another section of the training session involved preparing participants without disabilities to play with and to assist the campers with handicaps. Each nondisabled child was told that he or she would be paired with a disabled companion. Children were told to begin a leisure activity by giving their companion a simple verbal direction, then proceed by demonstrating the task or activity, and finally, if necessary, to help their companion through the activity with gentle hand-over-hand guidance. Campers were told to offer assistance rather than force participation. Their roles as friends, rather than as teachers or tutors, were emphasized repeatedly (Voeltz et al., 1983). Following the session, two groups of four campers (1 with severe disabilities and 3 without disabilities) and one group of three campers (1 with severe disabilities and 2 without disabilities) were organized.

Activities

A typical day began with campers preparing breakfast on a wood stove in their lodge. After morning meal cleanup, children participated in a craft activity in their groups. Campers ate lunch in the central dining hall. Afternoon activities included hiking, boating, fishing, and swimming. Groups took turns preparing dinner and doing chores at the farm. Evening activities included games, hay rides, folk dancing, ice cream making, and campfire programs.

Such activities as clearing dishes from the table after meals and placing them in the dishwasher and preparation for swimming were targeted as instructional tasks for the campers with disabilities. These activities were selected for instruction for several reasons. Both activities were chronologically age-appropriate and occurred at least once every day. Many of the component steps of both activities could, potentially, generalize to home, social, or employment settings. For example, clearing a table and loading a dishwasher are domestic skills useful at home; diners in school or employee cafeterias often bus their own dishes.

During the morning craft activity, such as wool or woodcraft, and an afternoon activity such as hiking or boating social behaviors of the campers with disabilities and interactions between them and their nondisabled peers were observed and measured.

Experimental Design

A quasi-experimental (A-B), single subject research methodology was used to examine the effects of behavior-specific positive reinforcement and cooperative learning training on the social behavior and skill acquisition of children with severe disabilities. The effects on their social interactions with nondisabled peers were also examined.

Intervention

Reinforcement of appropriate behavior in campers with disabilities and reinforcement of social interactions between campers with and without disabilities commenced immediately following the training session. Each group sat together at a table during breakfast and dinner meals in the lodge. A rotation system was instituted during the craft activity during which campers without disabilities took turns within their small groups in assisting peers with disabilities to complete a craft project. The same grouping arrangements were used to assign groups to dinner preparation, farm chores, or free time. Contingent reinforcement procedures, such as pats on the back, verbal praise, and smiles, were used throughout the day.

The domestic and self-help skills that were selected for instruction utilized separate task analyses. Adult leaders began training the campers with disabilities on the task-analytic steps that they were unable to complete independently. A cue hierarchy consisting of verbal prompts, modeling, and physical assistance was implemented. Campers were reinforced with social praise following successful performance of each step of the task analysis. Training of table clearing skills took place during both the breakfast and dinner meals in the lodge. Following the noon meal in the dining hall, campers received training on a small portion of the task analysis: they cleared their dishes and carried them to a counter where kitchen staff placed them in a dishwasher.

Results

The purpose of this program was to successfully integrate three children with severe disabilities and eight children without disabilities in a 2-week residential camping program. Participant behavior targeted for change included: 1) the acquisition of leisure and daily living skills, 2) increases in social interactions between campers, 3) increases in socially appropriate behavior, and 4) changes in attitudes. The impact of the integrated camp on staff members' attitudes was also assessed.

Skill Acquisition For John, Molly, and Mary, low and stable rates of independent and appropriate behavior were exhibited during the baseline phase of the study: 12%, 10%, 15% on clearing the table, and 11%, 57%, 9% on swimming preparation, respectively, as compared to mean performances during intervention (78%, 61%, 46% on clearing the table, and 82%, 76%, 51% on swimming preparation, respectively).

A rapid and steady increase in the percentage of steps of the task analyses performed independently was exhibited throughout the skill acquisition phase of the camping program. By the termination of the 2-week camping program, all three participants with severe disabilities had acquired at least 70% of both activities, with the exception of swimming preparation for Mary, who acquired 50% of the task. However, even those gains were significant in light of the lack of Mary's skill on this activity during baseline, where she averaged only 9% mastery of the activity.

Social Interaction Data for the three participants with severe disabilities were combined. A t-test showed a significant increase ($p < .0001$) ($t[27] = -4.29$) in the frequency of social interactions per minute observed from the baseline phase to the intervention phase of the craft activities. Social interactions also increased significantly ($p < .0001$) ($t[31] = 4.56$) from the baseline to the intervention phase of the afternoon outdoor activities. In regard to socially appropriate and inappropriate behavior, the participants with severe disabilities showed a slight, but not statistically significant, reduction in socially appropriate behavior from baseline to intervention. Campers' appropriate behaviors averaged 92% during baseline activity, and 83% during intervention.

Attitude Attitude data were collected through two sources. The first source was a rating scale completed each day by nondisabled participants, intended to assess their feelings about interacting with disabled peers in terms of perceived friendship, self-confidence and enjoyment. The second source was a prepost survey instrument that was given to staff members of the outdoor education environment who were either involved directly or indirectly with campers. The survey was intended to assess staff members' perceptions of operating an integrated camping program versus a segregated program. Elements such as logistical ease or difficulty, benefits to both disabled and nondisabled campers, and desire for more or less integration were measured in the survey.

On the attitude scale, ratings at the positive end of the scale (4's or 5's) predominated, though not to an extent that produced statistically significant differences between baseline and final-day ratings.

Regarding staff ratings of the integrated camping experience (1: low to 5: high) on a pre-post basis, respondents received questions that were designed to solicit feelings about the program. Staff members who were either directly involved, such as residential camp counselors, and the nurse who visited the campers on a daily basis, or who were indirectly involved, such as kitchen and maintenance staff members, generally showed more positive attitudes toward the integration of the residential camp following the intervention.

Responses to two of the questionnaire items were found to be significantly different on a pre-post basis across indirectly involved staff, but not across staff involved directly in the integrated camp. Additionally, one item (i.e., "Ease of operating an integrated camp versus a segregated one") was rated in a less positive manner before and after intervention among the directly involved staff; no changes in attitude were found among the indirectly involved staff. Also, this particular item received among the lowest ratings in both pre- and postresponses across both groups.

CONCLUDING REMARKS

The results of the study were encouraging. Evidence of increased positive attitudes of campers without disabilities toward peers with disabilities, increased skill acquisition in campers with severe disabilities, and of generally positive, and increasing, posttest ratings by staff members support the argument for utilizing integrated outdoor education programs rather than the segregated programs that are relatively common for children with disabilities. However, operating an integrated program is not free of challenges. For example, nondisabled participants were, at times, perplexed by the inability of one of the severely retarded participants to converse on topics typical of nondisabled campers of his age.

The challenges associated with operating an integrated camp are also reflected in staff members' ratings of the ease with which an integrated program can be operated. Despite the fact that the 13 staff members showed increased desire for integrated camping, they also revealed feelings that an integrated camp is more difficult to operate than a segregated one. The authors judge these feelings to be valid and comparable to the authors' own perceptions. Such reactions signal a need to not only plan, structure, and monitor integration programs very carefully, but to identify service delivery models and administrative practices (e.g., adding an additional staff member or volunteer) that will facilitate the smooth and effective operation of an integrated camp.

These findings bode well for professionals in recreation, outdoor education, and special education who are concerned about providing age-appropriate, challenging, and socially valid activities to persons with and without disabilities in integrated environments. Also, the benefits to the nondisabled participants of this study, as manifested in attitudinal enhancement and interactional increases, should not be taken lightly: that campers without disabilities were prepared to participate socially with their peers with severe disabilities is a significant achievement. However, it is important to remember that it was the preprogram orientation efforts by parents and investigators that contributed to the socially valid changes in all campers' behaviors. Indeed, demonstrating benefits to both disabled and nondisabled participants, in the same integrated setting and at the same time, could be increasingly important to the growth and development of the integration movement itself.

EXEMPLARY PROGRAM IV

Developing an On-Call Guide Network to Enhance Cross-Country Ski Opportunities for Persons With Visual Impairments

M. Tipton Ray and Stuart J. Schleien

For over 2 decades, in Norway, sighted and visually impaired individuals have cross-country skiied together, the former serving as an "on-snow guide" to the latter. Imported to the United States in 1974, this concept of pairing individuals with and without disabilities in the sport of cross-country skiing has been realized through an outreach program sponsored by the Sons of Norway fraternal organization. The program is called Ski For Light, Inc. (Rostad, 1985). The primary goal of this program is to socially integrate participants with and without disabilities, thus enhancing formation of friendships, trust, and understanding. Each year, several hundred individuals with and without visual impairments gather at national and regional locations to participate in weekend and week-long programs that introduce persons with visual impairments to cross-country skiing. Training is provided to sighted skiers to become instructor/guides.

Even though a rationale exists for inclusion of persons with disabilities into active, healthful, leisure experiences such as cross-country skiing (Leon & Amundson, 1979; Opel, 1982), few opportunities for participation in these activities exist for the person with visual disabilities, even if that person has gained skiing experience through previous participation in special events and segregated programs (e.g., Ski For Light, local ski clubs). Also, these persons must continue to rely on experienced, sighted cross-country ski guides to assist them on the snow by giving verbal directions and information regarding terrain features, appropriate ski technique, and trail configuration. Community support systems must be created to give persons with visual impairments outdoor recreation opportunities throughout the year. Such opportunities are especially valuable during the winter months, when mobility and transportation can be especially difficult for persons with disabilities. The primary intent of this program, therefore, was to develop an on-call network of locally trained and sighted instructor/guides, who could be contacted conveniently by persons with visual impairments who wish to ski at local parks and other public and private open spaces. Sighted skiers who have received guide training would have their names, addresses, and phone numbers added to a referral list created and maintained by the local park or ski area personnel. These guides would be "on call" for visually impaired persons who need a guide in order to ski.

METHODS

Guide Training Program

Initially, a guide training program was provided to sighted persons wishing to learn skills to cross-country ski with persons with visual impairments. The program was similar to the training provided by Ski For Light, Inc. (Norbie, 1983), a program wherein participants are introduced to principles and practices of guiding persons with visual impairments.

The cross-country ski guiding principles and practices introduced in the training sessions included:

1. Role of the instructor/guide, particularly in developing a trusting relationship with the person with visual impairments through a mutual exchange of thoughts, feelings, and opinions
2. Proper cross-country ski technique
3. Methods of instruction, including: explanation method; show/feel method; correction method
4. Progressions of instruction (i.e., beginning skills to advanced skills, such as introduction of new skier to equipment and clothing, simple stepping exercises on skis, etc., to lane changing and uphill/downhill techniques)
5. Principles and techniques of guiding in tracks, on downhills, and in races
6. Safety issues

Setting and Participants

The guide training program took place in Minnesota at a conveniently located (i.e., accessible by public transportation, near large residential area) community recreation setting in metropolitan Minneapolis. The recreation area had facilities to accommodate many winter recreation activities, including: sledding hills, tracked and groomed cross-country ski trails, a downhill ski area with rope-tow, an ice-skating pond, and a large warming-house and snack bar. Services provided at the area included inexpensive ski equipment rentals.

Potential participants for the guide training program were solicited through a recreation agency information brochure, local newspapers, flyers, and by word of mouth. Each training session lasted approximately 3 hours. Persons with visual impairments were invited to participate in the sessions to understand how sighted individuals receive guide training. Guide training sessions served a variety of functions. They provided sighted participants with the perspective of a person with visual impairments by giving them an opportunity to guide a visually impaired skier on the snow. The training sessions also enabled recreation staff to evaluate and improve program content by soliciting feedback from participants with and without visual impairments.

Following the 1½ hour indoor training, an on-snow training session of equal duration took place in which the instructor demonstrated guide skills and gave participants an opportunity to practice, on skis and with each other, newly acquired skills. Participants teamed-up, 1-to-1 with each other, and alternated being blind-folded to simulate visual impairment while the other partner practiced being a guide. Several participants were able to ski with one or the other of the visually impaired participants.

After the session, a master list of guide training participants was developed that included names, addresses, and phone numbers. The recreation agency distributed the list and served as a liaison between sighted guides and visually impaired persons who wished to cross-country ski. Participant information could be alphabetized or ordered by geographic region, for example, by using the telephone prefix or street address. Advocacy groups serving persons with visual impairments were then informed of the guide training program and the development of the on-call guide network system. Potential skiers with visual impairments could call the recreation agency, receive one or more names of potential guides, and then initiate the contacts with these guides.

Results

Guide training sessions were offered once per year for 2 years at this community recreation site. Twenty persons, ranging in age from late teens to middle age attended the indoor and on-snow sessions. Their skiing ability ranged from beginner to advanced level. Two persons with visual impairments, age 21 and 23, possessing beginner to intermediate skiing ability, attended the sessions. The recreation center director and a part-time staff member also attended to gain skills as guides, and to evaluate the program. An informal evaluation of training session participants revealed that all participants, with and without disabilities, felt positive about the program and that similar programs should be conducted in the future. The sighted participants all agreed to register on the on-call guide network list. The participants with visual impairments seemed particularly enthusiastic about the future potential of other persons with visual impairments to successfully engage in this outdoor winter sport.

CONCLUDING REMARKS

By administering the on-call guide network, the Minneapolis Park and Recreation Board serves an important role as facilitator of accessible and integrated community leisure services for persons with disabilities. This network ties in neatly with other local segregated activities (e.g., Ski for Light programs, local club-sponsored ski outings) that teach visually impaired persons how to cross-country ski. Persons with visual impairments are able to take advantage of an outdoor environment in a season, winter, that is generally not hospitable to most persons with disabilities. This increases their opportunities to participate in an active, popular sport with nondisabled peers. Additionally, use of this on-call guide network has good potential for year-round use (e.g., running, biking, long term friendships) and should be explored by community recreation professionals.

EXEMPLARY PROGRAM V

Integrating Children With Moderate to Severe Cognitive Deficits into a Community Museum Program

Stuart J. Schleien, M. Tipton Ray, Marcie Soderman-Olson, and Kathy McMahon

A number of authors (Copeland, 1984; Dalke, 1984; Lowenfeld & Brittain, 1970; Sherrill, 1979) have discussed the potential benefits of art education for children with and without disabilities. Broudy (1984) argued that art education is not only a benefit, but that aesthetic education in the visual arts is fundamental to cognitive development, and especially to the development of verbal skills. Art education instructs individuals in the fundamental language of the visual arts, and provides opportunities to practice and develop skills in manipulating art materials. One of its most important functions is to provide students with opportunities for personal expression. In order to be complete, art education should also present children with examples of the highest quality works of art while teaching that art is an expression of the values of the culture and the historical period in which the artist lived.

Since art education can provide training to increase perceptual discrimination, cognitive and motor skill development, and the development of self-identification and self-confidence (Lowenfeld & Brittain, 1970), it might also serve as a powerful tool to promote successful integration. When art instruction is provided in a nonjudgmental, noncompetitive, and integrated context, it can become an activity in which all children could receive a personally satisfying experience. For example, children with and without mental retardation can experience the satisfaction of personal expression while learning to participate socially with peers.

Through a collaborative effort between the St. Paul Public Schools, the Minnesota Museum of Art, and the University of Minnesota, nine children with moderate to severe mental retardation and a class of 27 regular education same-age peers participated in a 6-month integrated art education program at the Museum's KIDSPACE Gallery. The program offered participants opportunities to gain experience in the visual arts, as well as skill in manipulating art materials, chances for self-expression, and first-hand exposure to museum-quality art. Through the use of time samplings and multi-variable analyses, participants' social behaviors and interactions during the integrated art experience were analyzed. Also, attitudes of nondisabled peers acting as "Special Friends" (Voeltz et al., 1982) were assessed from pre- to post-program using a standardized acceptance scale (Voeltz, 1982).

METHODS

Setting and Participants

Children chosen for this study were from second grade classrooms (i.e., one special education, one regular education) in two different schools within the same educational jurisdiction. Prior to enrollment, it was determined by the art educators that students at this grade level would be likely to gain from those learning experiences mentioned previously. The gender mix was approximately equal within each classroom, with ages ranging from 7–10 ($\overline{X} = 7.7$). The nine students from the special education classroom performed at varying levels of cognitive and motor achievement, and were functioning in the moderate to severe ranges of mental retardation. An informal assessment of special education students' abilities to identify color, manipulate line through drawing, and their general level of fine motor skills was conducted by program staff. This assessment information was useful in generating activity adaptations to facilitate at least partial participation by the students. While all students were ambulatory, one student had a severe mobility impairment requiring him to wear protective headgear and to receive frequent physical assistance to move about the museum environment.

The community museum setting used for this art education program was the Minnesota Museum of Art in St. Paul. In 1983 the Minnesota Museum of Art opened KIDSPACE Gallery, an interactive art exhibition designed especially for elementary-age children. KIDSPACE is based on the premise that children's interest in art will be generated more readily when they are actively involved in manipulating works of art. The KIDSPACE art integration project was designed to provide interactive experiences for all children regardless of level of ability. The materials and art objects within the gallery could be approached and manipulated by individuals with mobility impairments, and, in fact, the gallery was designed to accommodate children with physical disabilities. The theme of the 1984–1986 KIDSPACE exhibition, which changes biannually, was "Architectural Illusions." The exhibition included works of art representing variations on familiar architectural elements such as windows and columns, but with an unfamiliar twist (e.g., windows with holograms inside, columns encircled with flashing neon lights). Because classrooms were within the same school district, a cooperative agreement was made to share bus transportation to the museum. This enabled project participants and staff to overcome transportation inaccessibility, an obstacle often cited as a barrier to participation in community leisure settings by members of special populations (Schleien & Ray, 1986; Vaughan & Winslow, 1979).

Procedure

The KIDSPACE art integration project took place over a period of 6 months with both classrooms meeting jointly once each month. The overall art concept to be learned from this exhibition was that architectural design involves the manipulation of line, shape, and color transferred into three dimensions. Each basic element of architectural design was broken down into single tasks (i.e., art education activities) to provide the students with repeated learning experiences. Sequential units of study were planned to permit students to build on experiences learned the previous session, culminating in the creation and exhibition by students of a final art product, a "Fantasy City," which illustrated the overall concept of the art education project. A gallery experience enabled students to learn about design elements through participatory gallery tours and "hands-on" interaction with works of art such as holograms, light columns, velcro-backed wall panels of different designs, and murals. Opportunities to create individual and group works of art (each group included three non-disabled and one disabled student) through the manipulation of art materials (e.g., construction and tissue paper, paste, paints, boxes, scissors) were provided in the studio phase of the program. The gallery and studio experiences, coordinated during all six sessions, lasted approximately 45 minutes each.

It was assumed by the investigators that regular education students would play a vital role in the successful integration of their peers from the special education classroom into the KIDSPACE program environments. Thus, regular education students were brought to the museum prior to the first joint meeting to become acquainted with the gallery and studio program areas. This preintegration visit to KIDSPACE permitted regular education students to focus their initial interactions on their special education peers rather than focusing attention on the new and unusual museum environment. Following the preintegration visit, a baseline assessment of students' attitudes toward persons with disabilities was administered. A "Special Friends" (Voeltz et al., 1982) sensitivity training session with nondisabled participants was conducted using a slide-tape presentation and group questions and answers.

To enhance social integration and skill acquisition among students, cooperative groups were formed. Nine groups of approximately four students each were created with one special education student teamed with three regular education students (N = 36). Cooperative grouping arrangements were established to enhance the potential for art education and socialization between students with and without disabilities. To facilitate group identity and socialization, each member had a name tag with a construction paper color strip attached, with a different color for each group. Positive social reinforcement was used by staff, teachers, and observers to help students maintain groupings and to encourage students who were observed interacting appropriately.

Data Collection

A multi-variable analysis was used to examine participant involvement in the museum program. Three dependent variables were considered for investigation in this study. The first concerned the attitudes and general levels of acceptance by regular education students toward their peers with handicapping conditions. To assess this variable, Voeltz' (1982) Acceptance Scale, Lower Elementary Level, was administered pre- and postprogram to the regular education students. Scores from the pretest were tabulated at the conclusion of the KIDSPACE special education project to prevent teacher and trainer bias toward students. The other two dependent variables, social interaction and appropriate and inappropriate social behaviors in the museum, were measured using time samplings.

Results

In order to determine whether the children with and without disabilities were successfully integrated into the museum program, the following variables and research questions were considered and approached statistically.

Social Interactions The initiation and reception of positive social interactions between retarded and nondisabled participants increased substantially throughout the duration of the art integration program. Specifically, using a one-way analysis of variance (ANOVA), the number of social interactions received by the retarded participants from their nondisabled "Special Friends" increased significantly ($p < .015$).

Again, using a one-way ANOVA, the number of social interactions initiated by the retarded participants with their nondisabled "Special Friends" was found to increase markedly, but not at a statistically significant level ($p < .053$).

Social Behavior Rates of appropriate and inappropriate social behavior exhibited by the retarded participants in the gallery and studio showed nonsignificant changes across time. However, using t-tests, it was found that the percentage of socially appropriate behavior within environments was significantly higher than inappropriate behavior throughout the 6-month study. Differences in their rates of appropriate ($\overline{X} = 45.9$) to inappropriate ($\overline{X} = 14.1$) social behaviors were significant in the gallery environment ($p < .002$). Similarly, significant differences in rates of appropriate ($\overline{X} = 47.4$) and inappropriate ($\overline{X} = 12.5$) social behaviors were exhibited in the studio environment ($p < .001$). No differences in the participants' rates of appropriate social behavior across environments (i.e., gallery versus studio) were found; in fact, the rates were very similar (i.e., $\overline{X}$ gallery $= 44.8$ vs. $\overline{X}$ studio $= 45.4$). Likewise, no significant differences in inappropriate behaviors were found when these two environments were compared.

PrePost Attitudes of Nondisabled Participants

A positive and significant attitude change ($p < .05$) from pre- to postprogram exhibited by the nondisabled "Special Friends" as measured on the Acceptance Scale (Voeltz, 1982) was found using t-tests. The mean score on the preattitude survey was 12.95, increasing significantly to a postprogram mean of 16.29.

CONCLUDING REMARKS

Nine children with moderate to severe mental retardation and 27 nondisabled same age peers participated successfully in an integrated community museum program. The program was judged to be successful by the positive changes in participants' appropriate interactions, by the high rates of socially appropriate behaviors, and by the attitude changes of the nondisabled peers. Additionally, it was demonstrated that through the use of a package of integration strategies and behavioral methods, children with mental retardation and nondisabled peers could participate successfully in a nontraditional community leisure environment.

In further support of the success of this integration program, interactions between participants with and without mental retardation were found to increase across sessions. Not only did the data reveal a marked increase in positive social interactions initiated by non-handicapped participants toward handicapped participants ($p < .015$), but mentally retarded subjects demonstrated a moderate increase ($p < .053$) in their initiation of these interactions toward their nondisabled "Special Friends."

The sessions in the museum's studio, which contained more student-initiated and hands-on craft activities than the gallery, consistently produced large rates of socially appropriate behaviors. The gallery experience, which was typically staff-directed and less conducive to sharing materials and peer interactions, also produced high rates of socially appropriate behaviors. It was anticipated that a combination of more cooperative activities, student generated activity outcomes (e.g., a craft project in the studio versus viewing holograms in the gallery), and increased opportunities for reinforcement (e.g., behavior specific positive feedback) by program staff in the studio would facilitate greater amounts of appropriate play behavior. However, high rates of socially appropriate behaviors were exhibited in both environments with nonsignificant differences found between them.

These data support previous studies documenting the positive and socially appropriate behavioral outcomes of cooperative grouping arrangements. Without the structure and reinforcement provided by the "Special Friends" and program staff in both environments, children with mental retardation would be less likely to exhibit socially appropriate behavior and interactions leading to successful integration. These findings could have implications for integrated programs within other museum and community leisure settings. It should be noted that rates of inappropriate behaviors remained unchanged across the studio and gallery settings and throughout the duration of the study. While it was encouraged to observe positive behavioral changes in the museum environment, we believe it is necessary to explore other behavioral methods which effectively bring inappropriate social behaviors in line with levels deemed acceptable for nondisabled peers.

The primary objective of this study was to successfully integrate children with and without mental retardation in a community leisure environment. The data support the attainment of this objective. Our secondary objective was to validate various methods to integrate children with mental retardation into after-school recreation environments. Although the specific effects of each of the individual components of our instructional "package" were not determined in this study, it seems likely that the integration procedures used were all necessary and reasonably effective. There is reason to believe that the instructional procedures used in this study could be applied to a wide variety of other community recreation environments with similar outcomes.

EXEMPLARY PROGRAM VI

After-School Programs to Enhance Community Recreation Integration: Minneapolis Exemplars

Stuart J. Schleien and M. Tipton Ray

The city of Minneapolis, Minnesota is renowned for the quality of its urban parks, lakes, and other open spaces. This city of approximately one-half million residents has an extensive system of 42 established parks and community and neighborhood recreation centers.

Many of the parks and recreation centers are linked to a 20-plus mile "greenway" and chain of lakes that permit most residents ease of access by motor vehicle, bicycle, or by foot. However, there is an important communication link in addition to the physical proximity of parks and recreation centers and neighborhood schools. In these instances, it is not uncommon to have recreation professionals and school personnel collaborating by sharing resources to address the unique recreation needs of all students with and without disabilities.

As a consequence of federal legislation that mandates an appropriate education for all children with disabilities in least restrictive, community-based environments (e.g., PL 94-142 and its amendments), many of these neighborhood schools have mainstreamed students with disabilities. Therefore, these students are also having their leisure and recreation needs met through special recreation and integrated programming at these adjacent park sites. For schools that offer segregated services, student recreation needs are being met both on-site and through select after-school programming in the students' home communities.

RECREATION SERVICE MODELS

The purpose of this discussion is to present several exemplars, or models of service, that have been implemented through the collective efforts of the Minneapolis Public Schools, the Minneapolis Park and Recreation Board, and the parents and teachers of students with disabilities. During its 2-year grant period, 1984–1986, the Project for Integrated Recreation in the Community (PIRC) made community recreation programs and sites accessible to students with disabilities by applying the strategies outlined in this book. The authors believe that the lessons learned from the following three exemplars have positive implications for recreation programming for students with disabilities in other communities.

Emerson After-School Program

Emerson is a segregated school that provides intensive functional skills (e.g., activities of daily living, vocational, leisure, domestic) training to students with developmental disabilities. It is located near the center of the city and is bounded by (but separate from) a small hospital, commercial businesses, and several older apartments. A large park, with a small pond, walking paths, and a recreation shelter, is located two blocks away. The majority of the students do not live in the immediate vicinity and, therefore, must be bused to school. For many years, school personnel and parents had desired the provision of high quality recreation services for these students. To achieve this, the parents and school personnel contacted various park and recreation staff to investigate the best means of providing these services to the students at Emerson School. Table 8.1 provides a brief historical overview detailing these contacts and efforts.

The focus of the Emerson After-School Program evolved from a segregated, special recreation alternative for a limited number of students, most who are classified in the mild to moderate range of mental retardation, to a program that stresses age-appropriate activities in integrated settings proximal to the student's home community. Persons with varying degrees of disability are currently involved in a variety of recreational pursuits throughout Minneapolis. Staff at recreation centers receive annual inservice training on techniques to integrate such students into community recreation environments, thereby relying less on the skills of part-time teachers and classroom aides to administer programs. Ongoing communication and collaboration meetings between the schools, recreation agency, parents, and interested others, (at least two to three times per school year), ensure that barriers such as transportation and funding will continually be addressed and met with workable and realistic solutions. While this program addressed, on a community level, the recreation

TABLE 8.1.   Emerson after-school program: historical overview

1973–76	• Due to efforts of parents and the parent-teacher-student association, after-school programs in libraries are established; parents provide car pools.
	• Individuals are grouped by their functional levels.
	• Park personnel are reluctant to try programming because of their lack of experience with persons with disabilities.
1977	• Title IV-C Project: After-School program federally funded for 3 years as an ESEA (Elementary/Secondary Aid).
	• Three levels of students are to be served: 1) multiply disabled, 2) moderately mentally retarded, 3) mildly mentally retarded. One hundred-twenty students attend Emerson School, ages 5–16 years.
1978–79	• School refers inidividuals (e.g., teachers, classroom assistants) to serve as instructors in park sites with 15–20 participants involved in the Emerson After-School Program.
	• Programs serving Level I participants (i.e., severely disabled) dropped due to lack of funding.
1979–80	• Four park sites with 30 participants total are involved in the Emerson After-School Program.
	• Each after-school park site receives a Resource Manual: 268-page book describing the program including over 150 games and recreational activities.
	• Transportation becomes a problem, due to lack of funds.
1981–82	• Seven park sites with 65 students total participate in the Emerson After-School Program.
	• Transportation is funded and provided by Minneapolis Public Schools.
1982–83	• Sixty-six students attend after-school program in eight park sites.
	• Individuals who use wheelchairs participate for the first time.
	• Individuals are grouped by age, leisure interest, and geographical area.
1983–84	• Sixty-four students attend after-school program in eight sites; age-appropriate activities are implemented.
	• Persons who are multiply disabled attend programs.
	• Social integration is encouraged by staff.
	• Division of Recreation, Park, and Leisure Studies at the University of Minnesota becomes a resource for volunteer advocates.
1984–85	• Sixty-six students attend the programs in eight sites.
	• Persons with severe hearing impairments and persons with behavior disorders attend the program.
	• PIRC staff become involved in program planning and evaluation.
	• Revision of application form is implemented to include more personal background information (e.g., special considerations, concerns).
	• Efforts toward social integration in the after-school program continue and are systematically applied using techniques developed by PIRC, school, and park staff.
	• Joint effort is officially established between the University of Minnesota and the Minneapolis Park and Recreation Board to provide maximum opportunity for persons with disabilities to participate in community recreation settings.
1985–86	• Seven programs at seven park sites are attended by 53 students.
	• Individuals with visual impairments participate in the program.

The authors wish to express their appreciation to the following persons who assisted with developing this historical overview: Diane Tornes, Minneapolis Public Schools; Dale Johnson, Minneapolis Park and Recreation Board; Angela Larson, PIRC Graduate Research Assistant; Jeanne Colburn, Student Assistant, Division of Recreation, Park, and Leisure Studies, University of Minnesota.

needs of students with developmental disabilities who attended a segregated school, the next exemplar illustrates the efforts of recreation staff and school personnel to optimize recreation participation of students labeled autistic attending a mainstreamed school setting.

After-School Programs In Mainstream Settings

As was noted earlier, several park and recreation centers are located adjacent to school settings. In this case, school and recreation personnel, along with a PIRC grant project staff person, developed a process for including elementary-age students with disabilities in integrated recreation activities to be conducted after school at the adjacent park site. The pilot program was an ice-skating activity to be held 1 day per week, 1½ hours per session, for 6 weeks. Ten children without disabilities and two children labeled autistic would participate together in the program. Ice skates were donated to participants in need. Also, before program implementation, and within the classrooms, recreation staff would discuss with the children the proper clothing to wear while ice-skating.

Prior to program implementation, recreation staff were invited by teachers to the classroom setting to observe the two students with autism. This was helpful to the recreation staff who feared that negative behaviors were often exhibited by persons with this label. Eliminating unnecessary stereotypes allowed the recreation staff to facilitate a positive, successful ice-skating program. Additionally, a volunteer advocate was involved to bridge gaps between students with and without disabilities, thus enhancing social integration at the park site.

Based upon the collective efforts of school, recreation, and grant project personnel, a model process for including persons with disabilities into after-school recreation programs was developed. As described in Table 8.2, the process has implications for system-wide use by the various schools and recreation centers that share park sites. This process was disseminated throughout Minneapolis by the respective agencies involved.

Leisure Education and Future Park Users

This final exemplar highlights the efforts of PIRC grant staff and recreation and school personnel to provide to 38 elementary-age students with learning disabilities a leisure education program on how to successfully use a community recreation setting. The program was implemented at a neighborhood park that was located approximately 200 feet from the school. The participants were students in the kindergarten through third-grade special education classrooms within a mainstream school setting. Each student's involvement in the leisure education program consisted of four 75-minute sessions, teaching the functional use of a community recreation center. Professional staff agreed that a segregated, large group leisure education program might be the most effective and efficient way to prepare the students for future integrated programming within the park and recreation leisure service system.

Various school and recreation staff met to develop the 4-week leisure education program. (This curriculum appears in Table 8.3.) Recommendations for future leisure education programs serving persons with disabilities were made following the program. These recommendations included the following:

1. Do not adapt recreation activities unless a child cannot participate otherwise.
2. Teach participants the independent and functional use of the park. Do not set up special recreation activities prior to their arrival.
3. Provide an organized, quality program so the participants will return and recreation staff will continue to offer future programming opportunities.
4. Remember that this group of children may not be using this facility in the future. Provide them with an experience that is generic to many community recreation centers located throughout the city and in their respective neighborhoods.

TABLE 8.2.   A process for including persons with disabilities in after-school recreation programs

Step 1. School Personnel:
    a. Contact recreation personnel for class and registration information.
    b. Inform recreation personnel of the general abilities and interests of their students with disabilities who may be potential participants.

Step 2. Recreation Personnel:
    a. Highlight programs that would provide the most appropriate, successful, and enjoyable integrated experiences.
    b. Send class and registration materials.

Step 3. School Personnel:
    a. Send registration materials home with students, along with highlighted recommended programs.

Step 4. School Personnel:
    a. Once received from students and/or parents, send registration information to the appropriate staff person for processing.

Step 5. School Personnel or Recreation Personnel:
    a. Call recreation personnel or school personnel to arrange meeting to discuss participant characteristics with program instructor(s) and/or complete Environmental Analysis Inventory.

Step 6. Recreation Personnel:
    a. Contact program instructors for meeting established in Step 5.

Step 7. The meeting agenda should address, but not be limited to:

	Content	*Provided by*
a.	Description of participant's abilities	School personnel
b.	Need for volunteer advocate	School personnel
c.	Expectations and basic skills needed in class	Instructor
d.	Anticipated modifications or adaptations	All
e.	Date and time of follow-up meeting (either during or at conclusion of program) to address following questions:	All

       1. Could process be improved? How?
       2. Is there a resource to solicit and train volunteer advocates?
       3. Is there a need for more staff training?
       4. Other:

5. Do not allow participants to "bend the rules" because one individual thinks that he or she is "special." This will only hinder participants' full, independent participation at other community recreation centers.

6. Choose chronologically age-appropriate activities in which their peers would most likely participate at other community recreation centers.

7. Allow time for free play to enhance the participants' abilities in decision-making, sharing equipment, and self-initiated activity.

CONCLUDING REMARKS

The intent of introducing these three exemplars is to provide the reader with some positive and workable processes for enhancing community leisure services and opportunities for children and youth with disabilities. The collaborative efforts of school and recreation agencies provides support for the conclusions reached by Schleien and Werder (1985) in their study on perceived responsibilities of special recreation services to persons with disabilities. Specifically, these programs address many of their recommendations regarding trans-agency relationships, shared responsibility for programming, expansion of activity offer-

TABLE 8.3.   Leisure education curriculum for the functional use of a community recreation center

Goal: To teach the functional use of a community recreation center.

Strategies:
1.   Increase child's awareness of the community recreation center and its recreational opportunities.
2.   Teach standard rules of the community recreation center.
3.   Teach the correct procedure for "checking out" and returning community recreation center materials/equipment.
4.   Provide children with an enjoyable experience at the community recreation center.

aSession 1:
   Focus:
   1.   Establish positive rapport with the participants.
   2.   Provide an overview of the facility, including rules and equipment.
   3.   Review check-out and return procedure.
   4.   Offer a positive recreational experience.

   Curriculum:
   1.   Greet students. Distribute name tags.
   2.   Introduce park staff involved in the leisure education program.
   3.   Define the purpose of the program.
   4.   Tour the facility and describe various recreation opportunities available.
   5.   Discuss equipment check-out.
   6.   Role play the equipment check-out and return procedures.
   7.   Play a simple game (e.g., kickball, basketball).
   8.   Group departs.

Session 2:
   Focus:
   1.   Provide awareness of the variety of structured/unstructured recreational activities available at the community recreation center.
   2.   Encourage decision-making and free play for independent use of the community recreation center.

   Curriculum:
   1.   Greet students. Distribute name tags.
   2.   Review recreation opportunities at the community recreation center.
   3.   Review equipment check-out and return procedures.
   4.   Divide the group into two small groups.
   5.   One group checks out materials necessary to play a group recreational activity (e.g., floor hockey). The other group is given access to various "free-play" equipment and materials and is instructed to check out equipment of personal preference (e.g., board game, table tennis).
   6.   After 30 minutes, both groups alternate activities.
   7.   Group departs.

Session 3:
   Focus:
   1.   To encourage independent use of the community recreation center, and to provide less specific directions regarding equipment check-out and return procedures.

   Curriculum:
   1.   Greet students.
   2.   Divide the group into two smaller groups.
   3.   One group checks out equipment for group recreational activity.
   4.   The alternate group participates in self-initiated leisure (e.g., equipment check-out and free-play).
   5.   After 30 minutes, both groups alternate activities.
   6.   Group departs.

(continued)

TABLE 8.3. *(continued)*

Session 4:
Focus:
1. Without guidance or reinforcement, recreation staff allow the children to use the facility independently. Prompts are offered only when necessary.

Curriculum:
1. Greet students.
2. Review overall programming opportunities at the community recreation center.
3. Provide an overview of this session's format of self-initiated play at the recreation center.
4. Allow the children to use the entire facility without guidance from staff.
5. Provide supervision only when necessary.
6. Provide the classroom teachers with materials (e.g., Community center brochures) for their students' future participation in their respective neighborhood recreation centers.

ᵃEach session is approximately 75 minutes in duration.

ings and opportunities, and community recreation integration. Additionally, recreation and school personnel have successfully addressed common obstacles that typically prevent or limit recreation participation (Schleien & Ray, 1986; Smith, 1985; Vaughan & Winslow, 1979) related to transportation, scarce financial resources, untrained staff, and lack of clear lines of communication. Another positive consequence of these collaborative efforts is a successful bridging between recreation agencies and families of children with disabilities. Often, it is difficult for the recreation agency to identify community residents who have disabilities and, therefore, to assess their needs and activity preferences. Because of various legal and ethical implications behind releasing information on students being served in special education classrooms, recreation agencies could communicate with these students and/or their families through a direct linkage with the classroom teacher or special education administrator. Finally, a communication process and leisure education curriculum, both intended to enhance participation opportunities for persons with disabilities, was depicted.

FINAL COMMENTS

A substantial legal base has been established to support the right of all citizens to equal opportunity to participate in leisure/recreation experiences. However, by the nature of their disabilities, special characteristics, and needs, persons with disabilities are often victims of discrimination. Often, the individual with disabilities is required to master prerequisite skills or to receive training in a sheltered environment prior to his or her participation in enjoyable and age-appropriate activities and settings with nondisabled peers.

The literature is replete with pleas for educational programming for special populations in least restrictive environments. Arguments against segregated service delivery include a *lack of exposure* to nondisabled peer role models, the presence of *poorly trained staff* due to high turnover, and large amounts of *dead time* that encourage counterproductive and inappropriate behavior. Recreational programs in integrated community leisure environments must be advocated for and developed. The inclusion of persons with disabilities in community recreation settings and activities is more likely to have greater long-term value for them and to be more consistent with the principle of normalization.

The six exemplary programs described in this chapter were attempts to investigate the benefits accrued by persons with disabilities, nondisabled peers, and staff in integrated community recreation environments. Without additional expenditures, a majority of the children and adults participated in the programs with a great degree of success. Investments in staff training and development in the recreation agency could improve the quality of the programs, and could subsequently increase the degree of participation, success, and enjoyment experienced by all citizens of a locality. The costs involved in training are minimal in comparison to the return to the community. It is recommended that future programs and research efforts be initiated to further investigate the use of the strategies described in this book for integrating persons with disabilities into regular community recreation environments.

The least restrictive environment principle should be applied to recreation, as well as to educational services. In the past, when recreation was considered to be a form of therapy for persons with disabilities, the services were often delivered in a therapeutic milieu, such as a hospital or rehabilitation center. Many persons with disabilities still participate in segregated recreation activities in special settings, such as "therapeutic recreation" or "motor rooms" in recreation centers, schools, hospitals, and developmental learning centers. Given the adaptations, prosthetic devices, and environmental modifications that are presently available to facilitate full participation in community recreation activities, there is little justification for limiting the activity participation of persons with disabilities to segregated and potentially restrictive environments.

It is apparent that the responsibility for leisure services does not solely lie with any one agency or professional group, but is instead the responsibility of all organizations involved in the delivery of human services. The responsibility for improving and expanding leisure/recreation programming rests with service providers and families in home, school, and community environments. Maximizing cooperation and coordination among community recreation departments, families, schools, human service agencies, and universities is an important goal that will facilitate recreation participation across settings. However, if responsibilities are spread too widely among agencies, it is possible that no one organization will ensure they are carried out. Once again, it is recommended that municipal recreation and park departments may be designated by the community to assume overall programming responsibility.

Not all leisure experiences in least restrictive environments need to be successful. But the ability to try and achieve, or fail, is part of a learning process that for too long has been denied individuals with disabilities. The recent federal and state legislation, supportive of the principles of normalization and programming in the least restrictive environment, has at times been unclear and inconsistent in statements concerning the form and degree of support needed to fulfill these mandates. In the final analysis, it is up to consumers with disabilities, parents, community recreation professionals, and other key players to ensure that community leisure services are available and accessible to all members of the community. As was successfully demonstrated in the exemplary programs described in this final chapter, human services professionals must continue to change traditional community leisure service systems and to experiment to find the most successful means of achieving integration into least restrictive recreation environments. Additional opportunities for participation in integrated community recreation programs and environments will increase the chance that persons with disabilities will live their lives as normally and as meaningfully as possible.

Appendix A

THE ACCESSIBLE
COMMUNITY LEISURE SERVICE PROCESS
A Process Analysis of Community
Leisure Services for Persons with Disabilities

Social planning process[a]	"Accessible process"	Process tasks
I. Develop philosophic/ideologic framework	*Guidelines for Decision-Making* 1. Right to engage in recreation 2. Freedom of choice 3. Allows for individual differences 4. Access to quality leisure environments 5. Consistent, nondiscriminatory service delivery	*Accessibility Checklist* — a. physically accessible — b. age-appropriate — c. integrated (when appropriate) — d. addresses needs and preferences — e. affordable — f. convenient
II. Identify Needs	A. Gather Information: 1. Leisure Attitudes, Values	A.1.1 Examine attitude research in professional literature 1.2 Talk with potential consumers of services, with and without disabilities
	2. Demographic data	2.1 Contact advocacy agencies and schools to ascertain "who, what, where" 2.2 Visit neighborhood to observe environmental and residential modifications signalling "disabled live here" 2.3 Informally interview area residents 2.4 Consult census tables
	3. Available resources	3.1 Consult accessibility survey 3.2 Identify staff skilled in therapeutic recreation 3.3 Note existing programs by other agencies (e.g., community education, schools) 3.4 Determine if existing leisure materials are adaptable by persons of varying abilities 3.5 Determine budget allocations for recreation program services
	4. Leisure behavior	4.1 Examine existing studies conducted by leisure researchers, advocacy groups

4.2 Co-sponsor survey with advocacy agency, parent groups, and/or special education classrooms in schools to determine current leisure involvement by persons with disabilities

B. Identify Needs
   1. Conduct preference assessments with constituents of service area
      B.1.1 Administer formal needs/preference assessment (mail out survey) of neighborhood residents with disabilities and their parents/careproviders
      1.2 Conduct informal needs/preference assessment (interview) with same groups as B.1.1
      1.3 Contact advocacy groups to determine the general needs of special population group

C. Identify Programs
   1. "Brainstorm" creative ideas considering A & B, above
   2. Choose alternatives
      C.1.1 Consider accessibility issues related to A.3.1 and A.3.4, above
      2.1 Base decisions on determined needs and preferences in B, above
      2.2 Coordinate program selections and time with advocacy or special recreation groups to avoid duplication or conflicts

D. Publicize Programs/Recruitment
   1. Develop/implement marketing plan
      D.1.1 Contact advocacy agencies, parent groups, schools regarding program offerings
      1.2 Include nondiscrimination statements on all written and verbal advertising and promotion
      1.3 Utilize photographs of participants with disabilities alongside nonhandicapped participants (must obtain photography release)
      1.4 Portray disabled participants positively: as role models for *everyone*, not just for other disabled persons
      1.5 Access cable TV networks

III. Plan Program Intervention

169

2. Develop/distribute program brochure

    2.1 Eliminate all references to "special," "adaptive," or "handicapped" programming

    2.2 Distribute program offerings via brochures door-to-door and through neighborhood/community media, advocacy agency newsletter, community bulletin boards, computer clubs, and school classrooms

E. Conduct Registration

    1. Participant completes and submits form and pays fee, if appropriate

        E.1.1 Include response area for persons who may have special considerations on standardized registration forms; Include contact number for further information

        1.2 Establish consistent protocol for registering participants (e.g., mail, telephone, on-site, combination)

        1.3 (Refer to Environmental Analysis, Chapter 4, for complete detailing of Process Tasks)

        1.4 Determine appropriate adaptations and modifications

IV. Implement Programs/Interventions

F. Implement Programs

    1. Conduct organized programs

        F.1.1 Implement program modifications and adaptations specified in Environmental Analysis Inventory, Parts 2 and 3

V. Evaluate Programs/Interventions

G. Evaluate Programs

    1. Specify type and method of evaluation

    2. Conduct ongoing (Formative) and final (Summative) evaluations of program

        G.1.1 Collect data on interactions between persons with and without disabilities, social behaviors, acquisition of skills, etc.

        2.1 Collect qualitative (natural observation), as well as quantitative data

H. Summarize Findings and Report

    1. Write narrative of evaluation data

    2. Present summary findings to administrative personnel; include

        H.1.1 Analyze data and graphics and summarize findings

        2.1 Present findings to "significant others" (parents/careproviders)

critique of program design and implementation

3. Consider presentation to professional peers at workshops and conferences

2.2 Critique modifications/adaptations chosen to facilitate accessibility such as grouping arrangements, volunteer advocates, equipment/material/setting modifications, or behavioral approaches

3.1 Present findings to appropriate advocacy agencies, parent groups, schools

3.2 Collaborate with other personnel to report significant findings to allied health professional groups

VI. Feedback, Modification

I. Provide Appropriate Feedback
1. Provide constructive criticism to affected persons throughout all phases of programming

I.1.1 Provide reinforcement to volunteer advocates, instructors, and non-handicapped participants throughout program implementation phase

2. Make necessary modifications, as needed

2.1 Develop and evaluate adaptations as needed to ensure successful experience for participant with disabilities

J. Determine Future Programs/Interventions
1. Make decisions based on evaluation information and feedback

J.1.1 Be proactive versus reactive

1.2 Make appropriate modifications in leisure service delivery to persons with disabilities

2. Modify program philosophy or orientation as needs of constituency change

2.1 Participate actively on a Community Advisory Board that provides support for persons with disabilities in leisure service delivery

2.2 Advocate on behalf of participants with disabilities

2.3 Provide technical assistance to advocacy agencies, parents, schools

3. Modify programs, interventions, other service delivery

3.1 Modify and upgrade staff training program

Source: Edginton, Compton, and Hanson (1980).

Appendix B

LEISURE INTEREST SURVEY

Sample

Date _____

Name _____ Age _____ Male _____ Female _____

Address _____

Home phone _____ Business phone _____

Marital status _____ Children's ages _____

PLEASE MARK AN "X" NEXT TO THE ACTIVITIES THAT BEST DESCRIBE YOUR COMMUNITY LEISURE INTERESTS.

Activity	Currently do	Interested in
Team sports		
Bowling	——	——
Softball	——	——
Basketball	——	——
Soccer	——	——
T-Ball	——	——
Football	——	——
Hockey	——	——
Other: (Specify) _____	——	——
_____		
Music		
Singing	——	——
Playing instruments	——	——
Attending concerts	——	——
Other: (Specify) _____	——	——
_____		
Dance		
Folk	——	——
Modern	——	——
Square	——	——
Aerobic	——	——
Tap	——	——
Ballet	——	——
Jazz	——	——
Other: (Specify) _____	——	——
_____		

Individual sports

Gymnastics ———— ————
Jogging/Running ———— ————
Tennis ———— ————
Archery ———— ————
Swimming ———— ————
Golf ———— ————
Badminton ———— ————
Horseback riding ———— ————
Horseshoes ———— ————
Fishing ———— ————
Bike riding ———— ————
Walking ———— ————
Other: (Specify) ———————————————— ————
————————————————

Arts and crafts

Painting ———— ————
Knitting ———— ————
Crocheting ———— ————
Latch hook ———— ————
Ceramics ———— ————
Other: (Specify) ———————————————— ————
————————————————

Table games

Cards ———— ————
Checkers ———— ————
Chess ———— ————
Dominoes ———— ————
Scrabble ———— ————
Puzzles ———— ————
Billiards ———— ————
Table tennis ———— ————
Other: (Specify) ———————————————— ————
————————————————

Outdoor leisure/social

Hiking ———— ————
Gardening ———— ————
Camping ———— ————
Barbeques/Picnics ———— ————
Skiing ———— ————
Canoeing ———— ————
Other: (Specify) ———————————————— ————
————————————————

Mini day trips

Historical ———— ————
Cultural ———— ————
Sporting events ———— ————
Shopping/Restaurant ———— ————
Other: (Specify) ———————————————— ————
————————————————

Social clubs

Scouts   ____   ____
Photography   ____   ____
Travel   ____   ____
Gourmet/Cooking   ____   ____
Card playing   ____   ____
Other: (Specify) _____   ____   ____

_____

My leisure experiences are usually:

____ Physical   ____ Individual   ____ Structured   ____ Active   ____ Planned   ____ Expensive
____ Mental   ____ Social   ____ Nonstructured   ____ Passive   ____ Long-term
____ Spontaneous   ____ Inexpensive

With whom do you usually engage in leisure experiences (actual names can be used)?

____ Alone   ____ A friend/s   ____ Family member/s

During what time of day do you participate in leisure time activities?

____ Morning   ____ Afternoon   ____ Evening

Are any of the following problems that might prevent you from participating in leisure activities?

____ Financial difficulties   ____ Lack of transportation   ____ Facility not accessible   ____ No one to participate with   ____ Geographic location   ____ Disability/Lack skill   ____ No motivation
____ Child care problems   ____ Others (specify) _____

Please check any special needs or considerations that may affect your participation.

____ Physical
____ Mental
____ Social
____ Other: (specify) _____

_____

Would you be interested in serving as a member of a Community Advisory Board on recreation for persons with disabilities?   ____ Yes   ____ No

Would you attend an open, organizational meeting to assist us in planning leisure services for persons in your commmunity?   ____ Yes   ____ No

Appendix C

SAMPLE NONDISCRIMINATION STATEMENTS

A. The (your municipality's name) Parks and Recreation Department works with a variety of individuals and agencies to ensure that recreational programs and services are available and accessible to all persons, regardless of age, sex, religion, socioeconomic status, and level of physical or mental ability.

   Our professional staff have the skills and experience to involve you, your friend, or your family member in any number of our recreation programs. Please contact us to let us know how we can make your recreation experience a safe, successful, and enjoyable one.

B. The (your municipality's name) Parks and Recreation Department actively seeks and supports participation by persons with disabilities in recreational programs and services. Please call us so that we will know how to serve you better.

C. The (your municipality's name) Parks and Recreation Department provides leisure/recreation programs which are open and accessible to all citizens in the community.

   If you feel that you, a family member, a friend, or a client have a special consideration that we should be made aware of prior to that person's involvement in any of our recreation programs, please do not hesitate to contact: 1) your local community recreation professional, or 2) the main recreation office.

Appendix D

**Networking Matrix:
Roles and Responsibilities**

Key Players: *Community Recreation Professionals*
Refers to persons employed by the municipal park and recreation agency or other organizations (e.g., special recreation agencies; in some cases, community education) that serve the principal role in providing community leisure services funded by local government(s). Persons in administrative or leadership positions are usually professionally prepared (i.e., minimum four year degree) to manage organized, comprehensive municipal park and recreation programs. Other recreation staff may be non-degreed, part-time, or volunteer. Community Therapeutic Recreation Specialists have specific responsibilities related to provision of leisure services to persons with disabilities, but not unlike those responsibilities held by other community recreation professionals.

Examples:
Municipal Park and Recreation Staff (e.g., Recreation Worker, Recreator, Director, Instructor, Leader); Community Recreator; Community Therapeutic Recreation Specialist.

Responsibilities:
The primary responsibilities of the community recreation professional within the networking and community leisure service delivery processes are as facilitator and enabler. That is, the recreation professional has the skills, knowledge, and experience to coordinate activities (e.g., information gathering, needs identification, program selection, etc.) which result in accessible community leisure services for persons with disabilities. No "special" background or training is needed to assume these roles; only a willingness and motivation to provide high quality leisure services to a group of individuals who traditionally have been denied access to appropriate opportunities to engage in a recreational experience. The community recreation professional should also note that these roles and responsibilities extend beyond any given program season into a year-round effort. Development of a Community Advisory Board, therefore, should be a high priority to increase the probability that accessible leisure services will have permanence.

Key Players: *Parents/Careproviders (Real or Surrogate)*
Individuals who, through their biological, foster, or paraprofessional relationships, have responsibility for the care of persons with disabilities within residential settings. These persons often assume a position of authority as guardians of the health and welfare of their children or residents, including making decisions regarding community leisure participation of these persons.

Examples:
Parents, Foster Parents, Guardians, Direct Care Workers, Child Care Workers, House Parents, Living Unit Staff.

Roles and responsibilities of key players correspond with the Accessible Leisure Service Process, Appendix A.

Responsibilities:

A. Information Gathering:
    A.1   Identify potential consumers; provide demographic data
    A.2   Identify potential volunteer advocates (e.g., self, sibling, friend, neighbor)
    A.3   Describe leisure behaviors and participation patterns of family member/client
    A.4   Identify current and subsequent nonschool environments (e.g., shopping malls, parks, community center) which will be accessed by person with disability)
    A.5   Provide information on the availability of leisure materials in the home
    A.6   Identify community leisure environments currently accessed by person with disability
    A.7   Provide information on the amount of time person with disability is able to spend in leisure activity
    A.8   Provide financial, transportation assistance
    A.9   Accumulate leisure resource file which notes accessibility, barriers, experiences, activities, etc.

B. Identifying Needs:
    B.1   Communicate preferences and expectations
    B.2   Assist consumer to communicate needs and preferences
    B.3   Be a liaison between other parents/careproviders

C. Selecting Programs:
    C.1   Identify programs and materials and activities which are chronologically age-appropriate, functional

D. Publicizing Programs/Recruitment:
    D.1   Disseminate program information to other parents/careproviders, advocacy agencies, community bulletin boards

E. Registration:
    E.1   Provide registration and orientation assistance to consumer, if necessary
    E.2   Assist with completion of *Environmental Analysis Inventory* and identification of special needs
    E.3   Assist in identification of appropriate program modifications and adaptations
    E.4   Assist with solicitation and training of volunteer advocates
    E.5   Identify appropriate behavioral methods

F. Provide Appropriate Feedback:
    F.1   Report opportunities for maintenance and generalization of skills to home and other community environments
    F.2   Provide positive social reinforcement to program staff
    F.3   Provide constructive criticism on program development and implementation

G. Determine Future Efforts:
    G.1   Provide to consumer leisure related support skills (e.g., opportunities to practice skills, family/staff training)
    G.2   Participate on Community Advisory Board
    G.3   Advocate for accessible community leisure services
    G.4   Ensure that leisure is an integral part of son's/daughter's or client's IEP/IHP
    G.5   Motivate and encourage consumer to continue participation in future programs

Networking Matrix:
Roles and Responsibilities

Key Players: *Consumers*

Individual residents of a community for whom park and recreation services are organized and administered. The range of individuals who will use these services may be characterized as young, teen, adult, elderly, handicapped, "special", female or male. For the purposes of this matrix, *consumers* will imply those individuals with physical and/or mental disabilities who have generally been denied full access to the range of leisure services provided by municipal park and recreation agencies for any of a variety of reasons.

Examples:

"Special Populations; Persons with Disabilities; Mentally Handicapped, Physically Disabled, Handicapped," etc.

Responsibilities:

A.   Information Gathering:
    A.1   Provide demographic data (e.g., age, address, residential setting, location)
    A.2   Relate past participation and current skills and abilities
    A.3   Identify possible volunteer advocates (e.g., friend, group home, staff, sibling)
B.   Identifying Needs:
    B.1   State leisure needs and preferences
    B.2   Identify obstacles (e.g., lack of transportation, funds, skills)
C.   Selecting Programs:
    C.1   Share ideas on preferred programs, activities, materials
D.   Publicizing Programs/Recruitment:
    D.1   Share program brochures with advocacy agencies, family, friends, neighbors, roommates
    D.2   Encourage others to participate
E.   Registration:
    E.1   Register for preferred programs
    E.2   Assist with completion of *Environmental Analysis Inventory,* including identification of special needs
    E.3   Identify intact strengths relative to skills needed for participation
    E.4   Assist in identification of appropriate program modifications and adaptations
    E.5   Assist with solicitation of volunteer advocates
F.   Provide Appropriate Feedback:
    F.1   Give constructive feedback to instructors, recreation staff on program modifications, adaptations
    F.2   Describe how skills learned in community recreation setting are used in other settings
G.   Determine Future Efforts:
    G.1   Be a self-advocate regarding need and desire to access community leisure services
    G.2   Continue participation in future programs
    G.3   Participate on Community Advisory Board

Networking Matrix:
Roles and Responsibilities

Key Players: *Advocacy Groups*

Public or private, usually non-profit agencies and their representatives, who have as their organizational mission a concern for the health and welfare of a particular constituency. Although not the primary service function of the agency, leisure/recreation services are one of a number of aspects considered in the context of the overall continuum of services to the constituency.

Examples:

Association for Retarded Citizens (ARC); Community Advisory Council on Persons with Disabilities; Multiple Sclerosis Society; Society for the Blind; Society for Children and Adults with Autism; Developmental Disabilities Council.

Responsibilities:

A.   Information Gathering:
    A.1   Identify potential consumers for accessible leisure services
    A.2   Be a liaison with other advocacy agencies, parent/careprovider groups
    A.3   Identify programs, services of a similar nature, offered by advocacy groups
    A.4   Identify possible volunteer advocates
B.   Identifying Needs:
    B.1   Give indication of general leisure/recreation, social needs of persons with disabilities

  B.2 Identify limitations of advocacy agency to provide community leisure services stressing need to collaborate with municipal park and recreation agency

C. Selecting Programs:
  C.1 Coordinate programs, including activities, times, settings, to avoid duplication of leisure services and to ensure that leisure needs of persons with disabilities are addressed

D. Publicizing Programs/Recruitment:
  D.1 Disseminate information to consumers, parents/careproviders
  D.2 Publish programs in agency newsletter
  D.3 Develop speaker's bureau to heighten public awareness regarding availability/accessibility of community recreation programs

E. Registration:
  E.1 Assist in identification of appropriate program modifications
  E.2 Assist with solicitation of volunteer advocates and their training and adaptations

F. Program Implementation:
  F.1 Provide volunteer advocacy to persons with disabilities

G. Provide Appropriate Feedback
  G.1 Provide constructive criticism on collaborative role
  G.2 Be liason between consumer, parent/careproviders, and recreation staff

H. Determine Future Efforts:
  H.1 Assist in development and implementation of staff, parent, consumer and volunteer inservice and preservice education
  H.2 Provide referral service for consumers wanting to be involved in leisure programs
  H.3 Participate on Community Advisory Board
  H.4 Author articles on integration for publication in agency newsletter

Networking Matrix:
Roles and Responsibilities

Key Players: *School/Day Program Personnel*
Individuals responsible for the education and training of persons with and without disabilities in a variety of curriculum areas including leisure/recreation. In the leisure domain, these instructors might focus on shaping attitudes, developing leisure skills, and providing opportunities for practicing skills. This learning usually takes place on-site at the school or day center, although adjacent parks, community centers, and other natural leisure environments are used frequently.

Examples:
Teachers, Administrators, Community Educators, Special Education Teachers, Adapted Physical Educators, Day Program Personnel, Sheltered Workshop Staff, Developmental Learning Center Personnel.

Responsibilities:
A. Information Gathering:
  A.1 Identify potential participants from student population
  A.2 Provide access/link to parents via student's communication book, school newsletters, parent/teacher meetings
  A.3 Supply recreation professionals and instructors with demographic information
  A.4 Provide demographic data on student (e.g., age, disability type, family/home status)
  A.5 Identify potential volunteer advocates (e.g., nonhandicapped peers from other classrooms)

B. Identifying Needs:
  B.1 Report findings from school-based assessments
  B.2 Identify leisure related needs that are part of students' IEP or IHP

C. Selecting Programs:
  C.1 Identify areas of skill training, leisure education in classroom

C.2   Establish link with park and recreation setting where school-based programs could be implemented

D.   Publicizing Programs/Recruitment:
    D.1   Place program brochure on school bulletin boards
    D.2   Disseminate information to parents/careproviders via students

E.   Registration:
    E.1   Assist in completion of *Part* I, *A.*, & *B.*, *Environmental Analysis Inventory*
    E.2   Provide additional information on special needs of participants and other considerations related to disability
    E.3   Assist with solicitation of volunteer advocates and their training in the schools
    E.4   Assist with identification of appropriate program modifications

F.   Provide Appropriate Feedback:
    F.1   Determine consistency of behavioral approaches, i.e., all behavioral changes being detected at school due to community leisure participation
    F.2   Determine generalizability of leisure skills to school and other natural settings
    F.3   Provide social reinforcement to students participating in community leisure programs

G.   Determine Future Efforts:
    G.1   Participate on Community Advisory Board
    G.2   Strengthen ties between school, home, community through Parent-Teacher-Student Organizations
    G.3   Incorporate leisure-related goals and objectives into IEP or IHP
    G.4   Conduct attitude assessment/sensitivity training to nonhandicapped students

Networking Matrix:
Roles and Responsibilities

Key Players: *Allied Health Professionals*
Individuals who provide therapeutic services to persons with disabilities usually in residential or clinical settings (e.g., Rehabilitation Hospitals, Intermediate Care Facilities for the Mentally Retarded). These services are provided by trained or licensed professionals who are typically endorsed by the medical community. Forms of services range from specific concentration on motor, language, or recreational skills development to the coordination of all services for an individual.

Examples:
Communication Disorders Specialist (Speech Therapist), Therapeutic Recreation Specialist, Physical Therapist, Occupational Therapist, Case Manager, Social Worker, Music Therapist, Vocational Rehabilitation Counselor, Psychologist, Activity Coordinator, Physician, Nurse.

Responsibilities:
A.   Information Gathering:
    A.1   Identify potential participants
    A.2   Provide transportation to community leisure settings/programs
    A.3   Accumulate leisure resource file
    A.4   Provide consultation services including teaching techniques/curriculum for leisure skill development, adaptations/modifications
    A.5   Provide information on positioning/handling techniques

B.   Identifying Needs:
    B.1   Conduct and share leisure, social skills assessment information

C.   Publicizing Programs/Recruitment:
    C.1   Disseminate program information to clients

D.   Registration:
    D.1   Assist with completion of various sections of *Environmental Analysis Inventory*
    D.2   Assist with identification of appropriate program modification
    D.3   Assist with solicitation of volunteer advocates and their training

E.   Provide Appropriate Feedback:
    E.1   Determine maintenance/generalization of leisure skills to other environments
F.   Determine Future Efforts:
    F.1   Provide leisure skills training in non-clinically-based environments
    F.2   Include leisure-related goals and objectives in IHP.
    F.3   Provide leisure-related support skills
    F.4   Provide referral services
    F.5   Participate on Community Advisory Board
    F.6   Assist with in-service training of staff, parents, consumers, volunteers, and others

Networking Matrix:
Roles and Responsibilities

Key Players: *Private Recreation Services*

Organizations and agencies which exist to provide a direct service for their membership. They are "member-centered" and respond to the unique interests of its membership. This group may be represented by commercial recreation organizations (e.g., video parlors, amusement parks), clubs and recreation associations and by industries and businesses who sponsor activities on behalf of their employees. Private recreation services are supported by member fees, profits or business capital rather than public monies. Public recreation organizations may contract with private services to use facilities, materials, settings, etc.

Examples:

Sports and health clubs; Country clubs; Swim and tennis clubs; Employee softball and bowling leagues; Amusement parks; Bowling alleys; Skating rinks; Restaurants; Aerobic workout studios.

Responsibilities:
A.   Information Gathering:
    A.1   Offer to share facilities, environments, materials
    A.2   Provide financial support through grants, endowments to persons with disabilities
    A.3   Share information on programs, activities
B.   Selecting Programs:
    B.1   Coordinate leisure services in order to integrate various programs in private recreation settings
C.   Publicizing Programs/Recruitment:
    C.1   Disseminate program information via bulletin boards, newsletters
D.   Registration:
    D.1   Assist with solicitation of volunteer advocates (i.e., could be company service project)
E.   Program Implementation:
    E.1   If facilities, settings physically accessible, permit programs to take place there
    E.2   Assist with implementation of those programs held in private recreation settings
F.   Evaluation:
    F.1   Assist with evaluation on those programs held in private recreation settings
G.   Provide Appropriate Feedback:
    G.1   Provide feedback on programs held in private recreation settings
    G.2   Be liaison between municipal park and recreation organization and business community
H.   Determine Future Efforts:
    H.1   Participate on Community Advisory Board
    H.2   Provide charitable contributions or assist in fundraising to support accessible community leisure services

Networking Matrix:
Roles and Responsibilities

Key Players: *Quasi-public Recreation Services*

Organizations basically dependent upon voluntary financial support and serving a distinctive clientele. Financial support may be through endowments, donations, member fees, grants, United Way funds, or voluntary contributions of time, materials, facilities, and personnel. These organizations are generally nonprofit and have the health and welfare of their constituency in mind. Clientele include youth, persons with disabilities, religious groups, and fraternal or patriotic societies. Public recreation organizations may contract with quasi-public services for use of facilities, materials, setting or volunteers.

Examples:
YMCA; YWCA; Boy Scouts; Girl Scouts; 4-H Club; Catholic Youth Organization; Boy's Club of America, Kiwanis International; Lions Club; American Lung Association; Special Recreation Clubs.

Responsibilities:
A. Information Gathering:
   A.1   Identify resources (e.g., financial, transportation, volunteers)
   A.2   Identify accessible programs and activities available to persons with disabilities
B. Identifying Needs:
   B.1   Provide rationale and support for activity participation by nonhandicapped persons and assist with relating needs to persons with disabilities
C. Selecting Programs:
   C.1   Identify programs complimentary to municipal park and recreation programs
   C.2   Discuss methods to collaborate on programs, settings
   C.3   Co-responsibility with park and recreation for activity offerings which serve as "stepping-stones" to quasi-public recreation programs
D. Publicizing Programs/Recruitment:
   D.1   Post program brochures on bulletin boards
   D.2   Referral for persons with disabilities to community leisure programs
E. Registration:
   E.2   Assist with solicitation of volunteer advocates (i.e., could be community service project)
F. Program Implementation:
   F.1   If facilities, settings physically accessible, permit programs to take place there
   F.2   Assist in programs held at quasi-public settings
G. Evaluation:
   G.1   Assist in program held at quasi-public settings
H. Provide Appropriate Feedback:
   H.1   Provide constructive feedback on program planning and implementation
I. Determine Future Efforts:
   I.1   Participate on Community Advisory Board
   I.2   Provide volunteer referral services

Networking Matrix:
Roles and Responsibilities

Key Players: *Professional and Educational Associations/Technical Resources*
Agencies and individuals not specifically organized as providers of leisure services but able to give consultation and/or technical resources in support of the delivery of leisure services within community settings.

Examples:
Recreation, Park, and Leisure Studies Departments in Universities; Publicly or privately funded research institutes; Leisure consultants; Professional Associations (e.g., National Recreation and Park Association; National Therapeutic Recreation Society; The Association for Persons with Severe Handicaps); Metropolitan Councils.

Responsibilities:
A. Information Gathering:
   A.1   Conduct formal research, data gathering, evaluation
   A.2   Compile and share demographic information
   A.3   Serve as a consultant to leisure service agency

A.4   Share mailing lists of agencies (e.g., group homes) serving members of special populations

B.   Identifying Needs:
  B.1   Present findings of research on recreation opportunities for persons with disabilities
  B.2   Train University students in Therapeutic Recreation to conduct preference assessments for persons with disabilities

C.   Selecting Programs:
  C.1   Make recommendations on appropriate and integrated program offerings

D.   Publicizing Programs/Recruitment:
  D.1   Advertise programs in educational settings and in agency newsletters (e.g., school newspaper, quarterly newsletter)
  D.2   Assist in outreach/networking between all groups

E.   Registration:
  E.1   Provide recommendations on program modifications

F.   Program Implementation:
  F.1   Assist with activity and/or task analysis of leisure activities and skills
  F.2   Provide volunteer advocates (e.g., student interns)

G.   Evaluation:
  G.1   Serve as independent observer at program
  G.2   Provide student interns to assist
  G.3   Analyze evaluative data concerning participant outcomes
  G.4   Assist in validation of data collection procedures and interobserver reliability

H.   Program Summary and Report:
  H.1. Report findings at workshops, conferences, and in journals and other written media
  H.2   Share evaluative data with community recreation professionals

I.   Provide Appropriate Feedback:
  I.1   Provide constructive feedback on integration approaches
  I.2   Solicit feedback from practitioner for future research and program evaluation

J.   Determine Future Efforts:
  J.1   Serve as central coordinating body and facilitator for Community Advisory Board
  J.2   Conduct longitudinal research on effects of integrated programs
  J.3   Develop new, improved integration technology
  J.4   Develop curriculum to educate/train community recreation professionals

Appendix E

NETWORKING REFERRAL LIST

Directions: 1. Make 9 copies of this form (i.e., one page per category) plus multiple copies of this or a similarly formatted page;
2. Designate a category for each sheet (See list immediately below);
3. When a contact is made, fill in appropriate information;
4. Put additional contacts on second and subsequent pages.

Category: ____ Community recreation professional
____ Parents/careproviders
____ Consumers
____ Advocacy groups
____ School/Day program personnel
____ Allied health professionals
____ Private recreation services
____ Quasi-public recreation services
____ Professional & educational associations/Technical resources

---

Name: _____ Title: _____
Agency: _____ Telephone: (w) _____
Address: _____ (h) _____
_____

Name: _____ Title: _____
Agency: _____ Telephone: (w) _____
Address: _____ (h) _____
_____

Name: _____ Title: _____
Agency: _____ Telephone: (w) _____
Address: _____ (h) _____
_____

Name: _____ Title: _____
Agency: _____ Telephone: (w) _____
Address: _____ (h) _____
_____

Name: _____ Title: _____
Agency: _____ Telephone: (w) _____
Address: _____ (h) _____
_____

Name: _____ Title: _____
Agency: _____ Telephone: (w) _____
Address: _____ (h) _____
_____

Name: _____ Title: _____
Agency: _____ Telephone: (w) _____
Address: _____ (h) _____
_____

Appendix F

BUILDING ACCESS SURVEY
(REVISED AUGUST 1986)
MINNESOTA STATE COUNCIL FOR THE HANDICAPPED

Metro Square, 7th & Robert Sts., Suite 208 • St. Paul, Minnesota 55101
Telephone (612) 296-6785 VOICE and TDD
TOLL-FREE HOTLINE 1-800-652-9747 VOICE and TDD

BUILDING _____

STREET ADDRESS _____

CITY/STATE _____ ZIP _____

SURVEYOR _____

TITLE _____ PHONE _____

BUILDING OWNER _____

DATE OPENED _____ ☐ NEW CONSTRUCTION   ☐ RENOVATION

MAJOR USE AND BRIEF DESCRIPTION _____

_____

HA-00003-05 (8-86)

The Building Access Survey (revised August 1986) is reproduced by permission of the Minnesota State Council for the Handicapped, St. Paul, Minnesota.

190

INSTRUCTIONS TO THE SURVEYOR

A circled item, for example ⑤ or ©, indicates that it is a specification of the Minnesota State Building Code Chapter 1340, or other statutory or regulatory requirement.

The Minnesota State Building Code Chapter 1340 establishes minimum requirements of accessibility for all new construction and structural renovation after November 18, 1975.

Even in those instances where it is not a legal requirement, these provisions present a good standard to strive for.

Recommendations of the Minnesota State Council for the Handicapped are also listed.

Surveyors are encouraged to use the comments section to give more detail when there is a discrepancy between the building's current status and the requirement.

PARKING

	Current Status	Requirement	Recommendation
1. How many off-street parking spaces are provided? If none, go on to question #7.			
② How many of these parking spaces are provided for use by disabled persons?		1 per 50 or a fraction of 50	
3. What is the surface of the parking area?			Paved and level
④ How many of the handicapped parking spaces are designated with upright, permanent signs?		All must be identified	
ⓐ Are the signs visible to a motorist inside a vehicle parked in the space?		Yes	
ⓑ Do the signs display the International Symbol of Accessibility?		Yes	
ⓒ Are the signs white characters on a blue background?		Yes	
ⓓ Do the signs require display of a state certificate or license?		Yes	

	Current Status	Requirement	Recommendation
(5.) How wide is the space reserved for use by disabled people?		Minimum of 12'	
(6.) Are the handicapped parking spaces located as near as possible to an accessible building entrance?		Yes	

Comments or Sketches:

EXTERIOR PATH

	Current Status	Requirement	Recommendation
7. Is the walk between the parking area & accessible entrance(s) paved?			Yes
8. Are there any curbs between the parking area & entrance? If no, go to #9.			
(a.) If yes, are curb cuts or curb ramps provided?		Yes	
(b.) What is the texture of the surface?		See page 4*	
(9.) Is there a continuous walkway to the main entrance without steps or abrupt changes in level? If no, describe in the comments section, including number of steps.			
10. Is there an inclined walkway (that is, external ramp) to the main entrance? If no or not applicable, go to #12.		Yes	

	Current Status	Requirement	Recommendation
a. What is the width of the inclined path?	_____	4' minimum	
b. What is the total rise of the level change?	_____		
c. What is the total horizontal length of the inclined path?	_____		
d. What is the ratio of the rise (b) to the horizontal length (c)?	_____	1:20 maximum slope	
e. Are handrails provided along the inclined path?			Yes, if there are dropoffs on either side
f. What is the texture of the surface?	_____	Concrete, asphalt, or similar permanent non-slip material	
11. If the walk has a cross-slope, indicate the degree of slope from side to side.	_____		1:50 maximum slope

*Aggregate is required on all state and municipal projects.

Comments:

ENTRANCE

	Current Status	Requirement	Recommendation
12. If there is an exterior entrance landing, what are the dimensions?		See UBC 3304	5' x 5'
13. Is the exterior entrance landing level?		Yes	
14. What is the rise of the threshold?		$1/2''$ maximum	
a. Is it abrupt or beveled?			Beveled
15. How much room is there next to the latch side of the door, so that a person in a wheelchair can approach and open it? (illustration below)		12'' minimum	18'' — 24''

	Current Status	Requirement	Recommendation
16. What is the width of the clear useable opening of the entry door (that is, from the face of the door when open at 90° to the face of the opposite door stop)?		31'' minimum 32'' (UBC)	34'' minimum
17. What is the height of the door latch hardware from the landing surface?		42'' maximum	
18. Describe the door latch hardware (e.g., round knob, lever handle, U-shape pull, push plate, etc.).		Lever handle	
19. Can the door latch hardware be operated with a single movement of one hand by persons having minimal grip strength?		Yes	

Comments:

194

	Current Status	Requirement	Recommendation

20. Is the building, facility or grounds designated as accessible by display of the International Symbol of Accessibility?

_____ Yes

INTERIORS

	Current Status	Requirement	Recommendation

21. Is there a level interior entrance landing?

_____ Yes

a. Is it level with or not more than ¹/₂" lower than the threshold?

_____ Yes

22. How much room is there next to the latch side of the door, so that a person in a wheelchair can approach and open it? (illustration below)

_____ 12" minimum   18" — 24"

23. Are there two sets of doors or doorways at the entrance that form a lobby, vestibule or foyer? If no, go on to #24.

a. What is the depth of the vestibule?

_____ 7' minimum

b. What is the clear useable opening of the second doorway (that is, from the face of the door when open at 90⁰ to the face of the opposite door stop)?

_____ 31" minimum   34" minimum
          32" (UBC)

Comments:

195

	Current Status	Requirement	Recommendation
24. If there is a security system, please describe (e.g., intercom, closed circuit TV, key or card controlled electronic lock). •			
ⓐ If yes, what is the height from the floor to the highest control?		60" maximum	36" – 48"
b. Is the "go ahead" signal audio, visual or both?			Both
㉕ Does the interior entrance landing provide access to the building's main floor or lobby?		Yes	
26. How many floors are there, including the basement?			
㉗ Which floors are not served by ramps or elevators?		Refer to section below*	
28. Do any of the floors have raised, lowered or terraced areas?			
ⓐ If yes, do ramps, elevators or lifts serve all of these levels? Specify means of access.		Refer to section below*	

* Access for disabled persons to other stories or levels of a building used by the general public and/or employees must be by elevator or ramp, except:

1. Hotels and apartment buildings not exceeding three stories in height.
2. Other buildings two stories or less in height which have an occupant load of less than 100 persons on floors, levels and mezzanines other than the floor of building access.

A lift may be installed in an <u>existing</u> building to provide access to another level, (refer to #31).

Comments:

196

29. Is there a working passenger elevator? If no, or not applicable, go to #30.

	Current Status	Requirement	Recommendation
a. What is the height of the top call button in the hallway?		60″ maximum	42″ maximum
b. What is the width of the clear useable opening of the elevator doorway from bumper to bumper?		32″ mimimum	
c. What is the height of the top floor button?		60″ maximum	48″ maximum
d. What is the height of the emergency stop, call button and/or phone box latch?		60″ maximum	48″ maximum
e. Are the elevator controls identifed by tactile labels?		Yes	Raised letters, numerals & characters
f. What is the height from the floor of the tactile floor numbers mounted on the elevator door jamb?		42″ — 54″	
g. Are there audio and visual signals for elevator direction and floor stops?			Both
h. Does the cabin have handrails on one side, both sides, rear wall or all three sides? Specify.			All 3 sides
i. What are the dimensions inside the cabin?			54″ deep x 68″ wide

Comments:

	Current Status	Requirement	Recommendation

30. Are ramps provided for access to all floors and levels not served by elevators? If no or not applicable, go to #31.

(a.) What is the width of the narrowest ramp?

Requirement: 36″ if occupant load is 50 or less, 44″ if more than 50*

b. What is the rise of the steepest ramp?

c. What is the horizontal length of the steepest ramp?

(d.) What is the ratio of the rise (b) to the horizontal length (c) of the steepest ramp?

Requirement: 1:12 maximum slope

(e.) What is the surface of the ramp?

Requirement: Non-slip

(f.) Are handrails provided on one or both sides of the ramp?

Requirement: Both sides if slope exceeds 1:15

(i.) How high is the handrail(s) above the ramp surface?

Requirement: 30″ — 34″

* Contact the local building official if there are questions concerning occupant load.

Comments:

	Current Status	Requirement	Recommendation
(ii.) How far do the handrails extend beyond the top & bottom of the ramp?	_____	6" minimum	12"
(iii.) Do the extensions return to the wall or terminate safely?	_____	Yes	
(g.) Is there a landing at the top and how long is it in the direction of the ramp?	_____	Yes, 5' minimum	
(h.) Is there a landing at the bottom and how long is it in the direction of the ramp?	_____	Yes, 6' minimum	
i. Is there an intermediate landing? (1.) How long is it in the direction of the ramp, excluding landings?	_____	5' minimum	
(2.) If the total rise (b) exceeds 3', what is the vertical height at the point of the landing?	_____	30" or less	
31. Are lifts provided for access to levels and areas not served by elevators or ramps? If no, go on to #32.	_____	See footnote on page 7	
(a.) How many sides are enclosed?	_____	All four sides	
(b.) Specify whether the surfaces leading to and from the lift are level, ramped at a 1:12 slope, or other.	_____	Level or ramped with 1:12 slope	

Comments:

199

	Current Status	Requirement	Recommendation

(c.) What are the inside dimensions of the platform? — 36"WX48"L min. 42"WX60"L max.

(d.) What is the total vertical traveling distance of the lift? — 54" maximum

32. Are stairs provided to any levels? If no, go on to #34.

(a.) Is the riser slanted to meet the tread or nosing edge (illustration #i), or does the tread extend beyond a vertical riser (#ii)? — Either

(b.) What shape is the nosing? — Rounded

(c.) How much does the nosing project beyond the riser? (Illustration below) — 1" maximum

ii

i

33. Are handrails provided on both sides of the stairs? — Yes

(a.) How high are the handrails above the nosing of the tread? — 30" — 34"

Comments:

	Current Status	Requirement	Recommendation

b. How far do the handrails extend beyond the top and bottom of the stairs? — Requirement: 6" minimum — Recommendation: 12" minimum

c. Do the extensions return to the wall or terminate safely? — Requirement: Yes

34. Do all interior doors provide at least 31" of clear useable opening (that is, from the face of the door when open at 90° to the face of the opposite door stop)? If no, give locations and clear openings of narrow doorways: — Requirement: Yes — Recommendation: 34" minimum

_____

_____

35. How much room is there next to the latch side of a typical door so that a person in a wheelchair can approach and open it? (illustration below) — Requirement: 12" minimum — Recommendation: 18" – 24"

36. What is the rise of the threshold of interior doors? — Requirement: 1/2" maximum

37. What is the height of the door latch hardware from the floor? — Requirement: 42" maximum

Comments:

	Current Status	Requirement	Recommendation
(38.) Describe the door latch hardware (e.g., round knob, lever handle, U-shape pull, push plate, etc.).		Lever handle	
(39.) Can the door latch hardware be operated with a single effort of one hand by persons having minimal grip strength?		Yes	
40. Are there doors to hazardous areas such as exit stairs, loading platforms, boiler rooms and stages?			
(a.) Do these doors have knurled or similarly marked handles?		Yes	
(41.) Is there tactile identification of doors to public spaces?		Yes	Raised numerals, letters & characters
(a.) What is the height from the floor?		54″ — 66″	
(b.) Is the tactile signage mounted to the wall on the latch side of the door?		Yes	
42. Are doors equipped with kickplates?			Yes
43. Are phones provided for public use?			
(a.) If yes, what is the height of the highest operable part of the lowest phone from the floor (i.e., handset, dial and coin receiver)?		54″	48″

Comments:

	Current Status	Requirement	Recommendation
b. How wide is the space in front of the phone?		30" in width	
c. How much room is there in front of the phone?		12" in depth	
d. Does any phone have a volume control for hearing-impaired persons?			Yes, at least one
e. Does any phone have special provisions for persons with hearing aids?			Yes, at least one
44. Are water fountains provided?			
a. If yes, what is the height of the spout of the lowest mounted water fountain from the floor?		33" maximum	
b. Describe the type of control and location.		Hand-operated, up front	Lever or push bar
c. If the fountain is in an alcove, how wide is the alcove?		32" minimum	
45. What is the working height of the following?			
a. Manual fire alarms		60" maximum	36" — 48"
b. Thermostats		60" maximum	36" — 48"
c. Light switches		60" maximum	36" — 48"

Comments:

	Current Status	Requirement	Recommendation
(d.) Electrical outlets	___	60" maximum	24" — 48"
(e.) Intercom controls	___	60" maximum	36" — 48"
(f.) Other: _____	___	60" maximim	36" — 48"
46. Do alarm signals have both audio and visual components?	___		Yes, both
47. Are there pedestrian aisles or lanes defined with directional barriers, rails, benches, tables, seats or fences? If no, go to #48.			
a. What is the minimum width of such aisles?	___	36" — 44" (UBC)	
(b.) If such aisles include check-out lanes or service lanes, does at least one such lane provide at least 31" clear width?	___	Yes	36" minimum
(c.) Is this lane identified for handicapped use?	___	Yes	
48. Describe the type of flooring (e.g., concrete, wood, tile, linoleum, low pile carpet, plush carpet, etc.)	___		Not plush carpet or slick flooring
49. Does the building have an auditorium, meeting, dining or other assembly room?			
(a.) Is it accessible by walk, ramp, elevator, lift or combination thereof, through a principal entrance?	___	Yes	

Comments:

	Current Status	Requirement	Recommendation

b. Does it have permanent fixed seating? _____

c. What is the seating capacity? _____

(d.) How many spaces are reserved for persons in wheelchairs? _____ Refer to table below

e. What are the dimensions of these spaces? _____ 33"W x 60"D minimum

(f.) Where are these spaces located? _____ Main floor & level surface — Scattered and not in aisles

VIEWING POSITIONS

MOTION PICTURE AUDITORIUMS	
Seating Capacity	Minimum Wheelchair Viewing Positions
500 and less	4
Over 500	8
OTHER ASSEMBLY OCCUPANCIES	
500 and Less	4
501 – 1,000	12
1,001 – 1,500	16
Over 1,500	16 plus 1 per 500 additional

50. Does this building house sleeping rooms, apartments, or residential suites for lease or rent? If no, go to #51.

a. If yes, specify hotel, motel, dormitory, apartment, other. _____

b. Give number of units. _____

	Current Status	**Requirement**	**Recommendation**

(c.) Give number of units equipped for disabled persons. _____ Refer to table below

Total Number of Dwelling Units/ Guest Rooms in Building	Number of Dwelling Units/Guest Rooms that must be Accessible
0 — 7	0
8 — 39	1
40 — 59	2
60 — 79	3
80 — 99	4
100 — 119	5
120 — 139	6
140 — 159	7
160 — 179	8
180 — 199	9
200 —	10 plus 1 per each 50 units exceeding 200

51. Specify if there are any special use areas in the building (e.g., community or recreation room, laundry, library, etc.). If no, go to #52. _____

   a. Is there a barrier free interior path of travel to each of these areas from the accessible entrance? If not, describe below. _____ Yes

Comments:

SANITATION FACILITIES

	Current Status	Requirement	Recommendation
52. Are there any toilet facilities? If no, go to #86.	_____		
53. If this is a hotel or apartment building, how many guest rooms or dwelling units are equipped for disabled persons?	_____	Refer to table on page 17	
54. How many toilet facilities are equipped for disabled persons?	_____	Refer below*	
55. Is the location of these equipped facilities listed in the room directory, if one is provided?	_____	Yes	
56. Are the facilities accessible from inside the building without leaving and re-entering?	_____	Yes	
57. Is there a continuous route of travel to the toilet rooms without steps or abrupt changes in level? If no, describe: _____		Yes	

* At least one toilet room for each sex or a private facility useable by either sex must be accessible. If a building has two or more toilet rooms for each sex or two separate facilities useable by either sex, at least two toilet rooms for each sex or two separate facilities useable by either sex must be accessible.

PLEASE ANSWER THE FOLLOWING QUESTIONS ABOUT FACILITIES EQUIPPED FOR HANDICAPPED PERSONS. IF THERE AREN'T ANY EQUIPPED FACILITIES USE A TYPICAL FACILITY. GIVE ANSWERS FOR BOTH WOMEN'S AND MEN'S OR SEPARATE FACILITIES, WHERE APPLICABLE.

	Women's	Men's or Unisex	Requirement
58. Is the door or entry identified as accessible?			Yes
59. What is the width of the clear useable opening of the door or doorway (that is, from the face of the door when open at 90° to the face of the opposite door stop)?	_____	_____	31″ minimum 34″ minimum
60. What is the rise of the threshold?	_____	_____	½″ maximum

207

	Current Status		Requirement	Recommendation
	Women's	Men's or Unisex		
61. What is the height of the door latch hardware from the floor?			42" maximum	
62. Describe the door latch hardware (e.g., round knob, lever handle, U-shape pull, push plate, etc.)			Lever handle	
63. Can the door latch hardware be operated with a single movement of one hand by persons with minimal grip strength?			Yes	
64. How much room is there next to the latch side of the door so that a person in a wheelchair can approach and open it? (illustration below)			12" minimum	18" — 24"
65. Are entry doors equipped with kickplates?				Yes
66. Is the entry through two doors or doorways that form a vestibule or foyer? (illustration below)				
(a.) If yes, what is the depth of the vestibule?			7" minimum	
(b.) What is the clear useable opening of the second door?			31" minimum	34" minimum

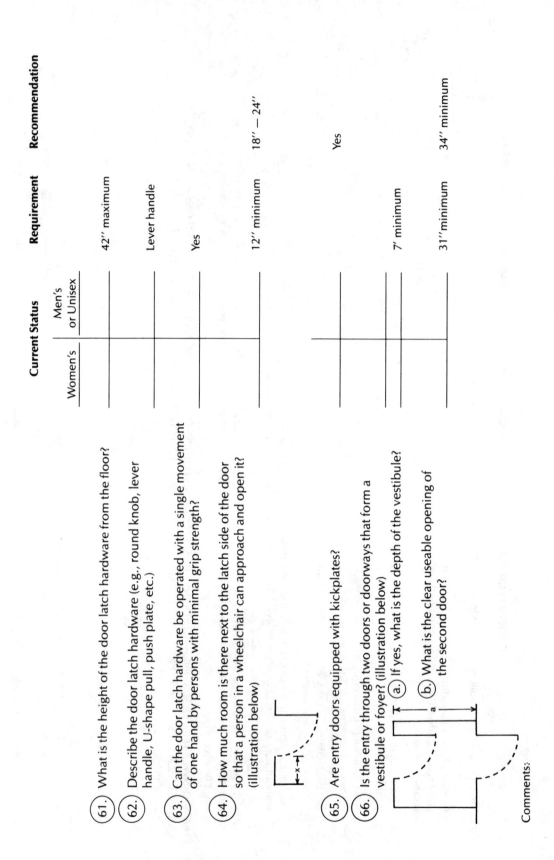

Comments:

	Current Status		Requirement	Recommendation
	Women's	Men's or Unisex		
67. Is the toilet room floor one common level?			Yes	
68. Is there a place that provides a full five foot diameter clear floor space in the toilet room?				Yes
69. Is there clear knee space under at least one sink for a person in a wheelchair?			Yes	
a. If yes, how tall is that space?			29″ minimum	
b. How wide is that space?			31″ minimum	
c. Not counting the drain pipes, how deep is that space?			12″ minimum	
70. What is the height of the top of the sink rim from the floor?			34″ maximum	
71. Specify the faucet hardware (e.g., lever handle, round knob, tip-tap, etc.)			Lever handles	
72. Are drain and waste pipes covered or insulated to prevent burns?				Yes
73. What are the working heights from the floor of the following:				
a. Soap dispenser control			40″ maximum	

Comments:

	Current Status		Requirement	Recommendation
	Women's	Men's or Unisex		
(b.) Towel dispenser control			40″ maximum	
(c.) Disposal unit's top edge			40″ maximum	
(d.) Mirror's lowest edge			40″ maximum	
(e.) Product dispenser control			40″ maximum	
(f.) Shelf top			40″ maximum	
(g.) Other _____			40″ maximum	
(h.) Are these accessories free of interference by grab bars, appliances or fixtures?	NA		Yes	
74. Are urinals provided?				
(a.) If yes, what is the height from the floor of the top of the lip of the lowest urinal?			18″ maximum	
(b.) How wide a space is there to approach the urinal?			31″ minimum	
(75.) How high is the toilet seat above the floor?			17″ – 20″	17″ – 18″
(76.) How much clear floor space is there between the front of the toilet bowl and the nearest obstruction (i.e., closed stall door, wall, heat register, etc.)?			36″ minimum	40″ minimum

Comments:

	Current Status		Requirement	Recommendation
	Women's	Men's or Unisex		
77. How wide is the approach area to the accessible toilet?			36" minimum	40"
78. Is the accessible toilet enclosed by privacy screens?				Yes, if more than 1 toilet
a. If yes, what is the clear opening of the door or doorway (that is, from the face of the door when open at 90° to the face of the opposite door stop)?			31" minimum	
b. If a 90° turn is required to enter the toilet compartment, how wide is the corridor?				42" minimum
c. If there is a door, which way does it swing, in or out?				Out
d. Specify the door latch hardware (e.g., lever, slide bolt, blade & slot, thumb screw, other).			Lever action	
e. Can the door latch be operated with a single movement of one hand by persons with minimal grip strength?			Yes	
f. Can the door be unlocked from either side?			Yes	
79. Are grab bars provided at the toilet?			Yes	

Comments:

211

	Current Status		Requirement	Recommendation
	Women's	Men's or Unisex		
80. Are they securely fastened with reinforcements in the walls, able to support a load of not less than 250 lbs.?			Yes	
81. If yes, are they on one side, both sides or rear wall?			Both sides or one side wall & rear wall	Both sides for front entry; side wall & rear wall for side entry
82. What is the outside diameter of these bars?			1-1/2"	
83. What is the clearance from walls or partitions?			1-1/2"	
84. On the side wall(s):				
a. Is there a horizontal component?			Yes	
b. What is the lowest point above the seat?			10"	
c. How far does it extend in front of the toilet bowl?			6" minimum	
d. How long is the bar?			12" minimum	42" minimum
e. Is there a vertical component?			Yes	

Comments:

212

	Current Status		Requirement	Recommendation
	Women's	Men's or Unisex		

f.) How far is it mounted from in front of the toilet bowl? — 12″

g.) How far is it mounted above the toilet seat? — 12″

h.) How long is the bar? — 18″

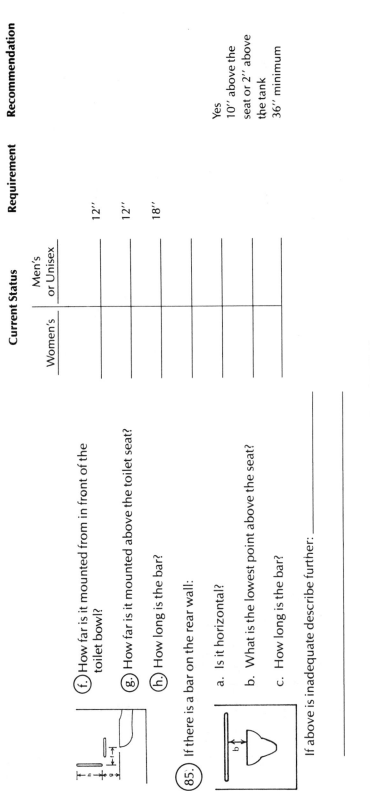

85. If there is a bar on the rear wall:

a. Is it horizontal?

b. What is the lowest point above the seat? — Yes 10″ above the seat or 2″ above the tank

c. How long is the bar? — 36″ minimum

If above is inadequate describe further: _____

BATHING FACILITIES

Current Status	Requirement	Recommendation
_____		

86. Are bathing facilities provided? If no, go to #108.

Comments:

	Current Status	Requirement	Recommendation
87. If this is a hotel or apartment building, how many guest rooms or dwelling units have bathing facilities equipped for disabled persons?		Refer to table on page 17	
88. If another type of building, how many bathing facilities are equipped for disabled persons?			
89. Is there a door or doorway to the tub room or shower compartment?			
a. If yes, what is the clear useable opening (that is, from the face of the door when open at 90° to the face of the opposite door stop)?		31″ minimum	34″ minimum
b. What is the threshold height?		½″ maximum	
90. Is there a fixed, folding or retractible seat available to use in the bathtub or shower? If yes, give dimensions of:		Yes	
a. Height from Floor		17″ − 20″	
b. Width			
c. Depth		15″ minimum	
91. Is it of water-resistive material?		Yes	
92. Is there a shower?			

Comments:

214

	Current Status	Requirement	Recommendation
93. Is the shower head hand-held with a flexible hose?		Yes, if no shower is provided	
a. If yes, how long is the flexible hose?	_____	6' minimum	
b. If there is a vertical height adjustment bar, how long is it?	_____	4' minimum	
94. Specify the type of water control valves (e.g., knob, lever, other).		Single Lever	
95. Are the controls reachable from the seat?	_____	Yes	
96. If there is a tub area, are grab bars provided? If no, go to #102.	_____	Yes	
97. Are they securely fastened with reinforcements in the walls, able to support a load of not less than 250 lbs.?	_____	Yes	
98. What is the outside diameter of these bars?	_____	1-1/2"	
99. What is the clearance from the walls?	_____	1-1/2"	
100. Is there a horizontal bar?	_____	Yes	
a. How high is it above the rim of the tub?	_____	4" – 6"	
b. How long is it?	_____	36" minimum	

Comments:

215

	Current Status	Requirement	Recommendation

101. Is there a vertical bar?

Requirement: Yes

  (a.) How far is it mounted from the end of the tub?

Requirement: 30"

  (b.) How high is the bottom of the bar from the rim of the tub?

Requirement: 9"

  (c.) How long is the bar?

Requirement: 33"

102. If there is a shower compartment, are grab bars provided? If no, go to #108.

Requirement: Yes

103. Are they securely fastened with reinforcements in the walls, able to support a load of not less than 250 lbs.?

Requirement: Yes

104. What is the outside diameter of these bars?

Requirement: 1-1/2"

105. What is the clearance from the walls?

Requirement: 1-1/2"

106. Is there a vertical bar?

Requirement: Yes

  (a.) On what wall is it mounted, in relation to the seat?

Requirement: On the wall opposite the seat

  (b.) How high is the bottom of the bar from the floor?

Requirement: 36"

  (c.) How long is the bar?

Requirement: 24"

Comments:

	Current Status	Requirement	Recommendation

107. Is there a horizontal bar? — Yes

   (a.) On what wall is it mounted, in relation to the seat? — On the wall adjacent to the seat

   (b.) How high is it above the seat? — 10"

   (c.) How long is it? — 18" minimum

KITCHEN FACILITIES

	Current Status	Requirement	Recommendation

108. Are kitchen facilities provided? If no, the form is complete.

109. If this is a hotel or apartment building, how many dwelling units have kitchens equipped for disabled persons? — Refer to table on page 17

110. What is the height of the top of the kitchen sink/counter? — 34" maximum

111. Is there clear knee space under a kitchen sink? — Yes

   (a.) If yes, how tall is that space? — 29" minimum

   (b.) How wide is that space? — 31" minimum

Comments:

217

	Current Status	Requirement	Recommendation
c. Not counting the drain pipes, how deep is that space?		12" minimum	
d. Are drain and waste pipes covered or insulated to prevent burns?			Yes
112. Specify the type of water control valves (e.g., lever handles, knob, other).		Lever handles	
113. Specify the location of the controls for the range (that is, on the front, side, or back of the unit).		On the front or side of the unit	
114. Is there a work surface with clear knee space for someone in a wheelchair?		Yes	
a. If yes, is it fixed, folding or retractible?		Either one	
b. Give the dimension of the surface width and depth.		4 square feet or 2' x 2'	
c. What is the height of the top of the work surface?		34" maximum	
d. How tall is the knee space?		29" minimum	
e. How wide is the knee space?		31" minimum	
f. How deep is the knee space?		12" minimum	

Comments:

Current Status	Requirement	Recommendation
	5' minimum between walls, cabinets, appliances or other obstructions	

(115.) How much clear floor space is there in the kitchen work area, including toe space under cabinets if that space is $8^3/4''$ high and 6'' deep?

Comments:

Appendix G

**DIRECTORY OF NATIONAL
ORGANIZATIONS SERVING PERSONS
WITH DISABILITIES**

DIRECTORY OF NATIONAL
ORGANIZATIONS SERVING PERSONS WITH DISABILITIES

American Foundation for the Blind, Inc.
15 West 16th Street
New York, NY 10011

Association for Children and Adults with Learning Disabilities
4156 Library Road
Pittsburgh, PA 15234

The Association for Persons with Severe Handicaps
7010 Roosevelt Way, N.E.
Seattle, WA 98115

Association for Retarded Citizens (ARC-US)
2501 Avenue J
Arlington, TX 76006

Council for Exceptional Children
1920 Association Drive
Reston, VA 22091

Epilepsy Foundation of America
4351 Garden City Drive
Suite 406
Landover, MD 20785

Information Center for Individuals with Disabilities
20 Providence St., Room 329
Boston, MA 02116

Muscular Dystrophy Association, Inc.
810 Seventh Avenue
New York, NY 10019

National Amputation Foundation
12–45 150th Street
Whitestone, NY 11357

National Association for Mental Health
10 Columbus Circle
New York, NY 10019

National Association of Developmental Disabilities Council
1234 Massachusetts Ave., N.W.
Suite 103
Washington, D.C. 20005

National Down Syndrome Society
141 5th Avenue
New York, NY 10010

National Easter Seal Society
2023 W. Ogden Avenue
Chicago, IL 60612

National Federation of the Blind
1800 Johnson Street
Baltimore, MD 21230

National Head Injury Foundation
280 Singletary Lane
Framingham, MA 01701

National Information Center on Deafness
Gallaudet College
Kendall Green
Washington, D.C. 20002

National Multiple Sclerosis Society
205 E. 42nd Street
New York, NY 10017

National Paraplegia Foundation
333 North Michigan Avenue
Chicago, IL 60601

National Society for Autistic Children
1234 Massachusetts Ave., N.W.
Suite 1017
Washington, D.C. 20005

National Spinal Cord Injury Foundation
369 Elliot Street
Newton Upper Falls, MA 02164

National Therapeutic Recreation Society
3101 Park Center Drive
Alexandria, VA 22302

United Cerebral Palsy Association
66 East 34th Street
New York, NY 10016

NATIONAL SPORTS AND RECREATION ASSOCIATIONS
SERVING PERSONS WITH DISABILITIES

American Blind Bowling Association
150 N. Bellaire Avenue
Louisville, KY 40206

American Wheelchair Bowling Association
Route 2, Box 750
Lutz, FL 33549

Disabled Outdoorsmen
5223 South Lorel Avenue
Chicago, IL 60638

**International Committee of the Silent
Sports Gallaudet College**
800 Florida Avenue and
7th Street, N.E.
Washington, D.C. 20002

**International Wheelchair Road Racers
Club, Inc.**
165 78th Avenue, N.E.
St. Petersburg, FL 33702

National Amputee Skiing Association
3738 Walnut Avenue
Carmichael, CA 95608

**National Council-Boy Scouts of America
Scouting for the Handicapped**
1325 Walnut Hill Lane
Irving, TX 75038-3096

**National Handicapped Sports &
Recreation Association**
4405 East-West Highway
Suite 603
Bethesda, MD 20814

National Recreation & Park Association
3101 Park Center Drive
Alexandria, VA 22302

National Wheelchair Athletic Association
3617 Betty Drive
Suite S
Colorado Springs, CO 80907

National Wheelchair Softball Association
PO 737
Sioux Falls, SD 57101

Ski for Light, Inc.
1455 W. Lake Street
Minneapolis, MN 55408

United States Association for Blind Athletes
Kiowa and Institute Streets
Colorado Springs, CO 80903

**United States Cerebral Palsy Athletic
Association**
34518 Warren Road
Suite 264
Westland, MI 48185

**United States Olympic Committee's
Committee on Sport for the Disabled**
1750 East Boulder Avenue
Colorado Springs, CO 80909-5760

Vinland National Center
3675 Ihduhapi Road
Loretto, MN 55357

Wilderness Inquiry II
1313 Fifth St., S.E.
Suite 327A
Minneapolis, MN 55414

Appendix H

**ENVIRONMENTAL ANALYSIS INVENTORY
EVALUATION FORMS**

On the following pages, blank copies of all forms are provided for you to reproduce and use as aids in your recreation programming efforts. Completed samples of the forms are included with explanations in the text.

ENVIRONMENTAL ANALYSIS INVENTORY
PART I: (A) APPROPRIATENESS OF RECREATION ACTIVITY/SETTING

When an activity or setting is being examined for recreation involvement, there are key areas that should be addressed prior to implementation of the program. These areas relate to the *appropriateness* of the activity or setting under investigation to an individual's needs, preferences, and skill level.

With such a wide variety of leisure-related activities and settings available to individuals with disabilities, the information gained from the following questions will assist the person with a disability, their care providers, and recreation staff in determining the appropriateness of the activity and setting for participation. In situations where a decision between two or more activities must be made, this information may assist in determining the best activity to meet the individual's needs and skill level.

Please record the participant's name, activity, setting, and date and check the correct response to the following seven questions. If the responses to the questions are affirmative (i.e., yes), proceed to the next step of the Environmental Analysis Inventory (PART II: ACTIVITY/DISCREPANCY ANALYSIS). If the responses to these questions fail to show positive results, an alternative recreation activity or setting should be selected for analysis and potential participation.

Name of Participant: _____   Date: _____

Name of Activity/Skill: _____

Community Leisure Setting: _____

1. Is the activity or setting selected appropriate for nonhandicapped persons of the same chronological age? _____ yes _____ no

2. Does the individual demonstrate a preference for this activity or could he/she benefit (i.e., individual has related goals/objectives stated in program plan, IEP, IHP, etc.) from participation in this particular activity or setting? _____ yes _____ no

3. Can the individual financially afford/receive financial assistance to access this specific activity/setting? _____ yes _____ no

4. If materials or equipment are necessary for participation in the activity or setting, does the individual own or have access to the necessary materials/equipment (i.e., borrow from recreation center, family, friend, etc.) _____ yes _____ no

5. If necessary, are material and/or procedural adaptations available for the individual with physical disabilities? _____ yes _____ no

6. Does the individual have access to some form of transportation to get to the leisure setting? _____ yes _____ no

7. If physical accessibility is a special consideration for participation, does the setting provide easy access (i.e., handicapped parking, curb cuts, ramp to entrance, etc.)? _____ yes _____ no

ENVIRONMENTAL ANALYSIS INVENTORY

PART I: (B) GENERAL PROGRAM AND PARTICIPANT INFORMATION

General Information

Recreation Program Experience: _____
Directions: Check or write in the requested information on the following items. If necessary, use space on back.

1. Dates: from: _____ to: _____
   Days/times: _____
   Number of sessions: _____

2. Registration required: ___ yes ___ no
   Procedure: ___ in person ___ mail ___ phone
   Deadline date: _____

3. Guardian permission required:
   ___ no ___ yes   Comment: _____

4. Fee charged or money required: ___ yes ___ no
   Amount: $ ___   Payment procedure: _____
   Are memberships available for free or reduced entrance fee?
   ___ no ___ yes;   Cost: ___ Good for how long? _____

5. Transportation provided: ___ yes ___ no
   If yes, is it handicapped accessible (e.g., wheelchair lift?) ___ yes
   ___ no
   Other comments: _____

6. Comment on type of dress worn: _____

7. List required equipment and materials:
   a. Facility owned: _____
   b. Participant owned: _____

8. Special rules related to this activity (e.g., appropriate dress): _____

Participant Information

Name: _____   Date: _____
Directions: Refer to item in left hand column. Check correct response for participant. Add comments when appropriate.

1. ___ Can participate
   ___ Any conflicts (i.e., arrive late, leave early?); Comment: _____

2. ___ Registration not required
   ___ Can register independently
   ___ Needs assistance; Comment: _____

3. ___ Permission not needed
   ___ Permission granted (consent form attached?)

4. ___ Participant can afford financial costs.
   ___ Other arrangements; Comment: _____

5. Participant's transportation choice(s):
   ___ Walk ___ Drive ___ Bus ___ Bike
   ___ Dropped off ___ Other: _____
   Assistance needed: ___ yes ___ no

6. ___ Participant has appropriate attire.
   ___ Other; Comment: _____

7. ___ Equipment/materials are supplied
   ___ Participant has equipment
   ___ Equipment/materials need to be purchased
   ___ Other; Comment: _____

8. ___ Participant can meet requirement
   ___ Other; Comment: _____

ENVIRONMENTAL ANALYSIS INVENTORY
PART II: ACTIVITY/DISCREPANCY ANALYSIS

Leisure Skill Inventory

Activity/Skill: _____

Leisure Setting: _____

Directions: Below, give a step-by-step breakdown of those *basic* and *vital* skills a nonhandicapped person would need in order to participate in the activity. Include all components (i.e., breaks, using restrooms, drinking fountain, telephone, etc.)

Inventory for Participant with Disability

Name: _____

Directions: Read the step(s) in left column. If participants can perform the step, mark a plus (+) in the center column. If the participant cannot perform the step, make a minus (−) in the center column. If the participant's performance is marked (−), identify a teaching procedure or adaptation/modification for that step in the right column. Upon completion, go to Part III: SPECIFIC ACTIVITY REQUIREMENTS.

STEPS (Activity Analysis):	+	−	Teaching Procedure, Adaptation/Modification, Strategy for Partial Participation
1.			1.
2.			2.
3.			3.
4.			4.
5.			5.
6.			6.

7.

8.

9.

10.

11.

12.

13.

14.

15.

16.

(continued)

7.

8.

9.

10.

11.

12.

13.

14.

15.

16.

(continued)

PART II: *(continued)*

STEPS (Activity Analysis):	+ −	Teaching Procedure, Adaptation/Modification, Strategy for Partial Participation
17.	17.	
18.	18.	
19.	19.	
20.	20.	
21.	21.	
22.	22.	
23.	23.	
24.	24.	
25.	25.	

(If needed, use additional space on back)

230

ENVIRONMENTAL ANALYSIS INVENTORY
PART III: SPECIFIC ACTIVITY REQUIREMENTS

Name: _____   Date: _____

Question: After completing and reviewing the ACTIVITY/DISCREPANCY ANALYSIS, if particular responses would be difficult for the participant to perform, would special material/procedural adaptations or teaching procedures be readily available to enable at least partial participation?

_____ yes _____ no

If yes, participate in the program.

If no, please check the area(s) of concern listed below. This allows for an in-depth analysis of the specific requirements needed for this activity in the identified area of concern (i.e., physical, cognitive/academic, social/emotional).

_____ Physical Skill Requirements: refer to ENVIRONMENTAL ANALYSIS INVENTORY PART IV (A).

_____ Cognitive/Academic Skill Requirements: refer to ENVIRONMENTAL ANALYSIS INVENTORY PART IV (B).

_____ Social/Emotional Skill Requirements: refer to ENVIRONMENTAL ANALYSIS INVENTORY PART IV (C).

ENVIRONMENTAL ANALYSIS INVENTORY

PART IV: FURTHER ACTIVITY CONSIDERATIONS—(A) PHYSICAL CONSIDERATIONS

Activity: _____

Name: _____ Date: _____

Directions: Comment if the following skills are necessary for participation. If checked "yes," *specify requirement(s)*. If needed, use additional space on back; signify this with the words "continued on back."

Directions: In relation to the physical considerations of the activity (left column), state whether the participant's level of functioning in these areas is less or the same as the specified requirement. If checked "less," comment if the participant has another means of accomplishing the skill requirements specified in the left column.*

1. Visual skills? ____ yes ____ no Requirement(s): _____	1. ____ less ____ same Comments:
2. Auditory skills? ____ yes ____ no Requirement(s): _____	2. ____ less ____ same Comments:
3. Gross motor skills? ____ yes ____ no Requirement(s): _____	3. ____ less ____ same Comments:
4. Fine motor skills? ____ yes ____ no Requirement(s): _____	4. ____ less ____ same Comments:
5. Locomotion, flexibility, or coordination skills? ____ yes ____ no Requirement(s): _____	5. ____ less ____ same Comments:
6. Strength or endurance skills? ____ yes ____ no Requirement(s): _____	6. ____ less ____ same Comments:
7. Speed or quickness skills? ____ yes ____ no Requirement(s): _____	7. ____ less ____ same Comments:
8. Other: _____ Skills? ____ yes ____ no Requirement(s): _____	8. ____ less ____ same Comments:

*If physical considerations have been met, proceed as planned. If not, an alternative activity or setting should be considered for investigation and potential participation.

ENVIRONMENTAL ANALYSIS INVENTORY

PART IV: FURTHER ACTIVITY CONSIDERATIONS—(B) COGNITIVE/ACADEMIC CONSIDERATIONS

Activity: _____

Name: _____ Date: _____

Directions: Comment if the following skills are necessary for participation. If checked "yes," *specify requirement(s).* If needed, use additional space on back; signify this with the words "continued on back."

Directions: In relation to the cognitive/academic considerations of the activity (left column), state whether the participant's level of functioning in these areas is less or the same as the specified requirement. If checked "less," comment if the participant has another means of accomplishing the skill requirements specified in the left column.*

1. Attention span? ____ great ____ little
   Requirement(s): _____
   _____
   _____

   1. ____ less ____ same
      Comments:

2. Time telling skills? ____ yes ____ no
   Requirement(s): _____
   _____
   _____

   2. ____ less ____ same
      Comments:

3. Time judgment skills? ____ yes ____ no
   (e.g., when to take a break)
   Requirement(s): _____
   _____
   _____

   3. ____ less ____ same
      Comments:

4. Other decisions (problem solving/judgments? ____ yes ____ no
   (e.g., where to sit, how to get instructor's attention, facility rules/policies to follow)
   Requirement(s): _____
   _____
   _____

   4. ____ less ____ same
      Comments:

5. Rate of learning/motivation level? ____ quick ____ slow
   Requirement(s): _____
   _____
   _____

   5. ____ less ____ same
      Comments:

(continued)

(continued)

233

PART IV (B): *(continued)*

6. Articulation skills? _____ yes _____ no
   _____ less _____ same
   Requirement(s): _____
   Comments: _____
   _____

7. Reading skills? _____ yes _____ no
   _____ less _____ same
   Requirement(s): _____
   Comments: _____
   _____

8. Writing skills? _____ yes _____ no
   _____ less _____ same
   Requirement(s): _____
   Comments: _____
   _____

9. Math skills? _____ yes _____ no
   _____ less _____ same
   Requirement(s): _____
   Comments: _____
   _____

10. Discrimination skills? _____ yes _____ no
    (e.g., color/symbol/object)
    _____ less _____ same
    Requirement(s): _____
    Comments: _____
    _____

11. Other _____ skills? _____ yes _____ no
    _____ less _____ same
    Requirement(s): _____
    Comments: _____
    _____

*If cognitive/academic considerations have been met, proceed as planned. If not, an alternative activity or setting should be considered for investigation and potential participation.

ENVIRONMENTAL ANALYSIS INVENTORY

PART IV: FURTHER ACTIVITY CONSIDERATIONS—(C) SOCIAL/EMOTIONAL CONSIDERATIONS

Activity: _____ Date: _____

Directions: Check, circle, or write in the correct information.

Directions: Refer to information in left-hand column. Answer yes or no as to whether the participant can participate at the level requested. If the answer is "no," comment on the assistance that is required.*

1. a. Does this activity occur: ____ alone ____ with 2 ____ in small group (3–8) ____ in large group (8 or more)

   b. This activity is structured:
      ____ class structure ____ no structure ____ combination

   c. Comment on the type and amount of supervision:
      _____

1. a.	____ yes ____ no
	Comments:
b.	____ yes ____ no
c.	____ yes ____ no
	Comments:

2. This activity involves: ____ females ____ males

   Age range: ____ preschool (under 5) ____ teens (13–19)
   ____ children (5–12) ____ senior citizens (65 +)
   ____ adults (20–64)

2.	____ yes ____ no
	Comments:

3. a. Check the social interactions listed below that pertain to this activity.
   ____ Share materials ____ Take turns ____ Compete
   ____ Communicate with other participants
   ____ Have physical contact with other participants

   b. Noise level: ____ quiet ____ medium ____ loud ____ mixed

3. a.	____ yes ____ no
	Comments:
b.	____ yes ____ no
	Comments:

4. List words or common phrases associated with or used during this activity (e.g., nice shot)
   _____
   _____
   _____

4.	____ yes ____ no
	Comments:

*If social/emotional considerations have been met, proceed as planned. If not, an alternative activity or setting should be considered for investigation and potential participation.

235

SKILL ACQUISITION EVALUATION

A. Name: _____   D. Program: _____   Date: _____

B. Goal Statement: _____

C. Verbal Cue: _____

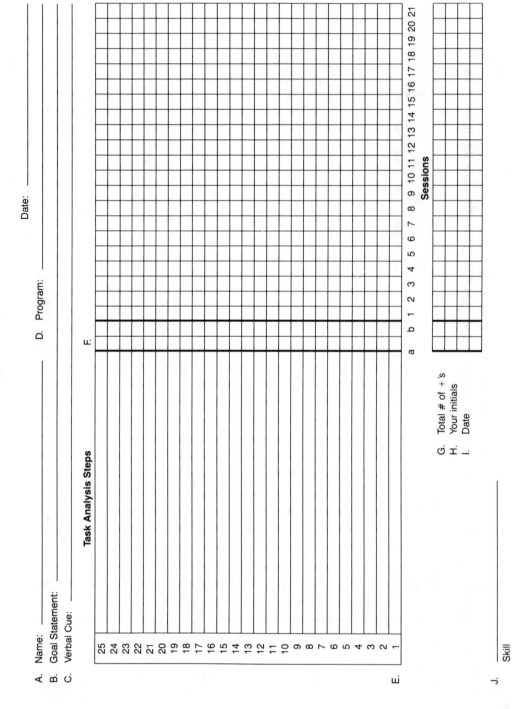

Task Analysis Steps

F.

E.

	25
	24
	23
	22
	21
	20
	19
	18
	17
	16
	15
	14
	13
	12
	11
	10
	9
	8
	7
	6
	5
	4
	3
	2
	1

a b 1 2 3 4 5 6 7 8 9 10 11 12 13 14 15 16 17 18 19 20 21

Sessions

G. Total # of +'s

H. Your initials

I. Date

J. Skill _____

SOCIAL INTERACTION EVALUATION FOR ONE PARTICIPANT

A. Program Title: _____

B. Program Goal: _____

C. Name: _____

   Evaluator: _____

D. Date: _____

E. Level of Interaction

Time (preset)	None	Staff	Dis. Part.	Nondis. Part.	Other	Activity	Comments

F.

G.

H. Totals

Key

A = Appropriate Social Interaction

I = Inappropriate Social Interaction

237

SOCIAL INTERACTION EVALUATION FOR TWO OR MORE PARTICIPANTS

A. Program Title: _____

B. Program Goal: _____

D. Date: _____

E. Times to Observe: 1. _____ 2. _____ 3. _____

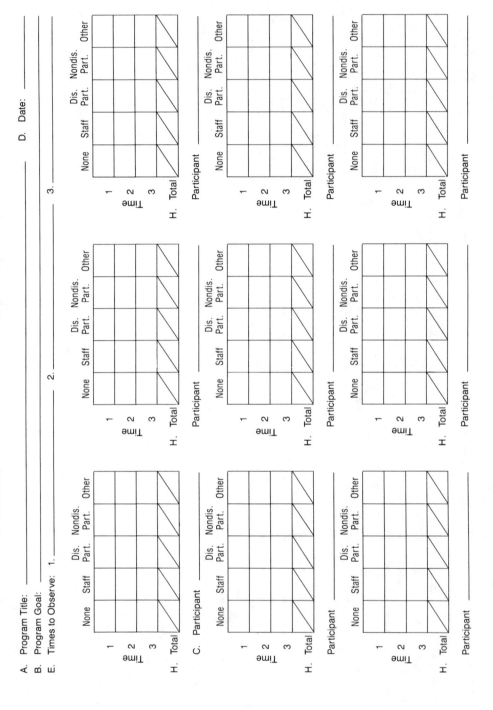

SOCIAL INTERACTION EVALUATION SUMMARY SHEET

A. Program Title: _____

B. Program Instructor: _____

C. Other Staff: _____

D. Duration of Program: _____   Date: _____

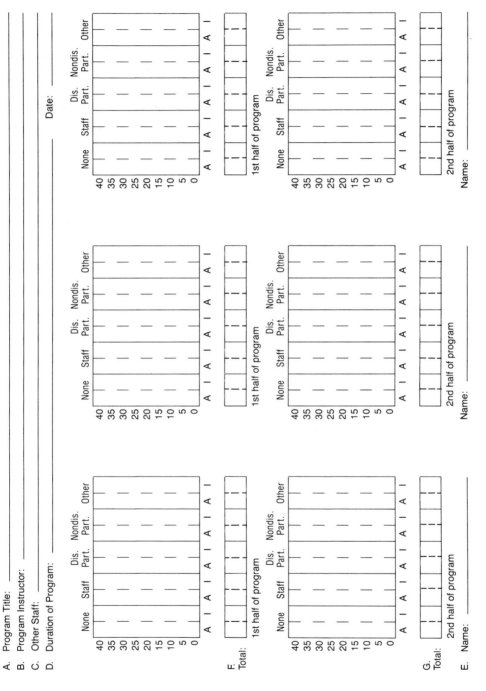

E. Name: _____

F. Total: _____

G. Total: _____

Key: A = Appropriate Social Interaction; I = Inappropriate Social Interaction

SOCIOMETRY EVALUATION INFORMATION FORM

A. Program Title: _____

B. Program Goal: _____

C. Date of Evaluation: _____

D.

Participant	Symbol	G. 1	2	3	4	5	6	7	8	9	10	11	12	13	14	15	16	17	18	19	20
1																					
2																					
3																					
4																					
5																					
6																					
7																					
8																					
9																					
10																					
11																					
12																					
13																					
14																					
15																					
16																					
17																					
18																					
19																					
20																					

TOTAL:

E. Question(s) Asked: _____

Symbol: $\bigcirc$ = Nondisabled participant; Δ = Person with a disability.

F. Evaluator: _____

SOCIOGRAM EVALUATION GRAPHING FORM

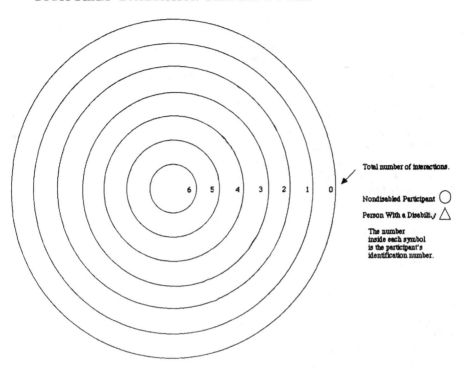

Total number of interactions.

Nondisabled Participant ◯

Person With a Disability △

The number
inside each symbol
is the participant's
identification number.

PEER ACCEPTANCE SURVEY

Name: _____

1. I don't have any friends who are mentally retarded or handicapped.
   Agree ____   Disagree ____   Undecided ____

2. If my sister or brother were retarded, I wouldn't talk about it to anyone.
   Agree ____   Disagree ____   Undecided ____

3. I have talked to people who use wheelchairs.
   Agree ____   Disagree ____   Undecided ____

4. If I found out that someone I hang around with is mentally retarded, I would still be his/her friend.
   Agree ____   Disagree ____   Undecided ____

5. I have talked with some mentally retarded people at the park.
   Agree ____   Disagree ____   Undecided ____

6. It snows in Minnesota in the winter.
   Agree ____   Disagree ____   Undecided ____

7. There is no reason for me to spend time with anyone who is handicapped.
   Agree ____   Disagree ____   Undecided ____

8. I think that a student who is deaf or blind could be in my recreation program.
   Agree ____   Disagree ____   Undecided ____

9. I wouldn't want a handicapped person to be my partner in an activity.
   Agree ____   Disagree ____   Undecided ____

10. I believe that I could become close friends with a person who is handicapped.
    Agree ____   Disagree ____   Undecided ____

11. I have helped some people who are in wheelchairs.
    Agree ____   Disagree ____   Undecided ____

12. Minneapolis is a large city in Minnesota.
    Agree ____   Disagree ____   Undecided ____

13. Persons who are retarded should not come to the park for activities.
    Agree ____   Disagree ____   Undecided ____

14. I wish I could become friends with a mentally retarded person.
    Agree ____   Disagree ____   Undecided ____

15. I would not like to be around a person who looked or acted different.
    Agree ____   Disagree ____   Undecided ____

16. If someone told me about a new TV program about handicaps, I would probably watch it.
    Agree ____   Disagree ____   Undecided ____

17. I have never talked with a person who is paralyzed or couldn't walk.
    Agree ____   Disagree ____   Undecided ____

18. I don't say "Hi" to people who are retarded.
    Agree ____   Disagree ____   Undecided ____

19. Minnesota has many lakes.
    Agree ____   Disagree ____   Undecided ____

20. I believe students with handicaps should participate with other people in the recreation department's programs.
    Agree ____   Disagree ____   Undecided ____

Finished! Thank you for completing the survey.

(This questionnaire was adapted from: Voeltz, L. [1980]. Children's attitudes toward handicapped persons. *American Journal of Mental Deficiency, 84,* 455–464.)

PEER ACCEPTANCE SURVEY ANSWER KEY

1. I don't have any friends who are mentally retarded or handicapped.
   Agree _0_   Disagree _2_   Undecided _1_

2. If my sister or brother were retarded, I wouldn't talk about it to anyone.
   Agree _0_   Disagree _2_   Undecided _1_

3. I have talked to people who use wheelchairs.
   Agree _2_   Disagree _0_   Undecided _1_

4. If I found out that someone I hang around with is mentally retarded, I would still be his/her friend.
   Agree _2_   Disagree _0_   Undecided _1_

5. I have talked with some mentally retarded people at the park.
   Agree _2_   Disagree _0_   Undecided _1_

6. It snows in Minnesota in the winter.
   Agree _2_   Disagree _0_   Undecided _0_

7. There is no reason for me to spend time with anyone who is handicapped.
   Agree _0_   Disagree _2_   Undecided _1_

8. I think that a student who is deaf or blind could be in my recreation program.
   Agree _2_   Disagree _0_   Undecided _1_

9. I wouldn't want a handicapped person to be my partner in an activity.
   Agree _0_   Disagree _2_   Undecided _1_

10. I believe that I could become close friends with a person who is handicapped.
    Agree _2_   Disagree _0_   Undecided _1_

11. I have helped some people who are in wheelchairs.
    Agree _2_   Disagree _0_   Undecided _1_

12. Minneapolis is a large city in Minnesota.
    Agree _2_   Disagree _0_   Undecided _0_

13. Persons who are retarded should not come to the park for activities.
    Agree _0_   Disagree _2_   Undecided _1_

14. I wish I could become friends with a mentally retarded person.
    Agree _2_   Disagree _0_   Undecided _1_

15. I would not like to be around a person who looked or acted different.
    Agree _0_   Disagree _2_   Undecided _1_

16. If someone told me about a new TV program about handicaps, I would probably watch it.
    Agree _2_   Disagree _0_   Undecided _1_

17. I have never talked with a person who is paralyzed or couldn't walk.
    Agree _0_   Disagree _2_   Undecided _1_

18. I don't say "Hi" to people who are retarded.
    Agree _0_   Disagree _2_   Undecided _1_

19. Minnesota has many lakes.
    Agree _2_   Disagree _0_   Undecided _0_

20. I believe students with handicaps should participate with other people in the recreation department's programs.
    Agree _2_   Disagree _0_   Undecided _1_

(This questionnaire was adapted from: Voeltz, L. [1980]. Children's attitudes toward handicapped persons. *American Journal of Mental Deficiency, 84*, 455–464.)

PEER ACCEPTANCE EVALUATION SUMMARY FORM

A. Name: _____

B. Program Title: _____

C. Program Goal: _____

D. Objective: _____ will increase his/her
   _(name)
   posttest score _____ points above his/her pretest score after attending _____ sessions
   _(number)   _(number)
   of _____ .
   _(program)

Total number of points possible = 40.

Date	Pretest Score	Date	Posttest Score	Difference between Pretest and Posttest Score
E.	F.	I.	J.	K. (J. − F.)

G. Number of program sessions _____ .

L. Number of sessions attended by the participant _____ .

Activities engaged in by the participant:

Date	Activity	Comment	Initial
H. _____	_____	_____	____
_____	_____	_____	____
_____	_____	_____	____
_____	_____	_____	____
_____	_____	_____	____
_____	_____	_____	____
_____	_____	_____	____
_____	_____	_____	____
_____	_____	_____	____
_____	_____	_____	____
_____	_____	_____	____
_____	_____	_____	____
_____	_____	_____	____
_____	_____	_____	____
_____	_____	_____	____

SELF-CONCEPT QUESTIONNAIRE

Name: _____

Date: _____

1.	I feel like I can improve how I look.	Never	Seldom	Sometimes	Often	Always
2.	Others think of me as a leader.	Never	Seldom	Sometimes	Often	Always
3.	I make friends easily.	Never	Seldom	Sometimes	Often	Always
4.	I learn how to play games fast.	Never	Seldom	Sometimes	Often	Always
5.	I consider myself smart.	Never	Seldom	Sometimes	Often	Always
6.	Others tease me.	Never	Seldom	Sometimes	Often	Always
7.	I want to be like someone else.	Never	Seldom	Sometimes	Often	Always
8.	I enjoy making decisions.	Never	Seldom	Sometimes	Often	Always
9.	I get picked last in games.	Never	Seldom	Sometimes	Often	Always
10.	I feel good when I learn something new.	Never	Seldom	Sometimes	Often	Always
11.	When I look in the mirror, I like myself.	Never	Seldom	Sometimes	Often	Always
12.	I am a leader when I am with kids my own age.	Never	Seldom	Sometimes	Often	Always
13.	I like to play alone.	Never	Seldom	Sometimes	Often	Always
14.	Others consider me smart.	Never	Seldom	Sometimes	Often	Always
15.	Others like playing games with me.	Never	Seldom	Sometimes	Often	Always
16.	Others ask me to be their friend.	Never	Seldom	Sometimes	Often	Always
17.	I feel bad when my team loses.	Never	Seldom	Sometimes	Often	Always
18.	Others tell me what to do.	Never	Seldom	Sometimes	Often	Always
19.	I can make up my own mind.	Never	Seldom	Sometimes	Often	Always
20.	I enjoy playing by myself.	Never	Seldom	Sometimes	Often	Always
21.	I only like to play if I win.	Never	Seldom	Sometimes	Often	Always
22.	I get mad when someone teases me.	Never	Seldom	Sometimes	Often	Always
23.	I get picked first in games.	Never	Seldom	Sometimes	Often	Always
24.	I like to play with others.	Never	Seldom	Sometimes	Often	Always
25.	I feel like I can get things done.	Never	Seldom	Sometimes	Often	Always
26.	I get what I can from others.	Never	Seldom	Sometimes	Often	Always
27.	I feel it's my fault when my team loses.	Never	Seldom	Sometimes	Often	Always
28.	Others enjoy being with me.	Never	Seldom	Sometimes	Often	Always
29.	I can choose what to do during my free time.	Never	Seldom	Sometimes	Often	Always
30.	Others like to be around me.	Never	Seldom	Sometimes	Often	Always

Finished! Thank you for completing the survey.

SELF-CONCEPT QUESTIONNAIRE ANSWER KEY

#	Statement	Never	Seldom	Sometimes	Often	Always
1.	I feel like I can improve how I look.	1	2	3	4	5
2.	Others think of me as a leader.	1	2	3	4	5
3.	I make friends easily.	1	2	3	4	5
4.	I learn how to play games fast.	1	2	3	4	5
5.	I consider myself smart.	1	2	3	4	5
6.	Others tease me.	1	5	4	3	1
7.	I want to be like someone else.	4	5	3	2	1
8.	I enjoy making decisions.	1	2	3	4	5
9.	I get picked last in games.	1	3	4	5	1
10.	I feel good when I learn something new.	1	2	3	4	5
11.	When I look in the mirror, I like myself.	1	2	3	4	5
12.	I am a leader when I am with kids my own age.	1	3	4	5	1
13.	I like to play alone.	1	4	5	3	1
14.	Others consider me smart.	1	2	3	4	5
15.	Others like playing games with me.	1	2	3	4	5
16.	Others ask me to be their friend.	1	3	4	5	1
17.	I feel bad when my team loses.	1	3	4	5	1
18.	Others tell me what to do.	1	3	4	5	1
19.	I can make up my own mind.	1	2	3	4	5
20.	I enjoy playing by myself.	1	4	5	3	1
21.	I only like to play if I win.	5	4	3	2	1
22.	I get mad when someone teases me.	5	4	3	2	1
23.	I get picked first in games.	1	3	4	5	1
24.	I like to play with others.	1	3	4	5	1
25.	I feel like I can get things done.	1	2	3	4	5
26.	I get what I can from others.	1	3	4	5	1
27.	I feel it's my fault when my team loses.	1	5	4	3	1
28.	Others enjoy being with me.	1	2	3	4	5
29.	I can choose what to do during my free time.	1	2	3	4	5
30.	Others like to be around me.	1	2	3	4	5

SELF-CONCEPT EVALUATION SUMMARY FORM

A. Name: _____

B. Program Title: _____

C. Program Goal: _____

D. Objective: _____ will increase his/her
   _(name)

   posttest score _____ points above his/her pretest score after attending _____ sessions
   _(number)   _(number)

   of _____ .
   _(program)

Total number of points possible = 150.

Date	Pretest Score	Date	Posttest Score	Difference between Pretest and Posttest Score
E.	F.	I.	J.	K. (J. − F.)

G. Number of program sessions _____ .

L. Number of sessions attended by the participant _____ .

Activities engaged in by the participant:

Date	Activity	Comment	Initial
H. _____	_____	_____	___
_____	_____	_____	___
_____	_____	_____	___
_____	_____	_____	___
_____	_____	_____	___
_____	_____	_____	___
_____	_____	_____	___
_____	_____	_____	___
_____	_____	_____	___
_____	_____	_____	___
_____	_____	_____	___
_____	_____	_____	___
_____	_____	_____	___
_____	_____	_____	___
_____	_____	_____	___

NUMERICAL EVALUATION INFORMATION FORM

A. Program Title: _____

B. Program Site: _____

C. Program Goal: _____

D. Program Information (include cost, meeting times, duration, day held, age of participants, etc.):

_____

_____

_____

	E. Number of nondisabled participants	F. Number of participants with disabilities	G. Program date	H. Comment
Session				
1	_____	_____	_____	_____
2	_____	_____	_____	_____
3	_____	_____	_____	_____
4	_____	_____	_____	_____
5	_____	_____	_____	_____
6	_____	_____	_____	_____
7	_____	_____	_____	_____
8	_____	_____	_____	_____
9	_____	_____	_____	_____
10	_____	_____	_____	_____

I. Total number of non-disabled participants

_____

J. Total number of participants with disabilities

_____

K. Total number of participants (nondisabled and disabled)

_____

L. Number of sessions conducted

_____

M. Average number of participants per session

_____

N. Number of participants registered

_____

Appendix I

VOLUNTEER ADVOCACY FORMS
Application for Volunteer Advocacy

Name _____ Date _____

Address _____

City/Zip _____

Home Phone _____ Business Phone _____

Birthdate _____ Age _____ Gender _____ Marital Status _____

Education _____

Employer _____

Special Skills/Interest _____

Have you taken Community Education/Community Recreation classes before?

Yes ____   No ____

Have you ever worked/volunteered with people with mental or physical disabilities?

Yes ____   No ____

How did you hear about this program?

_____ Local Newspaper(s). Specify: _____

_____ Radio Station. Specify: _____

_____ ARC Newsletter
_____ United Way Voluntary Action Center
_____ Other. Specify: _____

Please specify what age/gender you would prefer to participate with in recreation.

____ Child   ____ Teen   ____ Adult   ____ Senior   ____ Male   ____ Female

Do you have your own transportation?   Yes ____   No ____

Would you be willing to transport the participant to class?   Yes ____   No ____

How much time per week, on the average, would you be able to spend with a participant who has disabilities?

_____

Please list two personal and one work-related reference (name and day phone number).

1.

2.

3.

Please state the city/county locations you would be willing to travel to: _____

_____

Please indicate your areas of interest:

____ Sports/Fitness   ____ Health   ____ Other. Specify _____
____ Arts/Crafts/Hobbies   ____ Aquatics   _____
____ Finance/Budget Management   ____ Cooking   _____

Volunteer Advocate Call Sheet

Name _____

Address _____

Date called _____   Date material sent _____

Date material received in office _____

Date of personal interview _____

Date assignment given _____   Date of inservice training _____

Volunteer Advocate–Participant Match

Participant Name _____   Phone _____

Volunteer Name _____   Phone _____

Date of final confirmation _____   Date session begins _____

Date class ends _____   Session Title _____

Location of session _____

District _____   Is volunteer transporting student?   Yes ____   No ____

Additional Comments:

Volunteer Advocate Program Evaluation Form
(Sample Form)

Directions:

To be filled out by volunteer advocate. Return to community recreation professional.

1. Do you feel you received adequate orientation? If not, what do you suggest?

2. Was the program leader helpful to you?

3. In what ways was the experience beneficial to you?

4. Did you feel overworked during the program? If so, in what ways?

5. Did you enjoy the work? Explain.

6. Would you volunteer again?

7. Additional comments:

Volunteer Advocate Evaluation Form
(Sample Form)

Directions:

To be completed by community recreation professional or program leader.

1. Did the volunteer attend the scheduled training program?

2. Did the volunteer attend all program days as arranged? If not, why?

3. Did the volunteer offer any suggestions to improve the program? If yes, what were they?

4. How much supervision did the volunteer require?

5. Would you ask the volunteer back? If not, explain.

6. Additional comments:

Volunteer Advocate Job Description

Job title:

Job description:

Days needed:

Hours needed:

Length of program:

Location of program:

Immediate supervisor:

Special skills needed:

Description of participants and their needs:

Other considerations:

Appendix J

ANNOTATED BIBLIOGRAPHY

Austin, D. R., Peterson, J. A., & Peccarelli, L. M. (1978). The status of services for special populations in park and recreation departments in the state of Indiana. *Therapeutic Recreation Journal,
12*(1), 50–56.

This study determines the extent and level of local public recreation service for persons with
mental retardation, mental illness, physical disabilities, and for elderly persons. The study also examines recreation service provision for chemical abusers, economically disadvantaged persons, and
youth or adult correctional offenders. Questionnaires were mailed to 60 Indiana park and recreation
departments selected for the study. The special population group served by a large percentage of
Indiana park and recreation systems are the elderly. Although certain special population groups are
not served by many of the reporting park and recreation departments, a large percentage (80%) of the
respondents indicate it is their responsibility to do so. The primary source of funding for programs for
special population groups is the public tax funds. The lack of funds and services provided by other
agencies is given as a reason why departments did not offer programs for special population groups.

Baumgart, D., Brown, L., Pumpian, I., Nisbet, J., Ford, A., Sweet, M., Messina, R., & Schroeder, J.
(1982). Principle of partial participation and individualized adaptations in educational programs for
severely handicapped students. *Journal of The Association for Persons with Severe Handicaps, 8*(3),
71–77.

The authors define the principles of partial participation. They give specific guidelines for
consideration of individualized adaptations to enhance participation by persons with disabilities in
least restrictive, school and nonschool environments and activities. Types of adaptations are delineated. Also, an eight-phase strategy is presented, illustrating the use of the principles of partial
participation.

Bruininks, R. H., & Lakin, K. C. (1985). *Living and learning in the least restrictive environment.*
Baltimore: Paul H. Brookes Publishing Co.
Lakin, K. C., & Bruininks, R. H. (Eds.). (1985). *Strategies for achieving community integration of
developmentally disabled citizens.* Baltimore: Paul H. Brookes Publishing Co.

These companion texts offer the reader a state-of-the-art review of community services for
persons with mental retardation and developmental disabilities. *Living and Learning in the Least
Restrictive Environment* presents a rationale for programs in the least restrictive environment based on
empirical study, legislative support, and philosophical orientation. *Strategies for Achieving Community Integration of Developmentally Disabled Citizens* provides the reader several service models
and implementation strategies for achieving social and physical integration in community and other
least restrictive environments. A chapter in this text by Putnam, Werder, and Schleien details
guidelines for ensuring access to leisure settings and community-based environments. This chapter
investigates obstacles to community participation and presents recommendations for overcoming
these obstacles to achieve community recreation integration.

Certo, N. J., Schleien, S. J., & Hunter, D. (1983). An ecological assessment inventory to facilitate
community recreation participation by severely disabled individuals. *Therapeutic Recreation Journal, 17*(3), 29–38.

Severely disabled individuals have long been systematically excluded from actively participating in normalized recreation/leisure activities in integrated community settings. Severely disabled
individuals should be taught functional and age-appropriate skills, based upon the performance
characteristics of nonhandicapped peers. In order to present this position, typical assumptions of leisure skill instruction for severely disabled individuals are discussed and opposing points of view are
presented. The article presents a strategy, or inventory, that is divided into three interrelated areas,
including: skill selection and skill/facility description, component skills and adaptations for full/par-
tial participation, and supportive skills. The inventory can be used by therapeutic recreation specialists, community recreation professionals, educators, and others to develop functional and age-appropriate leisure skill instructional content. It is expected that this approach, coupled with longitudinal
planning, will facilitate the provision of opportunities for individuals with severe disabilities to actively participate in normalized recreation/leisure activities in integrated community settings.

Hayes, G. A. (1978). Philosophical ramifications of mainstreaming in recreation. *Therapeutic Recreation Journal, 12*(2), 5–9.

The author provides the reader with a provocative account of the problems inherent in setting up services for integrating individuals with disabilities into the community and into recreational settings. Hayes challenges recreation professionals and other persons providing services to examine their values and attitudes toward persons with disabilities and the systems set up to serve them.

Hutchison, P., & Lord, J. (1979). *Recreation integration: Issues and alternatives in leisure services and community involvement.* Ottawa, Canada: Leisurability.

The authors discuss the concepts of play, leisure and recreation, attitudes toward recreation, and "differences" in people. Steps to get integrated programs implemented in the community and strategies to improve social skills and community settings are outlined. Also, methods to educate consumers, volunteers, parents, and professionals concerning the development and evaluation of integrated recreation programs are described.

Kennedy, D. W., Austin, D. R., & Smith, R. W. (1987). *Special recreation: Opportunities for persons with disabilities.* Philadelphia: W. B. Saunders.

This book provides a comprehensive overview of leisure services for special population groups, specifically those implemented within community-based settings. The roles and responsibilities of recreation professionals in relation to program and facility planning and design are discussed. The authors provide a rationale and philosophical overview of special recreation services for persons with disabilities. Barriers to accessible leisure programming are detailed. Model recreation programs in a variety of recreation settings are also described.

Lord, J. (1983). Reflections on a decade of integration. *Journal of Leisurability, 10*(4), 4–11.

This article reviews the integration process and the accomplishments that have been made over a 10-year-period, beginning with the increased public awareness of integration that was manifested in the early 1970s. The author leads the reader through initial integration efforts, false alternatives to integration, improving integration options, and the importance of mediating structures or support systems. Future challenges to society are offered, including a concern for integrated services at both the societal level as well as the human service professional level.

Lundegren, H., & Farrell, P. (1985). *Evaluation for leisure service managers: A dynamic approach.* New York: Saunders College.

This book addresses the what, why, and who of program evaluation and management concepts. Evaluation designs and models, agency responsibilities concerning evaluation, administrative concerns, methods of collecting data, the treatment of data, and the evaluation report are also examined.

Martin, J., Rusch, F., & Heal, L. (1982). Teaching community survival skills to mentally retarded adults: A review and analysis. *The Journal of Special Education, 16*(3), 243–267.

This article reviews training procedures used to teach persons with disabilities 10 survival skills considered essential to successful community integration. Results of studies in the areas of travel, money management, meal preparation, clothing and personal care, telephone use, housekeeping, self-medication, leisure/recreation, social interaction, and conversation are reviewed. A second section of the article considers whether institutional training enhances community integration. The authors address the need to establish community-based training programs to enhance independent living skills of persons with disabilities. The conclusion discusses the need for future research on the long-term maintenance and generalization of community living skills, as well as social validation of what constitutes an essential skill for instruction.

Matthews, P. R. (1980). Why the mentally retarded do not participate in certain types of recreational activities. *Therapeutic Recreation Journal, 14*(1), 44–50.

One hundred eight elementary-age children were studied to determine why they do not participate in certain recreational activities and whether or not those differences are unique to persons with mental retardation. No differences were found between mentally retarded and nonretarded boys and girls for nine of 13 reasons. Of the four differences in recreation participation that were found, only two were attributed solely to mental retardation (i.e., lacking transportation and no opportunity to participate). Matthews summarizes that reasons for nonparticipation unique to persons with mental retardation were largely associated with access, ignorance of activities, and frequent adherence to culturally determined sex stereotypes.

McGill, J. (1984). Training for integration: Are blindfolds really enough? *Journal of Leisurability*, *11*(2), 12–15.

The importance of providing training to staff who are attempting to integrate people with various disabilities is the focus of this article. A case is made that inadequate staff training decreases the likelihood that integration efforts will be successful. To gain further insight into training needs and the extent of training that is currently being provided, a questionnaire was submitted to 400 local agencies serving individuals with mental retardation. Also, questionnaires were sent to 100 randomly selected municipal recreation agencies. The six primary concerns expressed in the questionnaires that were returned are discussed.

Nietupski, J., Hamre-Nietupski, S., & Ayres, B. (1984). Review of task analytic leisure skill training efforts: Practitioner implications and future research needs. *Journal of The Association for Persons with Severe Handicaps, 9*(2), 88–97.

Data-based task analytic instructional programs, recent position papers, and curriculum volumes aimed at teaching recreation/leisure skills to persons with moderate to severe mental and physical disabilities are reviewed in this article. Practical significance of research findings for direct service providers are discussed. Future research needs are addressed, including the need to: compare instructional strategies, examine and empirically verify leisure skill options for persons with severe disabilities, identify procedures to promote skill maintenance and generalization, increase access to integrated community recreation programs, and increase self-initiated leisure behaviors.

Putnam, J. W., Werder, J. K., & Schleien, S. J. (1985). Leisure and recreation services for handicapped persons. In K. C. Lakin & R. H. Bruininks (Eds.), *Strategies for achieving community integration of developmentally disabled citizens* (pp. 253–274). Baltimore: Paul H. Brookes Publishing Co.

Unfortunately, a gap exists between what is known about the short- and long-term benefits of participation in leisure activities and the current status of services to persons with disabilities. This chapter traces conceptual issues and assumptions in current leisure and recreational services for persons with disabilities, types of activities that are available in homes and schools, and obstacles that make participation in community recreation activities difficult. In the final section, the authors review programs designed to normalize the leisure and recreative activities of persons with disabilities, and provide guidelines for developing such programs.

Richler, D. (1984). Access to community resources: The invisible barriers to integration. *Journal of Leisurability, 11*(2), 4–11.

This article discusses the philosophy of integration and lists five basic prerequisites that must exist before integration can occur normally, rather than as a service exception. Some of the rights of individuals who are disabled are discussed with emphasis being placed on educating persons living in the community about these rights. The philosophy of the "Community Living Society" in Vancouver, B. C. is presented. This agency concentrates on enhancing social access and social integration of persons with disabilities. Six steps for incorporating ideology related to the normalization principle are listed; the steps range from "adoption-in-theory" to "adaption in practice."

Russell, R. V. (1982). *Planning programs in recreation*. St. Louis: C. V. Mosby.

This text is highly instructive for the recreation professional who desires to "travel the territory between the problem and a solution or between a need and a fulfillment" in the provision of community leisure services. The book presents a rational planning process that moves the professional through its major stages step by step, from identification of needs to evaluation. The book is described as a self-help guide on "how to get started" and a reference book on "how to keep going."

Rynders, J. E., Johnson, R. T., Johnson, D. W., & Schmidt, B. (1980). Producing positive interaction among Down syndrome and nonhandicapped teenagers through cooperative goal structuring. *American Journal of Mental Deficiency, 85*, 268–273.

Junior high school students with and without disabilities participated in cooperative, competitive, or individual recreational bowling activities using a cooperative goal structuring strategy. Interpersonal interaction and attraction are compared in the three conditions. Results indicate that the cooperative goal structured situation results in significantly more positive interactions between students with and without disabilities. The bowlers with Down syndrome are ranked substantially higher by their nondisabled peers on the basis of how much these peers enjoyed bowling in the cooperative condition than in either the competitive or individual goal structured conditions. Findings are discussed in terms of integrating students with disabilities into cooperatively structured, heterogeneous learning groups, resulting in increased expectations of positive interactions and interpersonal attraction between students with and without disabilities.

Salzberg, C. L., & Langford, C. A. (1981). Community integration of mentally retarded adults through leisure activity. *Mental Retardation, 19*(3), 127–131.

The leisure time pursuits of adults with mental retardation have traditionally consisted of segregated recreation programs, large group activities, and special events. The potential for community-based residences to promote the development of normalized adult leisure activities, and an alternative to the traditional model for recreation activities are presented. Based on a companion or friendship model, a program designed to match moderately or severely mentally retarded adults with non-disabled volunteers is described. Volunteers invited their companions with disabilities to accompany them on their usual leisure time outings or activities. The participants experienced various normalized leisure activities, and were provided a model to learn a variety of leisure skills, including using the salad bar in a restaurant, appropriate conduct in a night club, and paying for movie tickets. The relationship between the provision of opportunities to adults with disabilities to learn leisure skills and their independent functioning in the community is discussed.

Schleien, S. J., Olson, K., Rogers, N., & McLafferty, M. (1985). Integrating children with severe handicaps into recreation and physical education programs. *Journal of Park and Recreation Administration, 3*(1), 50–66.

This article reports the procedures and results of four pilot investigations that attempted to answer the question of whether children with severe handicaps could successfully participate in integrated community recreation and physical education programs. Without additional costs, staff training, or special modifications, these children successfully participated in the daily programs. Reports recorded using a naturalistic inquiry methodology and pre-post attitude survey revealed a positive change regarding nonhandicapped peers and staff willingness to include individuals with handicaps into future community recreation and physical education programs. Suggestions for future integrated community recreation efforts, including investments in staff training and development, are offered.

Schleien, S. J., & Werder, J. K. (1985). Perceived responsibilities of special recreation services in Minnesota. *Therapeutic Recreation Journal, 19*(3), 51–62.

To determine the quantity and quality of recreation programs and services throughout the state of Minnesota, the authors surveyed park and recreation departments, community education agencies, and schools by means of a needs assessment inventory. A 73% return rate enabled them to identify perceived responsibilities and the degree of coordination among agencies, and the extent and nature of special recreation services currently offered, including the integration of participants with and without disabilities. Based on these results, five recommendations for future special recreation program planning are offered.

Stanley, J., & Freedman, R. (1980). *A systematic approach to developing and implementing community recreation services for the disabled.* Trenton, NJ: Division of Community Resources, Office on Community Recreation for Handicapped Persons.

This manual provides information and guidelines on community recreation for administrators of public recreation agencies. Areas addressed include the implications of legislation concerning recreation service provision to persons with disabilities, a continuum of services designed to meet the needs of disabled persons and interests, and abilities of consumers with disabilities. Also, administrative procedures, techniques, and tools for designing and implementing community leisure services for persons with special needs are offered. The appendix offers a variety of assessment and survey instruments to use in a community recreation agency.

Thompson, G. (1979). Role changes of the therapeutic recreator and the community recreator in the mainstreaming process. *Expanding Horizons in Therapeutic Recreation VII*, 1–8.

This article describes the impact of community and school-based integration of persons with disabilities on the therapeutic recreation specialist and the community recreator. In his discussion of the continuum of leisure services, Thompson describes the therapeutic recreation specialist as the catalyst in the mainstreaming movement: assisting and advocating for persons with disabilities, and collaborating with community recreators. Thompson also lists skills he believes are essential for therapeutic recreation specialists and community recreators to master for integration to be successful.

Vaughan, J. L., & Winslow, R. (1979). *Guidelines for community based recreation programs for special populations.* Alexandria, VA: National Therapeutic Recreation Society.

The National Therapeutic Recreation Society (NTRS), a branch of the National Recreation and Park Association, created the Guideline Project Committee to develop specific standards for community-based recreation programming for members of special population groups. A total of 113 municipal park and recreation agencies completed a survey that had them rank by priority problems or barriers to recreation programming in their communities. The five main problem areas identified are: transportation, budget allocation, identification of persons with disabilities, lack of program personnel, and architectural barriers. Other less significant problem areas are also noted. Barriers are defined and specific solutions to alleviate them are offered. Guidelines are also provided regarding development and administration of recreation programs for special populations in communities of varying size.

Voeltz, L. M., Wuerch, B. B., & Wilcox, B. (1982). Leisure and recreation: Preparation for independence, integration, and self-fulfillment. In B. Wilcox and G. T. Bellamy, *Design of high school programs for severely handicapped students* (pp. 175–209). Baltimore: Paul H. Brookes Publishing Co.

This chapter examines leisure and recreation in the context of the developing secondary student with severe mental and physical disabilities. After the authors define the "leisure domain," as distinguished from vocational and independent living domains, they proceed to identify characteristics of leisure environments and pertinent issues of concern to leisure educators in secondary school settings. A rationale for leisure education of severely disabled students is presented, including strategies for leisure skills training in natural community settings. A complete literature review of state-of-the-art practices is also included. Also suggestions for future work in leisure education are offered.

Wehman, P. (1977). *Helping the mentally retarded acquire play skills: A behavioral approach.* Springfield, IL: Charles C Thomas.

This book provides a comprehensive collection of guidelines for developing play skills in persons who are severely and profoundly retarded. The text attends closely to the normal child development literature for the topic of play programming. The leisure time behavior development program model used by the author is based on behavior modification principles. It clearly describes how behavioral training methods may be applied to the play problems of persons with mental retardation, and provides specific instructional directions and an empirical rationale for program guidelines. The ideas and procedures detailed in this book will serve to reinforce the position that the use of behavioral programming to stimulate play skills in persons with mental retardation is both necessary and desirable.

Wehman, P. (1979). *Recreation programming for developmentally disabled persons.* Austin, TX: PRO-ED.

This book addresses the question: What do individuals with developmental disabilities do after school, after work, on the weekends, and during free time at home? The chapters in this text grew out of a need to provide specialized information on programming recreation and leisure skills. The author makes an effort to address the topical areas that have been discussed and inquired about most frequently by special education teachers. The areas of interest include: available curricular materials, methodology, and the outlook for community recreation programs. Also provided is a recreation curriculum for individuals with developmental disabilities of all ages and functioning levels.

Wehman, P., & Schleien, S. J. (1981). *Leisure programs for handicapped persons: Adaptations, techniques, and curriculum.* Austin, TX: PRO-ED.

This book is an easy-to-follow guide for teaching youngsters and adults how to make more of their leisure time, that is, how to make leisure time a learning time. Government policies and the increasing trend toward deinstitutionalization demand that persons with disabilities learn to use lei-sure time more creatively and constructively. The book presents the guidelines needed for effective planning—plus more than 100 sports, games, and hobbies in task analysis format.

This book provides explicit methods for helping persons with disabilities take meaningful part in normal and specially adapted recreational pursuits. The programs are for moderately, severely, and profoundly retarded persons, those with cerebral palsy, the seriously emotionally disturbed, and se-verely sensory-impaired individuals. The activities are sequenced, behavioral, and data-based. The text describes step-by-step: 1) how to assess levels of functioning, 2) how to translate behavioral goals into specific instructional steps, 3) how to choose and adapt age-appropriate activities, 4) how to select and modify materials to suit individual needs, and 5) how to evaluate programs. Teachers and therapists who work with persons with disabilities will find valuable advice and useful procedures for preparing IEPs and for developing instructional programs for both children and adults.

West, P. C. (1982). Organizational stigma in metropolitan park and recreation agencies. *Therapeutic Recreation Journal, 16*(4), 35–41.

West's article presents research results on organizational barriers to the implementation of accessible community recreation for persons with physical and mental disabilities. The role of "organ-izational stigma" and its effect on agency decision-making processes is emphasized. Two main bar-riers or types of organizational stigma are identified: organizational action reflecting stigmatized atti-tudes and negative reactions on the part of agency staff, and agency response to perceived community stigma. The author discusses ways to reduce organizational stigma in park and recreation agencies in order to improve the organizational climate, thereby increasing the opportunities for community rec-reation services for persons with disabilities.

West, P. C. (1984). Social stigma and community recreation participation by the mentally and phys-ically handicapped. *Therapeutic Recreation Journal, 18*(1), 40–49.

This article examines the results of a study on social stigma barriers perceived by persons with disabilities, and the affect of these barriers on rates of community recreation participation. The results indicate that the respondents with disabilities reported experiencing some type of negative com-munity response including staring, teasing, negative attitudes, and lack of respect. This perception of stigmatizing attitudes did prevent recreation participation for some individuals with disabilities; others had to use various coping mechanisms in order to participate. The author offers suggestions for future program direction and research.

Wolfensberger, W. (1972). *The principle of normalization in human services.* Toronto: National In-stitute on Mental Retardation.

Until 1969, the principle of normalization was not known to most workers in the human ser-vices. The concept was developed by Bank-Mikkelsen and was initially defined as "allowing mentally retarded persons to obtain an existence as close to normal as possible." In this text, Wolfensberger further defines this principle as the "utilization of means which are as culturally normative as possible, in order to establish and/or maintain personal behaviors and characteristics which are as culturally normative as possible." He expands this definition by stating that persons with special needs should be enabled to demonstrate behaviors and appropriate appearances within the culture for persons of simi-lar characteristics of age and gender as circumstances and the individual's behavioral potential permit. The text is divided into three sections: 1) principle of normalization defined and major implications, 2) application of principle to specific services areas such as architectural, residential, and sociosexual needs, and, 3) implementation strategies.

References

Adkins, J., & Matson, L. (1980). Teaching institutionalized mentally retarded adults socially appropriate leisure skills. *Mental Retardation, 18*(5), 249–252.

Anderson, S., & Ball, S. (1980). *The profession and practice of program evaluation.* San Francisco: Jossey-Bass.

Apolloni, T., & Cooke, T. (1978). Integrated programming at the infant, toddler, and preschool levels. In M. Guralanick (Ed.), *Early intervention and the integration of handicapped and nonhandicapped children.* Baltimore: University Park Press.

Austin, D. R., Peterson, J. A., Peccarelli, L. M., Binkley, A., & Laker, M. (1977). *Therapeutic recreation in Indiana: Health through recreation.* Bloomington, IN: Department of Recreation and Park Administration, Indiana University.

Austin, D. R., & Powell, L. G. (1981). What you need to know to serve special populations. *Parks and Recreation, 16*(7) 40–42.

Avedon, E. M. (1974). *Therapeutic recreation service: An applied behavioral science approach.* Englewood Cliffs, NJ: Prentice-Hall.

Azrin, N. H., Besalel, V. A., Hall, R. V., Hall, M. C., (Eds.). (1980). *How to teach series.* Austin, TX: PRO-ED.

Barrow, H. M. (1971). *Man and his movement: Principles of his physical education.* Philadelphia: Lea and Febiger.

Bates, P., & Renzaglia, A. (1979). Community-based recreation programs. In P. Wehman (Ed.), *Recreation programming for developmentally disabled persons* (pp. 97–125). Austin, TX: PRO-ED.

Baumgart, D., Brown, L., Pumpian, I., Nisbet, J., Ford, A., Sweet, M., Messina, R., & Schroeder, J. (1982). Principle of partial participation and individualized adaptations in educational programs for severely handicapped students. *Journal of The Association for Persons with Severe Handicaps, 8*(3), 71–77.

Bell, N. J., Schoenrock, C., & Slade, R. (1975). *Leisure activities of previously institutionalized retardates: A comparison with non-retarded community residents.* Paper presented at the Region V American Association on Mental Deficiency Meeting, St. Louis.

Belmore, K., & Brown, L., (1976). A job skill inventory strategy for use in a public school vocational training program for severely handicapped potential workers. In L. Brown, N. Certo, K. Belmore, T. Crowner (Eds.), *Papers and Programs Related to Public School Services for Secondary Age Severely Handicapped Students.* Vol. VI, Part I, Madison, WI: Madison Metropolitan School District. (Revised and republished: In N. Haring, and D. Bricker (Eds.) (1977). *Teaching the Severely Handicapped,* Vol. 111, Columbus, OH: Special Press).

Bender, M., & Valletutti, P. J. (1976). *Teaching the moderately and severely handicapped: Curriculum, objectives, strategies, and activities.* Vol. 2, Baltimore: University Park Press.

Beveridge, M., Spencer, J., & Miller, P. (1978). Language and social behavior in severely educationally subnormal children. *British Journal of Social and Clinical Psychology, 17*(1), 75–83.

Birenbaum, A., & Re, M. A. (1979). Resettling mentally retarded adults in the community—almost 4 years later. *American Journal of Mental Deficiency, 83,* 323–329.

Brinker, R. P. (1985). Interactions between severely mentally retarded students and other students in integrated and segregated public school settings. *American Journal of Mental Deficiency, 89,* 587–594.

Broudy, H. (1984). *Nature of aesthetic experience.* Lecture delivered at GIEVA, Los Angeles.

Brown, L., Branston, M. B., Hamre-Nietupski, S., Wilcox, B., & Gruenwald, L. (1979). A rationale for comprehensive longitudinal interactions between severely handicapped and nonhandicapped students and other citizens. *AAESPH Review, 4*(1), 3–14.

Byers, S. (1979). Wilderness camping as a therapy for emotionally disturbed children: A critical review. *Exceptional Children, 45*(2), 628–635.

Caplan, R. (1967). Tent treatment for the insane. *Hospital and Community Psychiatry, 18,* 145–146.

Carney, I., Clobuciar, A., Corley, E., Wilcox, B., Bigler, J., Fleisler, L., Pany, D., & Turner, P. (1977). Social interaction in severely handicapped students. In *The severely and profoundly handicapped child.* Springfield, IL: State Department of Education.

Carter, J. (1954). Camping together: Handicapped and nonhandicapped girl scouts. *Exceptional Children, 21*(4), 2–4.

Carter, M., & Farly, E. (1978). A literature analysis on camping for the handicapped. *Therapeutic Recreation Journal, 4*(2), 43–48.

Certo, N. J., & Schleien, S. J. (1982). Individualized leisure instruction. In P. Verhoven, S. Schleien, & M. Bender (Eds.), *Leisure education and the handicapped individual: An ecological perspective* (pp. 121–153). Washington, D.C.: Institute for Career and Leisure Development.

Certo, N. J., Schleien, S. J., & Hunter, D. (1983). An ecological assessment inventory to facilitate community recreation participation by severely disabled individuals. *Therapeutic Recreation Journal, 17*(3), 29–38.

Cheseldine, S., & Jeffree, D. (1981). Mentally handicapped adolescents: Their use of leisure. *Journal of Mental Deficiency Research, 25,* 49–59.

Chubb, M., & Chubb, H. (1981). *One third of our time?* New York: John Wiley & Sons.

Compton, D., & Goldstein, J. (1976). *The career education curriculum development project.* Arlington, VA: National Recreation and Park Association.

Copeland, B. (1984). Mainstreaming art for the handicapped child: Resources for teacher preparation. *Art Education, 37*(6), 22–29.

Crapps, J. M., Langone, J., & Swaim, S. (1985). Quantity and quality of participation in community environments by mentally retarded adults. *Education and Training of the Mentally Retarded, 20,* 123–129.

Dalke, C. (1984). There are no cows here: Art and special education together at last. *Art Education, 37*(6), 6–9.

Dattilo, J., & Rusch, F. (1985). Effects of choice on leisure participation for persons with severe handicaps. *Journal of The Association for Persons With Severe Handicaps, 10,* 194–199.

Decker, J. A. (1980). *Recreation and community education directors' perceptions of recreation services for the mentally retarded in Minnesota communities.* Unpublished doctoral dissertation, University of Minnesota, Minneapolis.

Descartes, R. (1955). Meditations on first philosophy. In D. J. Bronstein, Y. H. Krikorian, & P. P. Weiner (Eds.), *Basic problems of philosophy* (2nd ed.). Englewood Cliffs, NJ: Prentice-Hall.

Donder, D., & Nietupski, J. (1981). Nonhandicapped adolescents teaching playground skills to their mentally handicapped peers: Toward a less restrictive middle school environment. *Education and Training of the Mentally Retarded, 16,* 270–276.

Edginton, C. R., Compton, D. M., & Hanson, C. J. (1980). *Recreation and leisure programming: A guide for the professional.* Philadelphia: Saunders College.

Edginton, C. R., Compton, D. M., Ritchie, A. J., & Vederman, R. K. (1975). The status of services for special populations in park and recreation departments in the state of Iowa. *Therapeutic Recreation Journal, 9*(3) 109–116.

Ellis, G., Forsyth, P., & Voight, A. (1983). Leadership awareness of groups through sociometry. *Parks and Recreation, 18*(9), 54–57.

Eyman, R. K., & Call, J. (1977). Maladaptive behavior and community placement of mentally retarded persons. *American Journal of Mental Deficiency, 82,* 137–144.

Feldman, R., Wodarski, J., & Flax, N. (1975). Antisocial children in a summer camp environment: A time-sampling study. *Community Mental Health Journal, 11,* 10–18.

Fenrick, N., & Petersen, T. K. (1984). Developing positive changes in attitudes towards moderately/severely handicapped students through a peer tutoring program. *Education and Training of the Mentally Retarded, 19,* 83–90.

Flavell, J. (1973). Reduction of stereotypies by reinforcement of toy play. *Mental Retardation, 11*(4), 21–23.

Flax, N., & Peters, E. (1969). Retarded children at camp with normal children. *Children, 16*(4), 232–237.

Ford, A. Brown, L., Pumpian, I., Baumgart, D., Nisbet, J., Schroeder, J., & Loomis, R. (1984). Strategies for developing individualized recreation and leisure programs for severely handicapped students. In N. Certo, N. Haring, & R. York (Eds.), *Public school integration of severely handicapped students: Rational issues and progressive alternatives* (pp. 245–275). Baltimore: Paul H. Brookes Publishing Co.

Fredericks, H. D., Baldwin, V., Grove, D., Moore, W., Riggs, C., & Lyons, B. (1978). Integrating the moderately and severely handicapped preschool child into a normal day care setting. In M. Guralanick (Ed.), *Early intervention and the integration of handicapped and nonhandicapped children.* Baltimore: University Park Press.

Gibson, P. (1979). Therapeutic aspects of wilderness programs: A comprehensive literature review. *Therapeutic Recreation Journal, 13*(2), 21–23.

Goffman, E. (1963). *Stigma: Notes on the management of spoiled identity.* Englewood Cliffs, NJ: Prentice-Hall.

Gollay, E. (1981). Some conceptual and methodological issues in studying community adjustment of deinstitutionalized mentally retarded people. In R. H. Bruininks, C. E. Meyers, B. B. Sigford, & K. C. Lakin (Eds.), *Deinstitutionalization and community adjustment of mentally retarded people.* Washington, D.C.: American Association on Mental Deficiency.

Gronlund, N. (1959). *Sociometry in the classroom.* NY: Harper and Brothers.

Gunn, S. L., & Peterson, C. A. (1978). *Therapeutic recreation program design: Principles and procedures.* Englewood Cliffs, NJ: Prentice-Hall.

Hall, R. V. (Ed.). (1983). *Managing behavior series.* Austin, TX: PRO-ED.

Hamilton, E. J., & Anderson, S. (1983). Effects of leisure activities on attitudes toward people with disabilities. *Therapeutic Recreation Journal, 17*(3), 50–57.

Hamre-Nietupski, S., & Williams, W. (1977). Implementing selected sex education and social skills programs with severely handicapped students. *Education and Training of the Mentally Retarded, 12,* 364–372.

Handlers, A., & Austin, K. (1980). Improving attitudes of high school students toward their handicapped peers. *Exceptional Children, 47,* 228–229.

Hayes, G. A. (1969). The integration of the mentally retarded and non-retarded in a day camping program: A demonstration project. *Mental Retardation, 7*(5), 14–16.

Hayes, G. A. (1978). Philosophical ramifications of mainstreaming in recreation. *Therapeutic Recreation Journal, 12*(2), 5–9.

Hersen, M., & Barlow, D. (1976). *Single case experimental designs: Strategies for studying behavior change.* Elmsford, NY: Pergamon Press.

Hill, B. K., & Bruininks, R. H. (1981). *Family, leisure, and social activities of mentally retarded people in residential facilities.* Minneapolis, MN: Developmental Disabilities Project on Residential Services and Community Adjustment, University of Minnesota.

Horner, R. H., Meyer, L. H., & Fredericks, H. D. B. (Eds.). (1986). *Education of learners with severe handicaps: Exemplary service strategies.* Baltimore: Paul H. Brookes Publishing Co.

Howe-Murphy, R. (1980). The identification of guidelines for mainstreaming recreation and leisure services. *Journal of Leisurability, 7*(3), 36–41.

Hutchison, P., & Lord, J. (1979). *Recreation integration: Issues and alternatives in leisure services and community involvement.* Ottawa, Canada: Leisurability.

Karan, O., & Gardner, W. (1984). Planning community services using the Title XIX waiver as a catalyst for change. *Mental Retardation, 22,* 240–247.

Katz, S., & Yekutiel, E. (1974). Leisure time problems of mentally retarded graduates of training programs. *Mental Retardation, 12*(3), 54–57.

Kennedy, D. W., Austin, D. R., & Smith, R. W. (1987). *Special recreation: Opportunities for persons with disabilities.* Philadelphia: Saunders College.

Knapcyzk, D. R. (1975). Task analytic assessment of severe learning problems. *Education and Training of the Mentally Retarded, 10,* 74–77.

Krotee, M. L. (1980). The effects of various physical activity situational settings on the anxiety level of children. *Journal of Sport Behavior, 51*(9), 41–42.

Krotee, M. L., & Bart, W. M. (1986). A comparative and cross-cultural view of the quality of life. In M. Krotee & E. Jaeger, (Eds.), *Comparative physical education and sport* (pp. 59–67). Champaign, IL: Human Kinetics.

Kunstler, R. (1985). Emerging special populations and how they can be helped. *Adapted Physical Activity Quarterly, 2*(3), 177–181.

Lakin, K. C., & Bruininks, R. H. (Eds.) (1985). *Strategies for achieving community integration of developmentally disabled citizens.* Baltimore: Paul H. Brookes Publishing Co.

Lancaster, K. (1976). Municipal services. *Parks and Recreation, 18,* 18–27.

Laus, M. (1977). *Travel instruction for the handicapped.* Springfield, IL: Charles C Thomas.

Leisure Information Studies. (1976). *A systems model for developing a leisure education program for handicapped children and youth.* Washington, D.C.: Hawkins and Associates.

Leon, A. S., & Amundson, G. (Eds.) (1979). *Proceedings of the first international conference on lifestyle and health: Optimal health and fitness for people with disabilities.* Minneapolis: Department of Conferences, University of Minnesota.

Lord, J. (1983). Reflections on a decade of integration. *Journal of Leisurability, 10*(4), 4–11.

Lowenfeld, V., & Brittain, W. L. (1970). *Creative and mental growth* (5th ed.). New York: Macmillan.

Lupton, F. (1972). The effects of a behavior management training program on counselor performance in regular day camps which include children with behavior problems. *Dissertation abstracts international, 33*(6-A), 2780.

MacNeil, R. (1977). Opening minds and entryways at cultural centers. *Parks and Recreation, 12,* 41–44.

Matthews, P. R. (1977). Recreation and the normalization of the mentally retarded. *Therapeutic Recreation Journal, 11*(3), 112–114.

Matthews, P. R. (1982). Some recreation preferences of the mentally retarded. *Therapeutic Recreation Journal, 16*(3), 42–47.

McGill, J. (1984). Training for integration: Are blindfolds really enough? *Journal of Leisurability, 11*(2), 12–15.

McHale, S. M., & Simeonsson, R. J. (1980). Effects of interaction on nonhandicapped children's attitudes toward autistic children. *American Journal of Mental Deficiency, 85,* 18–24.

Meyer, H. D., & Brightbill, C. K. (1964). *Community recreation: A guide to its organization.* (3rd ed.). Englewood Cliffs, NJ: Prentice-Hall.

Meyer, L. H., & Kishi, G. S. (1985). School integration strategies. In K. C. Lakin and R. H. Bruininks (Eds.), *Strategies for achieving community integration of developmentally disabled citizens* (pp. 231–252). Baltimore; Paul H. Brookes Publishing Co.

Minneapolis Park and Recreation Board.(1984). [Statement of goals and objectives]. Recreation Division Procedural Manual, Vol. 1.

Minnesota State Council for the Handicapped. (1986). *Building access survey* (revised). St. Paul, MN: Author.

Mitchell, A., Robberson, J., & Obley, J. (1977). *Camp counseling.* Philadelphia: W. B. Saunders.

National Therapeutic Recreation Society. (1982). *Philosophical position statement of the National Therapeutic Recreation Society.* Alexandria, VA: National Recreation and Park Association.

Navar, N. (Ed.). (1981). Therapeutic recreation: An explanatory paper for the Joint Commission on Accreditation of Hospitals. In N. Navar & J. Dunn (Eds.), *Quality assurance: Concerns for therapeutic recreation* (pp. 145–159). Urbana-Champaign, IL: University of Illinois.

Newcomer, B., & Morrison, T. I. (1974). Play therapy with institutionalized mentally retarded children. *American Journal of Mental Deficiency, 78*(6), 727–733.

New Jersey Office on Community Recreation for Handicapped Persons. (1980). *A systematic approach to developing and implementing community recreation services for the disabled.* Trenton: New Jersey Department of Community Affairs.

Nietupski, J., Hamre-Nietupski, S., & Ayres, B. (1984). Review of task analytic leisure skill training efforts: Practitioner implications and future research needs. *Journal of The Association for Persons with Severe Handicaps, 9*(2), 88–97.

Nirje, B. (1969). The normalization principle and its human management implications. In R. Kugel and W. Wolfensberger (Eds.), *Changing patterns of residential services for the mentally retarded.* Washington, D.C.: President's Committee on Mental Retardation.

Norbie, R. M. (Ed.). (1983). *Ski for Light International instruction/guide manual.* Minneapolis: Ski for Light, Inc.

Opel, G. L. (1982). *Cross country skiing for persons with disabilities.* Loretto, MN: Vinland National Center.

Paloutzian, R. F., Hasazi, J., Streifel, J., & Edgar, C. (1971). Promotion of positive interaction in severely retarded young children. *American Journal of Mental Deficiency, 75*(4), 519–524.

Parten, M., & Newhall, S. (1943). Social behavior of preschool children. In R. Barker, J. Kovnin, & H. Wright (Eds.), *Child behavior and development,* (pp. 509–525), New York: McGraw-Hill.

Putnam, J. W., Werder, J. K., & Schleien, S. J. (1985). Leisure and recreation services for handicapped persons. In K. C. Lakin & R. H. Bruininks (Eds.), *Strategies for achieving community integration of developmentally disabled citizens* (pp. 253–274). Baltimore: Paul H. Brookes Publishing Co.

Ray, M. T., Schleien, S. J., Larson, A., Rutten, T., & Slick, C. (1986). Integrating persons with disabilities into community leisure environments. *Journal of Expanding Horizons in Therapeutic Recreation, 1,* 45–55.

Rehabilitation Act of 1973, Section 504. (PL 93-112), as amended, 29 U.S.C. 794.

Repp, Alan C. (1983). A history of mental retardation. *Teaching the mentally retarded,* Englewood Cliffs, NJ: Prentice-Hall (pp. 3–35).

Reynolds, R. P. (1981). A guideline to leisure skills programming for handicapped individuals. In

P. Wehman & S. Schleien (Eds.), *Leisure programs for handicapped persons: Adaptations, techniques, and curriculum* (pp. 1–13). Austin, TX: PRO-ED.

Reynolds, R. P., & O'Morrow, G. S. (1985). *Problems, issues, and concepts in therapeutic recreation*. Englewood Cliffs, NJ: Prentice-Hall.

Richler, D. (1984). Access to community resources: The invisible barriers to integration. *Journal of Leisurability, 11*(2), 4–11.

Robb, G. M. (1979). Transcript of past president Gary Robb's NTRS presentation to the NRPA board of trustees at the 1978 congress for recreation and parks, Miami, FL, 1978. *Newsletter.* National Recreation and Park Association.

Rosen, E. (1974). A special program of integrated summer camping and its effects upon emotionally disturbed adolescents and their normal peers. *Dissertation abstracts international, 35*(1-A), 288–289.

Rosen, H. (1959). Camping for the emotionally disturbed. *Children, 6*(2), 86–91.

Ross, C. D. (1983). Leisure in the deinstitutionalization process: A vehicle for change. *Journal of Leisurability, 10*(1), 13–19.

Rostad, B. K. (Ed.). (1985). If I can do this: The saga of Ski for Light. Minneapolis: Sons of Norway Foundation.

Russell, R. V. (1982). *Planning programs in recreation*. St. Louis: C. V. Mosby.

Rynders, J. E., Johnson, R. T., Johnson, D. W., & Schmidt, B. (1980). Producing positive interaction among Down Syndrome and nonhandicapped teenagers through cooperative goal structuring. *American Journal of Mental Deficiency, 85*, 268–273.

Sailor, W., & Mix, B. (1975). *The TARC assessment system*. Lawrence, KS: H and H Enterprises.

Salzberg, C. L., & Langford, C. A. (1981). Community integration of mentally retarded adults through leisure activity. *Mental Retardation, 19*(3), 127–131.

Schleien, S. J. (1984). The development of cooperative play skills in children with severe learning disabilities: A school-based leisure education program. *Journal of Leisurability, 11*(3), 29–34.

Schleien, S. J., Certo, N. J., & Muccino, A. (1984). Acquisition of leisure skills by a severely handicapped adolescent: A data based leisure skill instructional program. *Education and Training of the Mentally Retarded, 19*(4), 297–305.

Schleien, S. J., Kiernan, J., & Wehman, P. (1981). Evaluation of an age-appropriate leisure skills program for moderately retarded adults. *Education and Training of the Mentally Retarded, 16*(1), 13–19.

Schleien, S. J., Krotee, M. L., Mustonen, T., Kelterborn, B., & Schermer, A. D. (1987). The effect of integrating children with autism into a physical activity and recreation setting. *Therapeutic Recreation Journal, 21*(4), 52–62.

Schleien, S. J., Olson, K. D., Rogers, N. C., & McLafferty, M. E. (1985). Integrating children with severe handicaps into recreation and physical education programs. *Journal of Park and Recreation Administration, 3*(1), 50–66.

Schleien, S. J., Porter, J., & Wehman, P. (1979). An assessment of the leisure skill needs of developmentally disabled individuals. *Therapeutic Recreation Journal, 13*(3), 16–21.

Schleien, S. J., & Ray, M. T. (Eds.). (1986). *Integrating persons with disabilities into community leisure services*. Minneapolis: School of Physical Education and Recreation, University of Minnesota.

Schleien, S. J., Ray, M. T., Soderman-Olson, M. L., & McMahon, K. T. (1987). Integrating children with moderate to severe cognitive deficits into a community museum program. *Education and Training in Mental Retardation, 22*, 112–120.

Schleien, S. J., Rynders, J. E., Mustonen, T., Fox, A., & Kelterborn, B. (1987). Effects of employing activities representing four social levels of play on the appropriate play behavior of learners with severe disabilities. Manuscript submitted for publication in *Journal of Leisure Research.*

Schleien, S. J., & Wehman, P. (1986). Severely handicapped children: Social skills development through leisure skills programming. In G. Cartledge & J. Milburn (Eds.), *Teaching social skills to children: Innovative approaches* (2nd ed.) (pp. 219–245). Elmsford, NY: Pergamon Press.

Schleien, S. J., & Werder, J. K. (1985). Perceived responsibilities of special recreation services in Minnesota. *Therapeutic Recreation Journal, 19*(3), 51–62.

Schopler, E., & Reichler, R. (1979). *Individualized assessment and treatment for autistic and developmentally disabled children,* Volume I: Psychoeducational profile. Baltimore: University Park Press.

Sessoms, H. D. (1984). *Leisure services* (6th ed.). Englewood Cliffs, NJ: Prentice-Hall.

Shea, T. (1977). *Camping for special children.* St. Louis: C. V. Mosby.

Sherrill, C. (1979). *Creative arts for the severely handicapped, 2nd edition.* Springfield, IL: Charles C Thomas.

Sherrill, C., Rainbolt, W., & Ervin, S. (1984). Physical recreation of blind adults: Present practices and childhood memories. *Journal of Visual Impairment and Blindness.* 78(8), 367–368.

Shores, R., Hester, P., & Strain, P. S. (1976). The effects of amount and type of teacher-child interaction during free play. *Psychology in the Schools, 13,* 171–175.

Skinner, B. F. (1968). *The technology of teaching.* NY: Meredith.

Smith, R. W. (1985). Barriers are more than architectural. *Parks and Recreation, 20*(10), 58–62.

Stainback, S., & Stainback, W. (1985). *Integration of students with severe handicaps into regular schools.* Reston: The Council for Exceptional Children.

Strain, P. S., Cooke, T., & Apolloni, T. (1976). The role of peers in modifying classmates' social behavior: A review. *Journal of Special Education, 10*(4), 351–356.

Vaughan, J. L., & Winslow, R. (1979). *Guidelines for community based recreation programs for special populations.* Alexandria, VA: National Therapeutic Recreation Society.

Verhoven, P., & Goldstein, J. (1976). *Leisure activity participation and handicapped populations: An assessment of recreation needs.* Arlington, VA: National Recreation and Park Association.

Voeltz, L. M. (1980). Children's attitudes toward handicapped peers. *American Journal of Mental Deficiency, 84*(5), 455–464.

Voeltz, L. M. (1982). Effects of structured interactions with severely handicapped peers on children's attitudes. *American Journal of Mental Deficiency, 86,* 380–390.

Voeltz, L. M. (1983). *Why integration?* Minneapolis, MN: University of Minnesota Consortium Institute for the Education of Severely Handicapped Learners.

Voeltz, L. M., & Brennan, J. (1984). Analysis of interactions between nonhandicapped and severely handicapped peers using multiple measures. In J. Berg (Ed.), *Perspectives and progress in mental retardation,* Vol. I (pp. 61–72). Baltimore: University Park Press.

Voeltz, L. M., Hemphill, N., Brown, S., Kishi, G., Klein, R., Fruehling, R., Levy, G., Collie, J., & Kube, C. (1983). *The special friends program: A trainer's manual for integrated school settings.* Honolulu: Department of Special Education, University of Hawaii.

Voeltz, L. M., Kishi, G., & Brennan, J. (1981). *SIOS: Social interaction observation system.* Honolulu: Department of Special Education, University of Hawaii.

Voeltz, L. M., & Wuerch, B. B. (1981). Monitoring multiple behavioral effects of leisure activities training upon severely handicapped adolescents. In L. M. Voeltz, J. A. Apffel, & B. B. Wuerch (Eds.), *Leisure activities training for severely handicapped students: Instructional and educational strategies.* Honolulu: University of Hawaii, Department of Special Education.

Voeltz, L. M., Wuerch, B. B., & Wilcox, B. (1982). Leisure and recreation: Preparation for independence, integration, and self-fulfillment. In B. Wilcox & G. T. Bellamy, *Design of high school programs for severely handicapped students* (pp. 175–209). Baltimore: Paul H. Brookes Publishing Co.

Wehman, P. (1977). *Helping the mentally retarded acquire play skills: A behavioral approach.* Springfield, IL: Charles C Thomas.

Wehman, P. (1979). *Recreation programming for developmentally disabled persons.* Austin, TX: PRO-ED.

Wehman, P., & Schleien, S. J. (1980). Assessment and selection of leisure skills for severely handicapped individuals. *Education and Training of the Mentally Retarded, 15*(1), 50–57.

Wehman, P., & Schleien, S. J. (1981). *Leisure programs for handicapped persons: Adaptations, techniques, and curriculum.* Austin, TX: PRO-ED.

Wehman, P., Schleien, S. J., & Kiernan, J. (1980). Age appropriate recreation programs for severely handicapped youth and adults. *Journal of The Association for the Severely Handicapped, 5,* 395–407.

Wessel, J. (1976). *I Can Program.* Northbrook, IL, Hubbard Scientific.

West, P. C. (1982) Organizational stigma in metropolitan park and recreation agencies. *Therapeutic Recreation Journal, 16*(4), 35–41.

West, P. C. (1984). Social stigma and community recreation participation by the mentally and physically handicapped. *Therapeutic Recreation Journal, 18*(1), 40–49.

Wheeler, M. A. T., Lynch, J. M., & Thom, C. D. (1984). *Barriers to leisure: Identification and program implications.* Paper presented at the meeting of the American Association on Mental Deficiency, Minneapolis, MN.

Wilkenson, P. F. (1984). Providing integrated play environments for disabled children: A design or attitude problem? *Journal of Leisurability, 11*(3), 9–14.

Wolfensberger, W. (1972). *The principle of normalization in human services.* Toronto: National Institute on Mental Retardation.

Wolfensberger, W. (1975). *The origin and nature of our institutional models.* Syracuse, NY: Human Policy Press.

Wuerch, B. B., & Voeltz, L. M. (1982). *Longitudinal leisure skills for severely handicapped learners:* The Ho'onanea curriculum component. Baltimore: Paul H. Brookes Publishing Co.

Index

Note: Page numbers followed by t *or* f *indicate tables or figures, respectively.*